D0742825

Discourses of Disease

Discourses of Disease

Writing Illness, the Mind and the Body in Modern China

Edited by

Howard Y. F. Choy

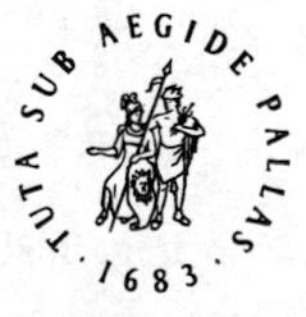

BRILL

LEIDEN | BOSTON

The Library of Congress Cataloging-in-Publication Data is available online at http://catalog.loc.gov
LC record available at http://lccn.loc.gov/2016011370

ISBN 978-90-04-31920-2 (hardback)
ISBN 978-90-04-31921-9 (e-book)

This book is printed on acid-free paper and produced in a sustainable manner.

For my wife, Shelley Wing Chan 陈颖, who has the proud ability to transform her disability into the love of all lives.

∵

Contents

PART 3
AIDS and Virus: From Film to Forum

Acknowledgments

The editor is grateful to the contributors and colleagues at many colleges and universities, whose support made this volume possible. The authors acknowledge the constructive comments and suggested changes by our peer reviewers, Marta Hanson at the Johns Hopkins University School of Medicine and Hu Ying 胡缨 at the University of California, Irvine, to whom we owe a debt that cannot be adequately expressed in words. Qin Higley, Victoria Menson, and Karen Cullen at Brill have been patient and indispensable with their editorial guidance. Working with them throughout the process has been a great pleasure. The editor is also pleased to acknowledge Wittenberg University for a sabbatical leave toward the editorial work of this project and Hong Kong Baptist University for a grant underwriting part of the copy-editing cost.

List of Figures

List of Contributors

Kevin Carrico
is a Lecturer in Chinese Studies at Macquarie University. He is currently completing an ethnography of the Han Clothing Movement (*Hanfu yundong* 汉服运动), a traditionalist majority nationalist movement in urban China. His research generally engages with popular culture, nationalism, ethnic relations, and notions of "pollution" in contemporary China. He has published articles in the recent volume *Critical Han Studies: The History, Representation, and Identity of China's Majority* (2012), the journal *Learning and Teaching in the Social Sciences*, and in recent edited collections on self-immolation in Tibet and ritual for *Cultural Anthropology*.

Shelley W. Chan 陈颖
is Associate Professor of Chinese Language and Cultural Studies at Wittenberg University. She earned her Ph.D. degree from University of Colorado-Boulder, her M.A. from University of Wisconsin-Madison, and her B.A. from Hong Kong Baptist University. She is the author of *A Subversive Voice in China: The Fictional World of Mo Yan* (2011) and the editor of *Mo Yan—Year 2000 Series: Close Readings on China* (1999). Her articles, translations, and book/film reviews on Chinese literature and culture have appeared in the United States, France, Germany, Australia, Sweden, China, Hong Kong, and Taiwan.

Howard Y. F. Choy 蔡元丰
is Associate Professor of Chinese Language and Literature at Hong Kong Baptist University. He is the author of *Remapping the Past: Fictions of History in Deng's China, 1979–1997* (2008) and the assistant author of *The Illustrated Encyclopedia of Confucianism* (2005). Currently editing a book of Liu Zaifu's selected essays, he has also published a number of articles and translations in major scholarly journals, including *positions*, *American Journal of Chinese Studies*, *Asian Theatre Journal*, *Transtext(e)s Transcultures*, and *minima sinica*. His ongoing research project is a comparative study of political jokes across mainland China, Hong Kong, Taiwan, and the United States.

Haomin Gong 龚浩敏
is Assistant Professor of Chinese at Case Western Reserve University. He is the author of *Uneven Modernity: Literature, Film, and Intellectual Discourse in Postsocialist China* (2012) and has published articles in *Modern Chinese Literature and Culture*, *Journal of Chinese Cinemas*, *Journal of Contemporary China*, *China*

Information, *Asian Cinema*, *Telos*, *Concentric*, and *Frontiers of Literary Studies in China*. In addition, he has also contributed chapters to a number of edited volumes.

Wendy Larson
is Professor Emerita of East Asian Languages and Literature at the University of Oregon. Larson's research monographs include *From Ah Q to Lei Feng: Freud and Revolutionary Spirit in 20th Century China* (2009), *Women and Writing in Modern China* (1998), and *Literary Authority and the Chinese Writer: Ambivalence and Autobiography* (1991). She translated Wang Meng's *Bolshevik Salute* (1989) and co-edited *Gender in Motion: Divisions of Labor and Cultural Change in Late Imperial and Modern China* (2005) and *Inside Out: Modernism and Postmodernism in Chinese Literary Culture* (1993). Her present project is on film director Zhang Yimou.

Li Li 李力
is an associate professor at the department of Literatures and Languages, and a joint faculty for Asia Studies, at the University of Denver. Having studied and compiled anthologies of Chinese translation of English language poetry in her earlier career, she has published a dozen of articles on modern and contemporary Chinese literature, popular culture and media studies in recent years. She is presently revising a manuscript on the politics of remembering and representing the Chinese Cultural Revolution in English-speaking countries. She is also working on co-editing a collection of critical essays on socialist culture/literature and its many intriguing incarnations in the postsocialist era.

Birgit Bunzel Linder
is Assistant Professor of Chinese and Comparative Literary Studies at City University of Hong Kong. Her research concerns presentations of madness in Chinese and comparative literature and issues of medical humanities in China. She has published a number of articles and translations in major scholarly journals, including *Renditions*, *Journal of Medical Humanities*, and *German Studies Review*.

Kun Qian 钱坤
is Assistant Professor of Chinese Literature and Film at the University of Pittsburgh. She earned her Ph.D. degree from Cornell University and has published articles in various journals. Her recently published book, *Imperial-Time-Order: Literature, Intellectual History, and China's Road to Empire* (2016), deals with the conception and representation of traditional Chinese empire in modern Chinese literature and media.

Stephanie Villalta Puig
is Assistant Professor of General Education at the Technological and Higher Education Institute of Hong Kong. She earns her Ph.D. degree in History from the Australian National University. Dr. Villalta Puig researches the History of the British Empire in China and, in particular, the British medical construction of the Chinese. She also has research interests in cultural history, social history and, more generally, global history. Dr. Villalta Puig has taught at the Chinese University of Hong Kong, the University of Hull, La Trobe University, Macquarie University, and Australian National University.

Introduction: Disease and Discourse

Howard Y. F. Choy 蔡元丰

From Freud's popularization of psychoanalysis to Foucault's formulation of bio-power, from traditional herbal treatments to modern scientific biomedicine, the meanings of disease have undergone such drastic changes with the introduction of modern Western medicine into China during the last two hundred years that new discourses have been invented to theorize illness, redefine health, and reconstruct classes and genders.[1] As a consequence, medical literature is rewritten with histories of hygiene, studies of psychopathology, and stories of cancer, disabilities and pandemics, etc. This edited volume is developed from an interdisciplinary panel bearing the same title at the 2011 joint conference of the Association for Asian Studies and International Convention of Asia Scholars in Honolulu.[2] Including studies of discourses about both bodily and psychiatric illness in modern China, it attempts to bring together groundbreaking scholarships that reconfigure the fields of film, literature, history, psychology, anthropology, ethnography, gender and cultural studies by tracing the pathological path of the "Sick Man of East Asia" (*Dong Ya bingfu* 东亚病夫) through the nineteenth and twentieth centuries into the new millennium.

Disease Concepts and Illness Metaphors

Throughout this volume, the terms "disease" and "illness" are often used interchangeably as synonyms since their strict institutional distinction has been deconstructed by Canadian sociologist Arthur W. Frank in the sense that illness as a social experience is an experience in and of disease as a physiological process.[3] In fact, Russian-American medical historian Owsei Temkin has

1 A landmark of the introduction of modern Western medicine into China was Dr. Alexander Pearson's (1780–1874) bringing in smallpox vaccination into Macao and Canton in 1805. See Louis Fu, "The Protestant Medical Missions to China: The Introduction of Western Medicine with Vaccination," *Journal of Medical Biography* 21.2 (May 2013): 112–17.

2 The book title phrase "Discourses of Disease" comes from this panel I organized in early Dec. 2009, two months prior to a call for papers with the exact same title for a special issue of *Modern Chinese Literature and Culture* 23.1 (Spring 2011) edited by Carlos Rojas, who also served as my panel discussant in Hawai'i.

3 Arthur W. Frank, *The Wounded Storyteller: Body, Illness, and Ethics* (Chicago: University of Chicago Press, 1995), 187n. Early on, in his "Framing Disease: Illness, Society, and History," Introduction to *Framing Disease: Studies in Cultural History*, ed. Charles E. Rosenberg and

 | DOI 10.1163/9789004319219_002

redefined "disease" as a spectrum from the ontological to the physiological since antiquity.[4] Researching on the history of disease concepts, British medical historian Adrian Wilson further distinguishes the naturalist-realist perspective of disease as ahistorical from the historicalist-conceptualist approach to disease as contingent.[5] Adopting the latter approach on "the premise that diseases are historically situated, socially defined, and culturally meaningful," American historian of Chinese medicine Marta Hanson relates disease concepts to individual illness narratives: "Disease concepts both structured patients' narratives of illness and led physicians to decide what part of what they said was objectively pertinent."[6]

As Wilson concludes his article with an aspiration for a comparative study of the Western and Chinese or Ayurvedic medical traditions,[7] the Chinese conception of disease remains an emerging field for further investigation beyond the scope of this volume. Where historian of Chinese medical literature Fan Xingzhun 范行准 (1906–98) has published two pioneering works in this regard in the 1980s,[8] here I just want to trace the modern compound word for

---

Janet Golden (New Brunswick, N.J.: Rutgers University Press, 1992), xxiii, Rosenberg distinguishes disease from illness in terms of "biological event versus socially negotiated construction." Yet later, in her *Lovers and Livers: Disease Concepts in History* (Toronto: University of Toronto Press, 2005), 5–14, Canadian medical historian Jacalyn Duffin differentiates illness, as subjective suffering on the part of individual patients, from the objective disease that conceptualizes illnesses as ideas—ideas that are governed by epistemology. As a matter of fact, the "illness/disease" dichotomy is so arbitrary that Adrian Wilson, in his "On the History of Disease-concepts: The Case of Pleurisy," *History of Science* 38 (2000): 311n69, aptly summarizes: "Both words are so elastic that it can be made in many different ways, or avoided altogether, according to one's *rhetorical* purposes" (my emphasis).

4 Such spectrum spans from the most general, metaphysical understanding of the nature of disease to the very individual, contextual characterization of the circumstances of sufferers. See Owsei Temkin, "The Scientific Approach to Disease: Specific Entity and Individual Sickness," in his *The Double Face of Janus and Other Essays in the History of Medicine* (Baltimore: Johns Hopkins University Press, 1977), 441–55. Duffin, *Lovers and Livers*, 28, explains that the ontological theory views the cause of an illness from outside the patient (e.g., a god, a germ), whereas the physiological theory attributes it to within the body (e.g., a gene, an imbalance).

5 Wilson, "On the History of Disease-concepts," 276.

6 Marta E. Hanson, *Speaking of Epidemics in Chinese Medicine: Disease and the Geographic Imagination in Late Imperial China* (New York: Routledge, 2011), 8–9.

7 Wilson, "On the History of Disease-concepts," 306.

8 Fan Xingzhun, *Zhongguo yixue shilüe* 中国医学史略 [A Brief History of Chinese Medicine] (Beijing: Zhongyi guji chubanshe, 1986); and his *Zhongguo bing shi xin yi* 中国病史新义 [New Significances for the History of Disease in China] (Beijing: Zhongyi guji chubanshe, 1989).

"disease/illness," *jibing* 疾病, to each character's oracle-bone and bronze inscriptions in antiquity. Philologist Luo Zhenyu 罗振玉 (1866–1940) analyzed the oracle-bone inscription of *ji*, which first appeared as a combination of the pictograph *shi* 矢 "arrow" and a drawing of "human" (大, instead of the "sickness" radical 疒), that it means "swift (like shooting)" and, by extension, "suffering (from being shot)."[9] Luo's in-law Wang Guowei 王国维 (1877–1927), also an epigrapher, explained the "illness" as a result of being shot in the context of ancient wartimes, but his most inspiring speculation is that *ji* may have originated from the graph *yi* 医 "doctor", which contains the same semantic element, *shi*.[10]

In respect to the oracle-bone inscription of *bing*, paleographer Zhu Fangpu 朱芳圃 (1895–1973) deciphered the graph, which consists of the archaic form of the "sickness" radical, i.e., *pan* 爿 or *pian* 片 "board/bed", and a "person" with some drops of blood around his/her body, as a haunted person lying in the sickbed.[11] Etymologist Xu Zhongshu 徐中舒 (1898–1991) identified the same graph simply as the later "sickness" radical 疒 and interpreted the dots on the sick person as sweat.[12] While Wang's relation of *ji* to *yi* implied a military need in the beginning of Chinese medical care, Zhu's reading of *bing* is reminiscent of its shamanistic practice.[13]

9 Luo Zhenyu, *Yinxu shuqi kaoshi* 殷虚书契考释 [A Study of the Scripts from the Yin Ruins] (Taipei: Yiwen yinshuguan, [1975]), 2.75a. However, Bernhard Karlgren, in his *Grammata Serica Recensa* (1957; repr., Göteborg: Elanders Boktryckeri Aktiebolag, 1972), no. 494, lists "sickness, pain" and "sufferance" as the primary meanings of *ji*. Xu Zhongshu 徐中舒, ed., *Jiaguwen zidian* 甲骨文字典 [A Dictionary of Oracle-bone Inscriptions] (Chengdu: Sichuan cishu chubanshe, 1989), 838–39, also agrees that "illness" is the original meaning.

10 Wang Guowei, "Mao gong ding ming kaoshi 毛公鼎铭考释 [A Study of Bronze Inscriptions on the Duke Mao Tripod]," in his *Wang Guowei yishu* 王国维遗书 [The Posthumous Works of Wang Guowei], 16 vols. ([Changsha]: Shangwu yinshuguan, 1940; Shanghai: Shanghai guji chubanshe, 1983), 6:3a, 8a (separate pagination). According to Karlgren's reconstruction of the archaic sounds of *ji* and *yi* in his *Grammata Serica Recensa*, nos. 494 and 958, the two graphs were pronounced as *dz'i̯ət* and *i̯əg*, respectively, with a common vowel that also points to a phonetic relationship between "illness" and "doctor" in ancient China.

11 Zhu Fangpu, *Yin Zhou wenzi shicong* 殷周文字释丛 [Collection of Explanatory Notes on Yin and Zhou Dynasties Characters] (Beijing: Zhonghua shuju, 1962), 119–20.

12 Xu, *Jiaguwen zidian*, 837–38.

13 For an introduction to the Chinese shaman doctor (*wuyi* 巫医), see Fan, *Zhongguo yixue shilüe*, 5–7, 12–13.

As Susan Sontag has demonstrated, one of the modern ways to frame diseases is by use of metaphors.[14] The metaphorization of disease as socio-cultural symptom and symbol of traumatic modernity emerged in modern Chinese literature from the late Qing to May Fourth periods according to Tan Guanghui 谭光辉, who observes that this "disease complex" has been suppressed by a certain ideology or discursive power and substituted with a healthy theme in contemporary Chinese fiction.[15] The writing of disease as a counter-discourse to the dominant Mao discourse had disappeared in the People's Republic of China (PRC) and only reemerged recently as a marginal voice against the mainstream of marketization. In effect, as indicated in Deng Hanmei's 邓寒梅 *A Study of Illness Narratives in Modern and Contemporary Chinese Literature* (*Zhongguo xiandangdai wenxue zhong de jibing xushi yanjiu* 中国现当代文学中的疾病叙事研究), the metaphorical approach to disease in modern Chinese literature has largely yielded to ethical concerns in the contemporary era for the sakes of harmony (*hexie* 和谐) and health (*jiankang* 健康).[16] In the end, Deng proposes five perspectives to study illness narratives, namely, literature, sociology, ethics, religion, and comparative literature, but disease per se is ignored.[17]

Medical Humanities and Illness Narratives

Medical humanities recently appeared as an academic field first in the West then in China, where a journal entitled *Chinese Medical Humanities Review* (*Zhongguo yixue renwen pinglun* 中国医学人文评论) has been published by Peking University Medical Press (Beijing daxue yixue chubanshe 北京大学医学出版社) since 2007, and the Peking University Institute for Medical Humanities (Beijing daxue yixue renwen yanjiuyuan 北京大学医学人文研究院) was established a year later.[18] Crossing the borders of nations, social sciences,

---

14 See Susan Sontag, *Illness as Metaphor and AIDS and Its Metaphors* (New York: Anchor Books, 1990).

15 Tan Guanghui, *Zhengzhuang de zhengzhuang: Jibing yinyu yu Zhongguo xiandai xiaoshuo* 症状的症状：疾病隐喻与中国现代小说 (The Symptom of Symptoms: Disease as a Metaphor in Modern Chinese Fiction) (Beijing: Zhongguo shehui kexue chubanshe, 2007), 7, 183, 280–81.

16 Deng Hanmei, *Zhongguo xiandangdai wenxue zhong de jibing xushi yanjiu* (Nanchang: Jiangxi renmin chubanshe, 2012), Chapters 2 and 3.

17 Ibid., 311–12.

18 See the institute's official websites in Chinese and English respectively: http://imh.bjmu.edu.cn/ybjj/ybjjz/index.htm; http://english.bjmu.edu.cn/friendshiplink/school/68915.htm (accessed Aug. 27, 2015).

literature and arts, discourses of disease have become more diversified. Books such as Angela Ki Che Leung's 梁其姿 *Leprosy in China: A History* (2009), her and Charlotte Furth's edited volume *Health and Hygiene in Chinese East Asia: Policies and Publics in the Long Twentieth Century* (2010), Marta Hanson's *Speaking of Epidemics in Chinese Medicine: Disease and the Geographic Imagination in Late Imperial China* (2011), Deng Hanmei's *A Study of Illness Narratives in Modern and Contemporary Chinese Literature* (2012), Anna Lora-Wainwright's specific fieldwork *Fighting for Breath: Living Morally and Dying of Cancer in a Chinese Village* (2013), Miranda Brown's *The Art of Medicine in Early China: The Ancient and Medieval Origins of a Modern Archive* (2015), and Andrew Schonebaum's forthcoming *Fictional Medicine: Diseases, Doctors and the Curative Properties of Chinese Fiction* are mushrooming.[19]

Among the various approaches to medical humanities is illness narratives. Two key figures from this emerging area of study in America are psychiatrist-anthropologist Arthur Kleinman of the Harvard Medical School and literary physician Rita Charon, founder and director of the Program in Narrative Medicine at Columbia University. Kleinman pioneers illness narratives through a literary inquiry towards the system of meanings that "thickens the [patient's] account and deepens the clinician's understanding of the experience of suffering."[20] Following Kleinman's steps, Charon borrows the literary methods of close reading, reader-response criticism and reception theory to broaden the vision of health care. In Charon's narrative medicine, "the telling and listening to stories of self…are themselves enabled by illness."[21] She suggests that "the body is heteroglossic," and doctors need to learn not only the language of symptom but also "the language of pleasure, the language of loss, the language of life, and [therefore] come to understand that these discourses, too, speak of health."[22] Indeed, illness narratives aim at both descriptions of symptoms and prescriptions of treatments, which are badly needed by a nation such as China

---

19 While Andrew Schonebaum's book uses Ming and Qing novels to approach medicine, health, and disease in the late imperial period, he has also published an article on tuberculosis in Republican-era fiction, i.e., "Vectors of Contagion and Tuberculosis in Modern Chinese Literature," *Modern Chinese Literature and Culture* 23.1: 17–46. I thank Marta Hanson for the reference to Schonebaum's forthcoming book.

20 Arthur Kleinman, *The Illness Narratives: Suffering, Healing, and the Human Condition* (New York: Harper Collins, 1988), 233.

21 Rita Charon, Afterword to *Psychoanalysis and Narrative Medicine*, ed. Peter L. Rudnytsky and Rita Charon (Albany: State University of New York Press, 2008), 287.

22 Rita Charon, "Where Does Narrative Medicine Come From? Drives, Diseases, Attention, and the Body," ibid., 24.

where many diseases remain taboos. Yet, it is precisely these taboos that generate a variety of discourses, particularly in the form of literature.

The narrativization of illness and textualization of the body reveal the politics of disease. If the mind and the body are the basic constituents of identity, discourses of disease probe into the psychosomatic politics of subjectivity by speaking about the sick person's mental and physical conditions in the socio-historical context. Linguistically, the relation between "discourse" and "disease" is embodied in the Chinese character for "diagnose," *zhen* 诊, which is categorized under the *yan* 言 "speech" radical. As a matter of fact, the four diagnostic methods (*si zhen* 四诊) in traditional Chinese medicine—observation, auscultation/olfaction, interrogation, pulse feeling and palpation (*wang wen wen qie* 望闻问切)—corresponding to looking/reading, listening/smelling, asking, and touching, are mostly related to language. Diagnosis on a disease can only be formed in the discourse of discussion and definition.[23] Diseases are definitely discursive; disease desires, indeed demands, discourse. Since disease is a condition in body and, according to Hwang Jinlin's 黄金麟 socio-historical study of body, "the existence of body is inevitably intermingled with the presence of many forces," such as those of politics, economics, society, and culture,[24] discourses of disease are not merely medical discourses, but also always already inter-discursive with imperialism, nationalism, marketization, revolutionary romanticism, socio-psychological crisis, social disorders, homo/sexuality, or political agenda as showcased in the nine chapters here.

Different Disciplines and Multiple Methodologies

Authors of this volume are from different disciplines and make multiple methodological contributions toward a common interest in the discourses of disease. The collection is organized chronologically and according to medical categories. It begins with the nineteenth-century medical missionary Dr. James Henderson's public health manual written for Britons in Shanghai. His influence on the early Chinese conception of hygiene is comparable to that

23 Rosenberg points out in his "Framing Disease," xix: "From the patient's perspective, diagnostic events are never static. They always imply consequences for the future and often reflect upon the past. They constitute a structuring element in an ongoing narrative, an individual's particular trajectory of health or sickness, recovery or death."

24 Hwang Jinlin, *Lishi, shenti, guojia: Jindai Zhongguo de shenti xingcheng* 历史、身体、国家:近代中国的身体形成 (1895–1937) [History, Body, and Nation: The Formation of Body in Modern China (1895–1937)] (2001; Beijing: Xinxing chubanshe, 2006), 6.

of Russian writer Maxim Gorky on an array of Chinese intellectuals from the Republican period (1912–49) through the end of the Cultural Revolution (1966–76), including Lu Xun 鲁迅, Guo Moruo 郭沫若, Ding Ling 丁玲 and others, whose painful search for revolutionary happiness has eventually led to the pathologization of "unhappiness." Against this historical background, however, Guo Lusheng 郭路生 (nom de plume Shizhi 食指) and Wen Jie 温洁, two poets from the 1970s and 1980s respectively, strive to poeticize their personal experience of mental illnesses.

With the rapid economic growth and the concomitant environmental pollution since the 1990s, Chinese people have become more concerned about their own physical wellbeing than ever. Female authors Xi Xi 西西 and Bi Shumin 毕淑敏 from Hong Kong and mainland China respectively have told their stories of being a cancer patient and a psychologist. Yet the real threat across the new millennium has changed from cancer to AIDS—just like cancer replaced tuberculosis in the last century—as both diseases are covered in Yan Lianke's 阎连科 fiction, which has inspired films, feature and documentary, about the moralized "plague" (even though it is actually spread by the "blood economy" rather than the sex industry) in the current decade. As Gu Changwei 顾长卫 and Zhao Liang 赵亮 expose the body politics of AIDS in their films, the fear of HIV infection is further transmitted through the internet to social networks.

The volume thus covers major public health problems, including mental illness, drug addiction, cancer, disabilities, and AIDS. The first part concerns hygiene and psychiatric disorder in both daily life and poetic form. Stephanie Villalta Puig's opening chapter, "James Henderson's *Shanghai Hygiene* and the British Constitution in Early Modern China," analyzes the function that hygiene had for British imperial medicine in early modern China as a discourse to prevent and caution against disease. After an outline of the origins and development of Western hygienic medicine from its expression as a private concern to a public matter, Villalta Puig reviews Henderson's *Shanghai Hygiene* as a unique work that reconciles classical and modern theories of British hygienic medicine in nineteenth-century China. Henderson issued numerous cautions to the British community in Shanghai and the rest of China in order to prevent the many diseases common to life in locations far away from the metropolis. In doing so, he mixed humoralist and public health principles with the racial, class, and moral prejudices prevalent in that period. The chapter ends with a study of selected reports from British doctors in the employment of the Imperial Maritime Customs Service in China between 1861 and 1884. These records reveal that the theory of hygienic medicine that informed *Shanghai Hygiene* was consistent with its practice by British doctors in China. The consistency between theory and practice showcases the importance of *Shanghai Hygiene* as an exemplar of a Chinese caution to the British constitution or, in other words, a British medical reaction to the prospect of the discourse of disease in late nineteenth-century China.

Entering into the modern times, when Chinese revolutionary culture reached its zenith in the 1950s and 1960s, Wendy Larson observes in her "Curing Unhappiness in Revolutionary China: Optimism under Socialism and Capitalism" that revolutionary optimism became a strongly encouraged emotional perspective, attitude, and expression. It was touted through literature, film, images, and virtually every aspect of daily life. Unhappiness, especially if publicly expressed, signaled personal and social dysfunction, which could be considered as mental illness in need of a cure. In literature, Maxim Gorky provided the theory that produced socialist realism and the positive hero who, under the influence of Maoist revolutionary romanticism, became the representative and purveyor of revolutionary optimism. As in the Soviet Union, where attempts to understand and manipulate the human mind through hypnosis, suggestion, and psychoanalysis had a long history, in revolutionary China a range of techniques and strategies were developed to encourage happiness and to cure—or penalize—unhappiness. However, the valorizing of happiness took place with equal fervency in the United States, where Émile Coué brought his theory of optimistic autosuggestion, inspiring influential figures such as Dale Carnegie, Norman Vincent Peale, and Robert H. Shuller. Larson argues that China and America can represent the extremes of socialist and capitalist societies, and both had similar, if not identical, strategic reasons for promoting and constructing happiness as the most acceptable public emotion. Emerging from the Enlightenment, socialism and capitalism embodied the modern ideals of progress and improvement characteristic of scientific rationalism, which drove their embrace of happiness as the most effective, efficient emotional state and pathologized unhappiness as a disease that must be cured.

After the fanaticism of revolution, Birgit Bunzel Linder investigates the postrevolutionary reception of poetry about mental illness in her "Metaphors unto Themselves: Mental Illness Poetics and Narratives in Contemporary Chinese Poetry." Linder's two cases are Shizhi (Guo Lusheng), diagnosed with schizophrenia since 1972, and Wen Jie, chronically depressed since childhood, both of whom have written poetry that courageously represents their sufferings. The chapter examines the relationship between mental illness and poetic composition in the two poets who have become metaphors of the struggle for identity and agency. Their poems, always markers of already achieved (temporal) wellness, reflect the complexity and vulnerability of trying to transcendent their illnesses. As such, they represent two notable contributions to the field of cross-cultural medical humanities and "illness poetics" from China.

Without the Cartesian split of the subject, the volume shifts its focus from the mind to the body in the second part on drugs and cancer as well as disabilities and AIDS. Gong Haomin 龚浩敏 examines the literary creation of drug addiction in his "Unmaking of Nationalism: Drug Addiction and Its Literary Imagination in Bi Shumin's Novel." Taking Bi's novel *Red Prescription* (*Hong chufang* 红处方) as a case study, he argues that nationalism, which used to be a central concern of the discourse of drug addiction in Chinese modernity, has become increasingly ineffective in charting this national "disease" in contemporary narratives. Postsocialist conditions, under which drug addiction is reimagined from a national crisis to a personal sickness, have rendered this discourse decidedly more heteroglossic than nationalistic. Also covering the Chinese writer-doctor Bi Shumin, Howard Y.F. Choy's 蔡元丰 "Narrative as Therapy: Stories of Breast Cancer by Bi Shumin and Xi Xi" focuses on the fictional writings about breast cancer by two contemporary Chinese women writers, namely, Bi's *Save the Breast* (*Zhengjiu rufang* 拯救乳房) and Xi Xi's *Elegy for a Breast* (*Aidao rufang* 哀悼乳房), to explore the therapeutic function of storytelling at the subjective level. In light of Australian family therapist Michael White's deconstruction practices of narrative therapy, Choy suggests that these masto-texts have emerged as investigative reports to rewrite fe/male fears of the malignant tumor that is not only incurable but also unspeakable because of its perceived relation to sexual characteristics. Though composed in different styles, both works examine the doctor-patient and author-reader power/knowledge relationships by seeking therapy in narrative and reinventing narrative as therapy.

Extending from cancer to other illnesses, Shelley W. Chan's 陈颖 "Narrating Cancer, Disabilities, and AIDS: Yan Lianke's Trilogy of Disease" studies three novels by Yan Lianke: *Streams of Light and Time* (*Riguang liunian* 日光流年), *Pleasure* (*Shouhuo* 受活), and *Dream of Ding Village* (*Dingzhuang meng* 丁庄梦). Chan discusses how the novelist sees humans' hopeless struggle with fate as well as with absurd phenomena, including lust, greed, and corruption, in the grotesque present-day China through writing about different kinds of sickness. The trilogy shows how, according to the stern satirist, the nightmare of being the "Sick Man of East Asia" is still haunting the nation even after its rapid economic developments.

The discourse of AIDS spreads from literature to film and the internet in the last part of this volume. Centering on an adaptation of Yan's *Dream of Ding Village*, Qian Kun 钱坤 observes in her "Reluctant Transcendence: AIDS and the Catastrophic Condition in Gu Changwei's Film *Love for Life*" that the feature film follows Yan's vision of AIDS as a metaphor for a vision of the catastrophic condition of a market society, but also paradoxically aestheticizes this situation by proposing love as a way of transcendence. The negotiation with social obligation, commercial concern, and political censorship results in a film that reluctantly projects a transcendent vision of love and hope, which points to the future in a phantasmagorical, magical manner.

Following Chan's study of Yan Lianke's fiction and Qian's chapter on Gu Changwei's film, Li Li's 李力 "Alone Together: Contagion, Stigmatization and Utopia as Therapy in Zhao Liang's AIDS Documentary *Together*" critically examines emerging Chinese independent director Zhao Liang's AIDS documentary *Together* (*Zai yiqi* 在一起), which was initially conceived as a companion piece for *Love for Life*. In addition to covering the individual agonies of the "straight" patients who become infected primarily from blood transfusions in some of China's poverty-ridden inland countryside, Zhao's stylistic documentary also brings to light, with the help of digital media technology, dreadful stories of "non-straight" HIV/AIDS patients, who are believed in popular imagination to be deviants and whose stories inspire fears and bizarre fantasies. Through showing how and why HIV/AIDS is not merely a medical problem, but also a social issue which reveals a collective socio-psychological crisis in present-day China, *Together* shows us that the biggest threats the AIDS epidemic has imposed on the society are secretive silence and public denial.

The proliferating discourse of AIDS continues with Kevin Carrico's "The Unknown Virus: The Social Logic of Bio-conspiracy Theories in Contemporary China," which is based upon a year of ethnographic research on a hypochondria or factitious illness known as "HIV-negative AIDS" (*yinxing aizibing* 阴性艾滋病) or "the unknown virus" (*weizhi bingdu* 未知病毒). In this epidemic, thousands of urban young people, following guilt-inducing visits to sex workers or ambivalent one-night stands, have come to the conclusion that they are infected with a gradually debilitating and fatal AIDS-like disease that nevertheless produces negative results on repeated HIV tests. Gathering online to exchange stories and symptoms, they eventually drew the attention of the media and the state, particularly the Ministry of Public Health that oversaw a clinical study of this illness in early 2011 and dismissively concluded that it was "simply AIDS-phobia." Acknowledging the fundamentally phobic and imaginary nature of this illness, yet contesting its resulting casual dismissal by the government, Carrico's interview-based research examines patients' illness narratives to trace the social and personal truths expressed through this highly contagious disease of discourse.

Disease Discourses and Discursive Diseases

Together, these collected critical essays examine the ways in which our knowledge about disease (be it sickness preventions, mental illness, drug addiction, cancers, disabilities, or AIDS) is produced through discourse. From medical practices of public health to symptomatic strategies of linguistic interrogation, both scientific language and literary metaphors are problematized in the contexts of cultural maladies, social disorders, political pangs, and economic epidemics. Meanwhile, these discourses of disease also reveal the "diseases" of discourse, that is, the problematics of illness writing. For instance, Villalta Puig's review of nineteenth-century British discourse of hygiene in China echoes the pseudo-science and Daoist art of *yangsheng* 养生, or "caring for life," so widely disseminated through table talks and social media and practiced by most, if not all, Chinese today that it has become paranoia in the face of the national crises of environmental pollution and food safety.[25] After all, in a country without democracy, people are powerless to change their unlivable living environment; all they can do is to keep in good health, which constitutes their immediate conditions and ultimate defense, because we live with/in our bodies; hence, health and happiness replaces liberation.[26]

Yet even the emotion of unhappiness, as Wendy Larson notices, was easily pathologized as unhealthy and penalized as abnormal during Mao's revolution. And if genre matters, further research of mental illness should turn to poetic discourses, as conducted by Birgit Bunzel Linder in this collection. While poets make use of poetic formalism to mirror social disorders, they also reveal

25 The term *yangsheng* is derived from the chapter titled "Yangsheng zhu" 养生主 (The Principle of Caring for Life) of the Daoist classic *Zhuang zi* and from the book *Su wen* 素问 (Basic Questions) in the medical canon *Huang di nei jing* 黄帝内经 (The Yellow Lord's Inner Classic). For a study of "Yangsheng zhu" and its relation to *Huang di nei jing*, see Chow Tse-tsung 周策纵, "*Zhuang zi* 'Yangsheng zhu' pian benyi fuyuan 《庄子·养生主》篇本义复原 (Recovering the Original Meaning of the 'Yang Sheng Chu' Chapter in *Chuang-tzu*)," *Zhongguo wenzhe yanjiu jikan* 中国文哲研究集刊 (Bulletin of the Institute of Chinese Literature and Philosophy) 2 (Mar. 1992): 13–50, esp. 14–21. One of the most popular social media in China nowadays is the mobile app WeChat (Weixin 微信) developed by Tencent (Tengxun 腾讯), whose users are extremely enthusiastic in exchanging information—often rumors—about Chinese medicine, hygienic taboos, healthy living, research findings, pharmaceutical alerts, food nutrition and, most importantly in Chinese culinary culture, daily dietotherapy.

26 This is my parody of Eileen Chang's essay "Chinese Life and Fashions," *The XXth Century* 4.1 (Jan. 1943): 60: "In an age of political disorder, people were powerless to modify existing conditions closer to their ideal. All they could do was to create their own atmosphere, with clothes, which constitute for most men and all women their immediate environments. We live in our clothes"; and of Michel Foucault's conclusion to his *The Birth of the Clinic: An Archaeology of Medical Perception*, trans. A.M. Sheridan Smith (New York: Vintage Books, 1994), 198: "Hence, too, its [i.e., the fundamental place of medicine] prestige in the concrete forms of existence: health replaces salvation, said Guardia."

the paradox that mental illness poetics per se manifests the very madness of civilization—just as disease discourses disclose discursive diseases.

Meanwhile, the allegorical and metaphorical discourses of disease in earlier literary studies and scholarship continue to be challenged as several chapters have showcased that the valance of nationalism is no longer adequate to appraise the theme of illness so familiar with Lu Xun's work in the construction of a modern Chinese nation; instead, individual subject formation and collective social-psychological crisis are attempted to address the topic of disease. With his Madman of the May Fourth New Culture Movement (mid 1910s–20s), Lu Xun is known for changing his career from a medical doctor to a psychosomatic writer, who concerned not only the problems of China but also the conditions in humans, including his own. For Lu Xun, the language of disease is no more figurative than literal. The tendency of diagnosing Lu Xun's moral burden as a mere "obsession with China" has overlooked other equally important facets of the discourses of disease in modern Chinese literature.[27] Literary scholar Gao Xudong 高旭东 reminds us that before becoming a doctor Lu Xun was a patient, who suffered from odontopathy, gastrectasis, enteroparesis, pleurisy, bronchial asthma, and tuberculosis throughout his life.[28] While Lu Xun did imbue his work with medical knowledge, his identity and experience as a patient have been ignored in the studies of him and, as a result, he was idolized.[29] The complexity of Lu Xun can only be seen when the dual characteristics of his spirit and madness, genius and sickness, as well as strength and weakness are read.

With regard to this, the nationalistic discourse of drug addiction, as shown in Gong Haomin's chapter, has been losing its relevance in the postsocialist context of China, while Howard Choy questions the interpretation of illness as national allegory and probes the therapeutic function of personal narrative. At the same time, Shelley Chan's reading of Yan Lianke's fiction expresses what Hwang Jinlin values as "the ultimate solicitude for humans and the human body that is lacking" in recent sociological study of the body, that is,

---

27 See C.T. Hsia, *A History of Modern Chinese Fiction*, 3rd ed. (Bloomington: Indiana University Press, 1999), 541–44.

28 Gao Xudong, "Lu Xun: Zai yisheng yu huanzhe zhijian 鲁迅:在医生与患者之间 [Lu Xun: Between a Doctor and a Patient]," in *Wenxue yu zhiliao* 文学与治疗 [Literature and Therapeutics], ed. Ye Shuxian 叶舒宪 (Beijing: Shehui kexue wenxian chubanshe, 1999), 159.

29 Ibid., 163–64. An early exception, as Gao has noted on p. 166, is C.T. Hsia's 夏志清 older brother, Hsia Tsi-an 夏济安, who saw the pathosis in Lu Xun's talent. See Hsia Tsi-an, "Aspects of the Power of Darkness in Lu Hsun," in his *The Gate of Darkness: Studies on the Leftist Literary Movement in China* (Seattle: University of Washington Press, [1968]), 146–62.

"humanistic and moral solicitude" in the age of market economy.[30] On the contrary, as Qian Kun points out, Yan's metaphorical critique of marketization is problematically compromised and "transcended" into a love story in its filmic adaptation, and yet Li Li suggests in her analysis of the documentary version of AIDS narratives that the epidemic cannot be coped with unless it is detached from its socially constructed metaphors of circulation, mutation, and contagion. Nor can the symptomatology of HIV be dealt with, for those who are tested negative in Kevin Carrico's survey, by reducing it to sheer phobia as reported by the government.

The dominant discourse by which the state defines diseases aims only at homogenizing the society by maintaining a healthy unity on a daily basis in order to meet a political agenda. In the end, in a nation obsessed with healthiness, these discourses of disease disturb the officially proclaimed social(ist) harmony with their mental and bodily heterogeneities. These are the discursive diseases that are seen as a threat against social stability in the eyes of the government and must be cured by controlling the individual(istic) sick voices.

References

Brown, Miranda. *The Art of Medicine in Early China: The Ancient and Medieval Origins of a Modern Archive*. New York: Cambridge University Press, 2015.

Chang, Eileen. "Chinese Life and Fashions." *The XXth Century* 4.1 (Jan. 1943): 54–61.

Chow Tse-tsung 周策纵. "*Zhuang zi* 'Yangsheng zhu' pian benyi fuyuan《庄子·养生主》篇本义复原 (Recovering the Original Meaning of the 'Yang Sheng Chu' Chapter in *Chuang-tzu*)." *Zhongguo wenzhe yanjiu jikan* 中国文哲研究集刊 (Bulletin of the Institute of Chinese Literature and Philosophy) 2 (Mar. 1992): 13–50.

Deng Hanmei 邓寒梅. *Zhongguo xiandangdai wenxue zhong de jibing xushi yanjiu* 中国现当代文学中的疾病叙事研究 [A Study of Illness Narratives in Modern and Contemporary Chinese Literature]. Nanchang: Jiangxi renmin chubanshe, 2012.

Duffin, Jacalyn. *Lovers and Livers: Disease Concepts in History*. Toronto: University of Toronto Press, 2005.

Fan Xingzhun 范行准. *Zhongguo bing shi xinyi* 中国病史新义 [New Significances for the History of Disease in China]. Beijing: Zhongyi guji chubanshe, 1989.

———. *Zhongguo yixue shilüe* 中国医学史略 [A Brief History of Chinese Medicine]. Beijing: Zhongyi guji chubanshe, 1986.

Foucault, Michel. *The Birth of the Clinic: An Archaeology of Medical Perception*. Trans. A.M. Sheridan Smith. New York: Vintage Books, 1994.

30 Hwang, *Lishi, shenti, guojia*, 10.

Frank, Arthur W. *The Wounded Storyteller: Body, Illness, and Ethics*. Chicago: University of Chicago Press, 1995.

Fu, Louis. "The Protestant Medical Missions to China: The Introduction of Western Medicine with Vaccination." *Journal of Medical Biography* 21.2 (May 2013): 112–17.

Gao Xudong 高旭东. "Lu Xun: Zai yisheng yu huanzhe zhijian 鲁迅:在医生与患者之间 [Lu Xun: Between a Doctor and a Patient]." In *Wenxue yu zhiliao* 文学与治疗 [Literature and Therapeutics], ed. Ye Shuxian 叶舒宪, 159–69. Beijing: Shehui kexue wenxian chubanshe, 1999.

Hanson, Marta E. *Speaking of Epidemics in Chinese Medicine: Disease and the Geographic Imagination in Late Imperial China*. New York: Routledge, 2011.

Hsia, C.T. *A History of Modern Chinese Fiction*. 3rd ed. Bloomington: Indiana University Press, 1999.

Hsia Tsi-an. *The Gate of Darkness: Studies on the Leftist Literary Movement in China*. Seattle: University of Washington Press, [1968].

Hwang Jinlin 黄金麟. *Lishi, shenti, guojia: Jindai Zhongguo de shenti xingcheng* 历史、身体、国家:近代中国的身体形成 (1895–1937) [History, Body, and Nation: The Formation of Body in Modern China (1895–1937)]. 2001. Beijing: Xinxing chubanshe, 2006.

Karlgren, Bernhard. *Grammata Serica Recensa*. 1957. Repr., Göteborg: Elanders Boktryckeri Aktiebolag, 1972.

Kleinman, Arthur. *The Illness Narratives: Suffering, Healing, and the Human Condition*. New York: Harper Collins, 1988.

Leung, Angela Ki Che 梁其姿. *Leprosy in China: A History*. New York: Columbia University Press, 2009.

——— and Charlotte Furth, eds. *Health and Hygiene in Chinese East Asia: Policies and Publics in the Long Twentieth Century*. Durham: Duke University Press, 2010.

Lora-Wainwright, Anna. *Fighting for Breath: Living Morally and Dying of Cancer in a Chinese Village*. Honolulu: University of Hawai'i Press, 2013.

Luo Zhenyu. *Yinxu shuqi kaoshi* 殷虚书契考释 [A Study of the Scripts from the Yin Ruins]. Taipei: Yiwen yinshuguan, [1975].

Rojas, Carlos, ed. *Modern Chinese Literature and Culture* 23.1 (Spring 2011).

Rosenberg, Charles E. "Framing Disease: Illness, Society, and History." Introduction to *Framing Disease: Studies in Cultural History*, ed. Charles E. Rosenberg and Janet Golden, xiii–xxvi. New Brunswick, N.J.: Rutgers University Press, 1992.

Rudnystsky, Peter L., and Rita Charon, eds. *Psychoanalysis and Narrative Medicine*. Albany: State University of New York Press, 2008.

Sontag, Susan. *Illness as Metaphor and AIDS and Its Metaphors*. New York: Anchor Books, 1990.

Tan Guanghui 谭光辉. *Zhengzhuang de zhengzhuang: Jibing yinyu yu Zhongguo xiandai xiaoshuo* 症状的症状: 疾病隐喻与中国现代小说 (The Symptom of Symptoms: Disease as a Metaphor in Modern Chinese Fiction). Beijing: Zhongguo shehui kexue chubanshe, 2007.

Temkin, Owsei. *The Double Face of Janus and Other Essays in the History of Medicine*. Baltimore: Johns Hopkins University Press, 1977.

Wang Guowei 王国维. "Mao gong ding ming kaoshi 毛公鼎铭考释 [A Study of Bronze Inscriptions on the Duke Mao Tripod]." In *Wang Guowei yishu* 王国维遗书 [The Posthumous Works of Wang Guowei]. 16 vols. [Changsha]: Shangwu yinshuguan, 1940; Shanghai: Shanghai guji chubanshe, 1983.

Wilson, Adrian. "On the History of Disease-concepts: The Case of Pleurisy." *History of Science* 38 (2000): 271–319.

Xu Zhongshu 徐中舒, ed. *Jiaguwen zidian* 甲骨文字典 [A Dictionary of Oracle-bone Inscriptions]. Chengdu: Sichuan cishu chubanshe, 1988.

Zhu Fangpu 朱芳圃. *Yin Zhou wenzi shicong* 殷周文字释丛 [Collection of Explanatory Notes on Yin and Zhou Dynasties Characters]. Beijing: Zhonghua shuju, 1962.

PART 1

Hygiene and Psychosis: From Routine to Poetry

∵

CHAPTER 1

James Henderson's *Shanghai Hygiene* and the British Constitution in Early Modern China

Stephanie Villalta Puig

Introduction

> Hygiene teaches the means of preserving health, and forms an important branch of moral as well as medical science.... A European with a tolerably good constitution has his health almost entirely in his own keeping on arriving in Shanghai; and if he is careful in regard to his diet, drink, exercise, and clothing, he need not fear the climate.
>
> JAMES HENDERSON, *Shanghai Hygiene*[1]

In the nineteenth century, China was a domain of the informal empire that Britain pretended to control over the Far Orient. British imperial ideology endeavored to legitimate the British exploitation of Chinese resources that came with the informality of its imperial control. The claim for legitimacy revolved around the British idea that the Chinese were stagnant and over-civilized. Medicine contributed to the propagation of that idea. Imperial ideology prejudiced the otherwise objective and empirical rationality of British medicine in China and persuaded British doctors to dismiss the Chinese as immoral, effeminate, filthy, distasteful, yellow, hairless, ugly, and sickly.[2] Nineteenth-century British medicine dismissed the Chinese as an inferior people lacking in a nervous system and logic and who, accordingly, happily lived in dirt, filth and unhygienic conditions.[3]

This chapter analyzes the effect that the Chinese periphery had on the constitution of the British body during the latter half of the nineteenth century. The theme, I argue, is one of caution, in the twofold sense of physical caution as well as civilizational caution. On the theme of caution, this chapter analyzes

1 James Henderson, *Shanghai Hygiene, or, Hints for the Preservation of Health in China* (Shanghai: Presbyterian Mission Press, 1863), 2–3.

2 For the development of the Chinese "yellowness," see Michael Keevak, *Becoming Yellow: A Short History of Racial Thinking* (Princeton: Princeton University Press, 2011).

3 Stephanie Villalta Puig, "British Medical and Imperial Ideology in China: Circa 1840s–1890s" (Ph.D. diss., Australian National University, 2009).

 | DOI 10.1163/9789004319219_003

British hygiene in China because hygiene is the branch of medicine that seeks to prevent and, therefore, caution against disease. It reviews *Shanghai Hygiene, or, Hints for the Preservation of Health in China* by James Henderson M.D. of the Customs Medical Service and published in 1863 as a unique work that reconciles classical and modern theories of British hygienic medicine in China. Henderson issues in *Shanghai Hygiene* numerous cautions to the British community in Shanghai and the rest of China in order to prevent the many diseases common to life in locations far removed from the metropolis. In doing so, he mixes humoralist as well as public health principles with the class and moral prejudices typical of that period. This book is unique in its content and serves as a definitive treatise on hygiene in China based on Dr. Henderson's experiences as a British medical practitioner posted to Shanghai. Whilst original, the manual does rely to some extent on the earlier work of two other English writers on tropical climatology, namely, Dr. James Johnson's *The Influence of Tropical Climates on European Constitutions* (1841) and Sir James Martin's *The Influence of Tropical Climates on European Constitutions* (1861).[4] Accordingly, the advice that Henderson gives to the British in China draws from experiences in other parts of the so-called British Empire, namely, India and Africa with occasional anecdotal references to experiences in Mediterranean climes. Nonetheless, *Shanghai Hygiene* is the only known work to have applied British hygienic medicine to the British in nineteenth-century China. As such, it is of great importance to the argument of caution that was applied during the early modern period.

Fear for the survival of the British constitution was the main concern of British medical practitioners who embarked on colonial service. To address that concern, they had to reconcile their understanding of constitution with their understanding of hygiene. At the time, hygiene was the oldest tradition of preventative medicine.[5] Until the reception of germ theory, hygienic medicine was the norm in the nineteenth century and incorporated such Galenic classifications as the naturals and the non-naturals.[6] This chapter asks: What was the role of traditional Western medical theory in the observation and

4 James Johnson and James Ranald Martin, *The Influence of Tropical Climates on European Constitutions*, 6th ed. (London: T. and C. Underwood, and Highley and Son, 1841); James Ranald Martin, *The Influence of Tropical Climates on European Constitutions, Including Practical Observations on the Nature and Treatment of the Diseases of Europeans on Their Return from Tropical Climates* (London: John Churchill, 1861).

5 *Companion Encyclopedia of the History of Medicine*, ed. William Bynum and Roy Porter (London: Routledge, 1993), s.v. "What Is Specific to Western Medicine?" by Arthur Kleinman.

6 Henderson, *Shanghai Hygiene*, 71. Henderson acknowledges his debt to classical writers. He states that the aim of medicine since Hippocrates has been to render medicine as an exact

experimentation of "health" in China? To what extent and how did these precepts change according to the pragmatic considerations of colonial life?

In response to these questions, this chapter consists of three parts. The first part considers the medical orthodoxy that the health of the constitution could be preserved only through the maintenance of hygiene, and the second applies this orthodoxy to the Chinese situation through a study of Henderson's *Shanghai Hygiene*; the third part examines reports by British medical officers in China in the period between 1861 and 1884 to determine whether British doctors in China put into practice the theories of hygienic medicine that Henderson so fervently prescribes.

Constitution and Hygiene

"Constitution" was the term coined in nineteenth-century British medicine to express a conception of the body as an organized and functioning structure. A person's constitution was conditioned, in part, by the place one was born, and where one resided. The structure was said to inherit certain traits, which would determine resistance or susceptibility to disease.[7] Hygiene, a developable trait, was said to be the other determinant of health.

In the classical period, "hygiene" was synonymous with "health." Thus, Galenic medicine drew a distinction between hygiene and therapeutics. Hygiene concerned the maintenance of health and prevention of disease whereas therapeutics, as the sum of physiology and pathology, concerned the treatment of disease.[8] Humoralism informed classical notions of hygiene until the nineteenth century. It was a system of medicine that considered illness to be the result of a disturbance in the natural balance of humors. The maintenance of balance, both within the body as a whole and within any one particular part of the body, was crucial.[9] Humoralism maintained that it was possible to identify the natural balance of health within an individual, and claimed the ability to restore the body to health as well as to maintain health. The natural balance of health was, therefore, paramount as it was constantly subject to potentially harmful influences from diet, lifestyle, and the environment.

science and despite much medical progress made since Hippocrates, medicine is still not yet an exact science.

7 *Companion Encyclopedia of the History of Medicine*, s.v. "Constitutional and Hereditary Disorders," by Robert C. Olby.

8 Ibid., s.v. "The History of Personal Hygiene," by Andrew Wear.

9 Ibid., s.v. "Humoralism," by Vivian Nutton.

The humoral framework formed the basis for all medical understanding, with diagnosis and treatments structured around the pattern of the six *non-naturals*.[10] The six non-naturals were, effectively, the categories of hygiene: air, food and drink, exercise and rest, sleep and waking, retentions and evacuations, and the emotions.[11] When the six non-naturals were used well, they improved the *naturals*—that is, the seven factors indispensable for a healthy constitution such as the elements (fire or earth), humors (blood or bile), or members (bones or nerves). When the non-naturals were misused, they turned into the three *contra-naturals*, that is, disease along with its causes and effects. In sum, then, physicians understood that health depended on the naturals (physiology), non-naturals (hygiene), and contra-naturals (pathology).[12]

From the classical period to the nineteenth century, hygienic medicine was concerned with lifestyle and the body's relationship with the environment around it. Accordingly, geographical location, climate, food, water, sexual activity, exercise, rest, sleeping and waking were determinants of cures and explanations of illness. Hygiene, then, was an individual, rather than a community responsibility.

Such a classical idea of hygiene influenced Europeans living in foreign lands and climates.[13] On the principle that one's constitution was partially determined by the place in which one was born and had resided, a move to a different land and climate implied a greater liability to ill health. Accordingly, one could regain one's natural balance through a gradual process of "seasoning" to new foods and drinks as well as climactic conditions. The influence of this classical notion of hygiene is evident in such seminal texts on tropical medicine as Dr. James Johnson's *The Influence of Tropical Climates on European Constitutions*. Johnson advised British residents in India to imitate the locals by eating vegetarian Hindu dishes, dressing in light clothing, and living in coolly kept houses.[14] Accordingly, such classical ideas of hygiene relating directly to the environment and lifestyle to health, allowed Europeans to settle into foreign environments.[15] This allowed Britons autonomy to control and direct one's health in the periphery.

---

10 Ibid.

11 Antoinette Emch-Deriaz, "The Non-Naturals Made Easy," in *The Popularisation of Medicine, 1650–1850*, ed. Roy Porter (London: Routledge, 1992), 135.

12 Ibid., 138.

13 *Companion Encyclopedia of the History of Medicine*, s.v. "The History of Personal Hygiene."

14 E.M. Collingham, *Imperial Bodies: The Physical Experience of the Raj, c. 1800–1947* (Cambridge: Polity Press, 2001).

15 David Arnold, *Colonizing the Body: State Medicine and Epidemic Disease in Nineteenth Century India* (Berkeley and Los Angeles: University of California Press, 1993); Phillip D. Curtin,

In the second half of the nineteenth century, humoralism began to become obsolete with the demise of Galenic medicine and its replacement with iatrochemistry and iatromechanics.[16] Hygiene reflected these broader changes in medicine, as documented by social and medical historians.[17] It became a community responsibility and nineteenth-century campaigns were concerned with the cleanliness of the poor.[18] Literary writers associated dirt with the poor, as many did with diseases like cholera. Andrew Wear writes how the poor, or the "great unwashed," "were the objects of the new hygiene.... They were given the means to become clean."[19] Public baths built in the latter half of the nineteenth century with housing, with personal cleanliness—sewage, and water regulations as the aim. The use of soap, toothpaste and toothbrushes was to spread to the working classes. Fear of infection was the driving force, for it was the idleness, ignorance, and indigence of the working classes who, reputedly, encouraged the defective lifestyles that bred disease.[20]

Cultural anxieties also set in, for with class conflict rife over a period of industrial revolution, a widespread feeling developed that it was the social body itself that was sick. The middle classes came to associate cleanliness, or the lack of it, with moral worth and immorality. Cleanliness campaigns foisted upon the working classes of Britain combined religious and social motives with medicine. Often, this attempt to impose cleanliness from above was the impetus for the development of public health. The introduction of state-enforced norms of hygiene on large groups of people was, in turn, a response to the development of theories of racial hygiene and progress.

These class anxieties had their racial counterparts. The Europeans saw themselves as clean while outside cultures were, allegedly, dirty.[21] By 1893, many argued filth to be a menace to Europe and proposals were made to invade countries in the Orient with missionaries of hygiene.[22] As Wear writes,

---

Disease and Empire: The Health of European Troops in the Conquest of Africa (Cambridge: Cambridge University Press, 1998).

16 *Companion Encyclopedia of the History of Medicine*, s.v. "The History of Personal Hygiene."

17 Mary Douglas, *Purity and Danger: An Analysis of the Concepts of Pollution and Taboo* (London: Routledge, 1996) and Mary Poovey, *Making a Social Body: British Cultural Formation, 1830–1864* (Chicago: University of Chicago Press, 1995).

18 Peter Stallybrass and Allon White, "The City: The Sewer, the Gaze and the Contaminating Touch," in *The Politics and Poetics of Transgression*, ed. Peter Stallybrass and Allon White (London: Routledge, 1986), 125–48.

19 *Companion Encyclopedia of the History of Medicine*, s.v. "The History of Personal Hygiene."

20 Ibid.

21 Ibid.

22 Edward S. Morse, "Latrines of the East," *American Architect*, Mar. 18, 1893, 1–18.

with the shift to high imperialism, "the non-whites races were viewed as analogous to poor whites: dirty, uneducated, and of a low moral and hygienic standard (and therefore dangerous)."[23]

James Henderson's *Shanghai Hygiene*

Published in 1863, James Henderson's *Shanghai Hygiene* serves as a pivotal and, at 100 pages in length, pithy contribution to the field of hygienic medicine. Its aim is to prevent disease among British residents in China.[24] As a book of advice, it draws from both the classical origins and modern development of hygiene and applies both traditions to the situation of the British expatriate community in Shanghai and the rest of China. Hence, *Shanghai Hygiene* is a work that applies classical and modern theories of preventative medicine to imperial practice. It cautions the British community against the health risks posed by the Chinese community that, like the great unwashed of the metropolis, was ignorant, dirty, and, consequently, immoral. While these cautions are testament to the modern approach to hygiene as a community responsibility, subject to class and moral prejudice, the work remains anchored in the classical approach to hygiene, providing advice that is invariably humoralist.

Henderson's arguments, derived from first hand observation and experiences, also rely heavily on the theoretical and empirical canon of other medical writers—classical, English and Continental authors. He quotes such disparate sources as Hippocrates, Galen, Cabanis, Abernethy and Lankester, as well as other doctors.[25] The development of tropical hygiene is also a focus of the text. Henderson frequently refers to Dr. Martin's *The Influence of Tropical Climates on European Constitutions, Including Practical Observations on the Nature and Treatment of the Diseases of Europeans on Their Return from Tropical Climates*. Martin had re-written the entire work of James Johnson, while retaining many

---

23 *Companion Encyclopedia of the History of Medicine*, s.v. "The History of Personal Hygiene."

24 Henderson, *Shanghai Hygiene*, iv.

25 Ibid., 50. In the Galenic tradition, Henderson defines nature as "an assemblage of causes, which are directed to perform certain operations, and produce certain effects or results, in the wisest manner—In other words, the great author of all wisdom and power, who directs the greatest and most minute proceedings throughout the whole frame of the universe; and who by fixed laws for suns and systems, as well as for grains of sand, and minute molecules of matter, makes every bodily organ operate, as if it were endowed with reason and intelligence."

of his observations. Both works are derivative of their experiences in British India.[26]

Shanghai Hygiene is organized under ten headings, all of which accord with classical hygienic medicine and some of which even overlap with the non-naturals of humoralism: diet, drink, exercise, clothing, bathing, perspiration, *lichen tropicus*, the liver, sleep, the passion.[27] The preface commences encouragingly that a European with a tolerably good constitution "has his health almost entirely in his own keeping on arriving in Shanghai" (3). Thus, his introductory caution was for one to be careful in relation to diet, drink, exercise, and clothing, such that one need not fear the climate. Climate, according to classical medicine, was the non-natural of air, and could profoundly affect the body. Nevertheless, given the reality of colonial expansion into less temperate zones, the balancing of the other non-naturals could assist in the maintenance of hygiene. For example, during the winter, the body's cold and wet qualities had to be countered by food and drink of opposing qualities.

Henderson also defines his understanding of the term "constitution," borrowed from medical author Dunglison:

> The Constitution of an individual is the mode of organization proper to him. A man for example is said to have a robust or a delicate, or a good or a bad constitution when he is apparently strong or feeble, usually in good health, or liable to frequent attacks of disease. The varieties in constitution are therefore as numerous as the individuals themselves. A strong constitution is considered to be dependent upon the due development of the principal organs of the body, on a happy proportion between these organs, and on a fit state of energy of the nervous system; whilst the feeble or weak constitution results from a want of these postulates. [6–7]

26 James Martin, "Review IX: The Influence of Tropical Climates on European Constitutions," *The Medico-Chirurgical Review, or, Quarterly Journal of Practical Medicine and Surgery* 18 (July–Oct. 1856): 126.

27 Henderson, *Shanghai Hygiene*, 53. Hereafter page references are given in the text. Henderson emphasizes the importance of balance in the non-naturals. For example, Henderson cites Sir J. Martin, who warned that, however useful medicine may be in moderate doses, "it is yet more on the proper selection of localities, the avoidance of day and night exposure, care in diet, clothing, exercise etc.; in short, on the adoption of all those well-known measures of avoidance, whether affecting individual habit of life, or those more general predisposing causes of disease, now so well understood, that the prevention of disease depends; and not on a system of self-quackery."

Diet

Henderson's first caution to the British constitution in Shanghai concerns diet. Here, the overlap with the humoralist classification of non-naturals is remarkable, for he considers that food qualities and quantities as well as meal times can be preventative measures for a balanced health (4).[28]

Henderson warns against certain foods. Newly arrived Englishmen to China, Henderson advises, should be wary when they voyage to a hot atmosphere to avoid rich foods while in transit. The result otherwise would be "the feeling of languor and prostration, resulting purely from over repletion," especially if one was previously accustomed to simple food in the metropole (5, 11–12).[29] He writes: "The marvel is that the system does not sink under such a pressure, or that the digestive organs do not suddenly stop, under such wanton abuse" (5). Upon arrival, passengers should eat only food that is light and nutritious, and avoid food that is too stimulating. Henderson uses himself as an example, in declaring that the lifestyle and habits he leads in Shanghai are identical to how he lives at home, "with the exception of rigidly abstaining from all kinds of vegetables and fruit during the summer and autumn months." As a result, he had not been sick for even one day in China (9).

Fruit and vegetables, warns Henderson, are not safe to consume in China. Almost every case of bowel complaints, diarrhea, dysentery or cholera occurring in Shanghai during the summer months, he traces directly or indirectly to the indulgence of Chinese fruit or vegetables (9). Although he is not certain as to why this may be the case, Henderson does append a footnote to speculate that it may be due to "the peculiar kind of manure used here, and all over China, in raising fruit and vegetables?" and that foreigners are certainly more susceptible to these complaints than the Chinese. With many case studies of his European patients, he declares: "I repeat, that indulgence in Shanghai fruit, during the summer and autumn months, is incompatible with *continued good health* among the residents." The only exception might be a "person who becomes habituated to Chinese fruit as one may with drugs" (10–11).

---

28 James Martin, cited as an authority for this point of view, based his experience in India and deemed that the enemy of good hygiene was the consumption of local dishes, such as spices and other condiments, and that the most important rule of hygiene concerned the quantity and simplicity of meals.

29 Henderson then quotes Dr. Abercrombie and Sir Francis Head as authorities on the dangers of consuming very rich foods on the digestive system, as well as on not having food properly masticated. Food indigestible with "the proper juices" would result "ultimately in a bilious attack" (11–12).

Only rice is "*absolutely safe*" to consume during hot weather, and Henderson recommends this food as sufficient for nutrition and good health. Ideally, then, residents should content themselves with rice and in order to avoid contracting diarrhea, dysentery, or disordered liver during the summer months in the East (11). Henderson's dietary prescriptions, then, are to eat simple food during hot weather: "roast mutton, beef, fowl, or fowl curry for dinner, while for breakfast a mutton chop, fresh eggs, curry, and bread and butter, with coffee or tea, or claret and water."

Henderson also warns against excessive quantities of food, particularly in the hot season (a constant concern of his). In the hot months, he writes, only half the quantity of food is required as compared with the cold months. Excess consumption of food oppresses the system with materials that the body cannot process, and, consequently, induces fever (6).[30] The dangers of over-eating in Shanghai, "and other parts of the East," are to overload the stomach, irritate the bowels, or derange the functions of the liver during very hot weather. Medically, he writes, the result of this excess of food is an enlarged and fatty liver, "languor, constipation, alternating with diarrhea, irritability, listlessness, and after a time, breathlessness, and a puffy appearance of the skin, or sallowness result according to individual temperament" (5). Medical treatment, therefore, would be required as well as "a change of air, or a more bracing climate for perfect recovery" (13).

Henderson is convinced that the British, who, while living in the West had always exercised moderation, somehow became complacent when moving to the East, and would lead a lifestyle of eating excessively, commonly, "six, eight or ten dishes during a meal" (6–7). Even those with "fine elastic constitutions," Henderson warns, "may *for a time* proceed with impunity and set all rules at defiance," but a time will arrive when more care will be required. Henderson is emphatic with his opinion:

> Why should a meal in Shanghai be so different from one in England? Why should a man partake of a greater quantity of viands at once here, than he used to do at home? Why should our palates be pampered by a greater variety of food, in the East, than in the West? The stomach cannot digest more, on the contrary, during the warm weather, Nature ever a kind and watchful mother, places as it were, her fingers on the wheels

30 Martin had issued that very warning to English residents in India and prescribed that those Europeans in the East should be wary of late and heavy dinners and should be content with a light and early principal meal, at six or seven o'clock. This would ensure an early rise in the morning with more vigor.

> of the digestive organs, and thus prevents them from turning so fast as to oppress the system and induce fever, apoplexy, and other evils. [13]

Henderson's last caution on diet is to do with meal times. The ideal time for breakfast, he writes, is 12 or 1 o'clock, as this time "adopted by many in Shanghai is good and wholesome" and should be "the most substantial meal of the day," while a light tea should only be partaken of during the hot weather "at seven or eight o'clock" (8–9), much later than teatime back in Britain.[31]

Shanghai Hygiene attacks, at great length, the dietary habits of foreigners in Shanghai as the cause of ill health, rather than to attribute disease to the climate. Controlling one's diet, then, is one of the reactive measures that foreigners can use to conquer their ability to survive in tropical climes:

> During Summer and Autumn here, the powers of the stomach and digestive organs are weak, and therefore it is a most injurious and dangerous practice to oppress them with too much, or too great variety of food; such practice is sure to result in mischief of some sort, and the most common result in Shanghai is diarrhea; and I am strongly inclined to blame errors in diet fully as much, if not more, for producing these and other disease at that season, than the Shanghai climate. [14]

Earlier, he had reported how:

> Instead, too many Europeans have heavy dinners—soup, then sherry, then one or two side dishes, champagne or beer, then rice and curry and ham, then game, then pudding, pastry, jelly, custard, more champagne, then cheese and salad, and bread and butter, a glass of port wine, then oranges, figs, raisins, walnuts, with 2–3 glasses of claret or other wine, then strong coffee and cigars. Now, in the name of reason and common sense, how *can* a man preserve his health, under such a system? [11]

Henderson concludes his prescriptions on diet with Abernethy's "Rules of Diet":

---

31 Henderson quotes an anecdote from Johnson's manual, which warned against heavy breakfasts in the East. One of Johnson's patients died following a heavy breakfast, and listed the "items of the last breakfast." "Let the fate of the dead prove a warning to the living." Extra caution, warns Johnson, must always be adhered for the purposes of good health "if the atmosphere is not bright and cold" (8–9).

1. Food should be nourishing and in readily digestible form;
2. Quantity should be moderate so that the stomach can digest it perfectly;
3. Meals should be eaten regularly—every 6 hours, three times a day; or four times in 24 hours (if sick);
4. Every meal to reduce naturally without additional fluids via mastication and liquids from the stomach;
5. Drink should be taken 4 hours after each meal to allow for digestion, and 2 hours for the conveyance of liquids from the stomach before more food is received;
6. Drink should not contain fermentable substances. Preferably, boiled water, flavored with toast, or with powdered ginger. [21–22]

Acknowledging that these rules may be too stringent to be observed by all, Henderson concludes with a simple dictum for readers to follow: "Never eat unless we are hungry; and never to drink unless we are dry; to observe great moderation in doing both" (22).

Drink

Temperance, in Victorian literature, is synonymous with drink. In China, temperance was of especial concern in the hot weather, where it was essential to balance one's body temperature and to keep cool. Those Europeans "who are temperate in the use of beer, wine and spirits, will be in the enjoyment of health and vigor, and capable to undergo the greatest fatigues, mental and bodily without injury" (24). Henderson, using both his own and other doctors' experience in foreign postings, warns of the danger of drinking excessive amounts of water and wine (22). Just as drunkenness might be the cause of "every crime," intemperance also promotes the invasion of every tropical or other disease, from a physical point of view. The abuse of alcohol consumption, he writes at a later point in the text, "is the next prolific cause of shattered health and general debility" (67). The consumption of wine, brandy and beer must be with moderation, for "taken in excess it is degrading and pernicious" (67). This has consequences for the family, and can lead to "idiocy ... brutality of disposition, and feebleness of procreative family" (68). In Sweden, as a singular caution for the interplay between individual and community health, Henderson quotes how "the existing people have, through abuse of alcohol, fallen in physical strength and stature, below the standard of their forefathers" (68).

Henderson addresses the question of what to drink. Wine, while "not essential to the welfare or health of a strong man in Shanghai more than in England," can be beneficial in small doses in the hot weather. In moderate quantities, wine "operates as a mild stimulant to the vascular and nervous system, diffuses an agreeable feeling of warmth over the body, quickens the action of the heart, increases muscular force, excites the mental powers, and dispels unpleasant thoughts" (29–30). Water, however, cannot be recommended in Shanghai, for it was very impure (28).[32] Shanghai water requires thorough distillation, then boiling. Excessively cold water, that is the use of ice, can also be injurious to health, especially as it could injure the process of digestion (28). Cold drink can further endanger the function of perspiration, he argues, "especially when fatigue or exhaustion has occurred" (25). Soda water and lemonade in moderate quantities may be good and refreshing, but could interfere with digestion (30–31).

Shanghai Hygiene recommends tea and coffee:

> Tea is far too little used, during hot weather. It has a peculiar and gently stimulating influence on the nervous system, which is not followed by a corresponding depression, as after wine or beer. Tea is also slightly astringent.... But when morbid, vascular, or nervous excitement exists, it generally proves an excellent tonic and sedative, procuring sleep, and diminishing both nervous and vascular disorder. In cases of asthenic vascular action attended by coma or lethargy, I have found it a most valuable restorative of both vital and cerebral power. [31]

In terms of humoral balance, then, Henderson acknowledges that while tea and coffee are not nutritious, their active agents are beneficial for the body. That is, that they delay the disintegration of useful bodily tissue, such that the body is sustained and supported. Without tea and coffee, the body would deteriorate faster (31). "I feel convinced," he writes, "that tea is the best, safest and most wholesome drink we could take here in the hottest weather" (32). Using as an example his own health during his time in Shanghai, he continues: "I may state, that during my first years in Shanghai, I drank nothing stronger than tea and coffee. During the hot weather I had two bottles of tea made in the morning with a little citric acid I used as a drink through the day, and found

32 In a footnote, Henderson adds: "Shanghai water should never be used as drink alone, unless it is both filtered and boiled; if thoroughly filtered, it may be drunk with wine or a little brandy without boiling; but it contains so much organic matter it should all be boiled" (28).

it both refreshing and agreeable" (32–34).[33] Coffee, Henderson agrees, has the same composition as that of tea and so concludes his advice on drink with this prescription to British residents: "let more tea and coffee be used in hot weather, and let the stronger wines and beer be used very sparingly, and let French and German wines take their place" (35).

Exercise

Henderson proceeds to the next of the non-naturals, that is, exercise. He continues to caution moderation. Exercise, under classical medicine, was essential to the regulation and maintenance of the constitution. Without exercise, the body would become languid and imbalanced between parts of the body. In Shanghai, Henderson's challenge for residents is to be able to undertake aerobic exercise without overheating:

> By exercise I do not mean a stroll along the Bund, or a walk out to the Race-course.... In order to be beneficial, exercise must be taken so as to stimulate all the bodily functions, the circulation should be quickened, respiration should be accelerated, more or less perspiration should be induced, and a healthy glow should be communicated to the whole system. [35]

Walking, for Henderson, is the best form of exercise, "as every organ or function is in action, all muscles are exercised and strengthened, especially in the back and lower extremities" (35). He scorns the hobby of driving in a carriage or riding in a chair, which "is only suitable for invalids, being far too passive for healthy people except in hot weather, when all active exercise should be modified or suspended" (35–36). He does, however, warn against walking "aimlessly" as it is "monotonous and tiring" (35), and against excessive exercise in hot weather. Accordingly, he recommends the performance only of *essential* exercise for one's daily duties, "except early in the morning, or after 6 pm, when a ride on horseback, a short walk, a drive or a pull on the river

33 Henderson also gives his own anecdote preceding his time in Shanghai to illustrate his predisposition to the merits of tea: "During my two last years at college, I used green tea and strong coffee freely, studying every night til 2–3 o'clock am. This with two light meals per day, one at half past 8 am and the other about 6 pm, I enjoyed excellent health, and could do almost any amount of work" (34).

may be beneficial" (36). While the aim of exercise in the north is to keep up a just balance in one's circulation in order to maintain the functions of the skin, the south, he warns European residents in tropical communities, holds more danger. With "perspiration, biliary, and other secretions being already in excess in equatorial regions, a perseverance in our customary European exercise, would prove highly injurious, and it often does so, by promoting and aggravating the ill effects of an unnatural climate" (36). Accordingly, any excess would lead to "debility," which diminishes the necessary actions of the body, and inequilibrium of the blood. Caution and judgment to preserve health and balance, then, is necessary to counteract these measures by passive or active exercise, climate permitting (36).

Clothing and Bedding

The temperature of the body could be moderated by clothing. To regulate the changes in temperature in Shanghai, Henderson cautions how:

> The cardinal rule to be observed, with regard to the changeable temperature of Shanghai, is, always to put on warm clothing as soon as the afternoons and evenings begin to be cool at the close of summer; and not to put on light summer clothing, until the warm weather has fairly set in. [37]

He attributes diarrhea, dysentery, and ague to insufficient clothing during the autumn, both during the day and evening, as well as the nights. Empirically, Henderson notes that the middle of September becomes very cold, and ordered the use of one or two blankets during such "chilly" nights and warned how changes in temperature can be very sudden: "I have traced more diseases of the bowels, and more functional derangement of the different organs to the neglect of this precaution, than to any other cause at that season" (37). A large number of cases of bowel complaints would follow, among natives and Europeans, as well as cases of cholera and jaundice. "At that season it is no uncommon thing to wake up at two or three o'clock cold and chilled, and with pain in the bowels, the precursors of diarrhea, dysentery, or cholera, and if one has to get out of bed at that time, matters are made worse" (37).

As an added precaution, Henderson recommends keeping an extra blanket over the feet, to pull over the body once the cold is felt. In line with another non-natural, the aim is that of slight perspiration, so that the body's fluids, which:

> by the cold, had been driven upon the inner organs and bowels, causing congestion and griping pains, are again attracted to the surface of the body, and instead of passing off by the bowels, escape by the skins; thus a reaction takes place, and the balance of the circulation is again restored, and disease is prevented. [38]

Henderson even recommends bed types. Beds with cane bottoms, he advises, are the best during the hot weather. Mattresses are not advisable; instead, he advises spreading a blanket over the cane work. This method keeps the body much cooler than sleeping on a mattress, such that "instead of rising in the morning, bathed in perspiration and feeling exhausted, we wake up comparatively cool and refreshed" (38). A blanket is to cover the bowels at all times, even during the hot seasons.

Another way to regulate bodily temperature is to control the fabric of one's clothes. Europeans should not wear linen, which Henderson considers unsafe and uncomfortable, in the tropics. Instead, he advises that cotton be worn, the cloth of the locals, despite socio-economic classes. Cotton dress is slow to conduct heat, and well adapted for tropical climate. The body is consequently more able to maintain an equilibrium of temperature, and therefore more able to perspire readily. Woolen and cotton dresses are also warmer than linen in low temperatures, and cooler in higher temperatures. Henderson does not recommend flannel, for he believes that it does not moderate the body's temperature as effectively as cotton (38–39).

Moderation, then, is again the key. Henderson writes how the "great object of tropical prophylactics" is to "*moderate without checking the cuticular discharge*" (40). He issues a caution, too, against changing one's clothing too frequently, a habit of many new-arrivals and a habit with no detrimental consequences at home. Changing clothes more than simply in the morning and evening in the tropics, however, is "simply injurious" (40). This is because the fluids on the body's surface, "already in excess, are thus powerfully solicited, and the action of the perspiratory vessels, with all their associations, morbidly increase, instead of being restrained" (40).

The hygienic caution relating to the non-natural issues of clothing, then, pertains to its centrality in maintaining bodily temperature, and thus of the avoidance of bowel related disorders. By regulating the blankets and materials in which a person sleeps, he believes, one can maintain a consistent body temperature when the body is at its weakest with any changes in temperature; by wearing cotton clothing can one regulate the essential function of perspiration. Henderson concludes: "Attention to the above subjects, is perhaps the most essential for the preservation of health in China …" (41).

Bathing

Bathing was a considerable hygienic consideration in maintaining balance and cleanliness in Shanghai. *Shanghai Hygiene* issues various recommendations as to the virtues of bathing, in particular, for warm baths, public baths, and the moral implications of taking baths.

Henderson cautions his readers on how bathing is a practice that is unknown among the Chinese as one of the differences that Chinese people share with others in the East and those peoples who live in "warm or temperate regions. They go unwashed literally, from the cradle to the grave. The only thing in the shape of a substitute observed, was a cloth moistened with hot water, and passed lightly over the face and hands by persons, of distinction!" (5)

Bathing with water, nevertheless, is of great hygienic significance and a practice with a long-standing tradition in Britain and the West. Henderson makes a plea for the merits of bathing, and for public bathing.

> Bathing is a powerful therapeutic agent and I feel convinced it does not occupy such a position as it is entitled to, in treating diseases in China. We lack those facilities, which are essential to the proper application of water as a remedial agent, in treating diseases here; and one great boon connected with a hospital for Foreigners here would be, that different kinds of baths for treating various diseases could be established. [42]

Bathing as a practice was clearly part of the classical model of hygiene. Henderson recounts how Homer "describes Achilles, on issuing from the bath, as looking taller and fairer, and nearer the gods" (43). Indeed, he claims how classical Rome, with a population of five million, had many baths but no hospitals; "and it was recorded that during a period of 500 years, there was no physician in that vast city" and illness plagued the city "as the thermae of the ancient Romans went out of general use" (43).

Henderson recommends bathing in warm water, however warm or cool the weather. Cold bathing is to invite intemperance in the body, which can upset the viscera (41–42).[34] Warm water contains therapeutic elements to assist with healing:

> It may be concluded for certain, that, to persons who have suffered from tropical diseases, or who are affected with visceral congestions, or with

34 Dr. Mosely is cited as Johnson's authority; Dr. Johnson maintains, too, that "the cold bath *is* death" (41–42).

> visceral enlargements, especially, the results of fevers of dysenteries, the warm bath is the only safe one *at all seasons*. The same rule applies to the dissipated, and to such as are in the habit of keeping late hours. In such persons the balance of circulation is already disturbed, and the effect of cold water is to throw the blood with force on organs already irritated by irregular courses of life, the abdominal viscera especially. [42]

Accordingly, then, Henderson highly recommends the warm Turkish bath, for its remedial agents and agitates for its use in Shanghai. Many letters appeared in the *North China Herald* and advocated its use in the treatment of disease. The bath's "importance can scarcely be overrated, but like every other powerful remedy, caution, and great discrimination are requisite in its application, especially when the patient is delicate, or much reduced by disease" (43).

For Henderson, in addition to the classical hygienic merits of the Turkish bath, many social and communal benefits are evident. The Turkish bath, he argues, is both social as well as sanitary. The warmth "destroys the craving for strong drinks. It is a Temple of Temperance. The illustrious Bacon lamented the loss of these baths to European nations" (45). Even the rich, "and Queen Victoria would institute a fourth class who would patronize, support and frequent, these Temples of Health ... as the badge of Temperance, Purity and Pleasure" (45).

On the basis of hygiene, community health, and even with class considerations, Henderson therefore concludes this section with an emphatic plea to the enterprising promoters of the General Hospital to make provisions for the Turkish bath (45).

Perspiration

The Turkish bath assisted with the balance of another non-natural, that of retention and evacuation, which Henderson classifies as perspiration. Classical hygiene maintained that the body must be able to drain the build-up of waste within the body. Henderson analyzes the composition of perspiration and points to all the impurities and traces of foreign materials. He asks what would happen to the constitution should such drainage be obstructed? Henderson accordingly advocates the use of the Turkish bath, "in order to keep the myriads of mouths of these drains clean and open" (46). Sweat, then, can eliminate the impurities of the body.

The function of perspiration, Henderson advises, is for the drainage of waste as well as the regulation of the body's temperature:

> An apparatus has been provided, for relieving the body of any superabundance of heat, which would accumulate where the atmospheric temperature equals, or exceeds that of the body. By perspiration also, a number of deleterious substances is removed from the body, which if allowed to remain and accumulate in the system, would destroy health and life. [46]

Medically, profuse perspiration is necessary in the hot season because blood stimulates the liver, "which has been to an unusual extent deprived of water, while the kidneys are affected in the same manner, by a large amount of saline impregnation" (47). The skin, during a Shanghai summer, is also very active. The effect is that an excessive flow of fluids and blood occurs towards the surface of the body, "for perspiration is essentially a *cooling process*" (47). Once more, Henderson stresses the classical principle of balance: to control body temperature in the hot weather with perspiration, as well as the importance of eliminating impurities from a constitution.

Repose, too, is of importance. Henderson advises how if, after walking in the sun extensively, one sweats excessively, one should rest for at least an hour. This period of rest will restore the appetite, until one drinks a stimulating fluid to "excite the energy of the stomach." If the appetite does not return, this "is Nature's caveat, to beware of eating at all." Such advice, Henderson concedes, may be difficult to follow, but "those who neglect or despise it may feel the bad consequences, or when it is too late to repair the error" (48). Though repose is an important hygienic concern for the community, Henderson does not make any alternatives for the poor.

Although not strictly a principle of classical medicine, *lichen tropicus* is a concern particular to residents of Shanghai. "Exercise, producing excessive perspiration is another cause of prickly heat, and hence perspiration should be modified" (49). Shanghai residents are particularly prone to this "annoyance," maintains Henderson, during the Shanghai summer (48). Prickly heat is a sensation that is:

> perfectly indescribable, being compounded of pricking, itching, tingling, and many other feelings for which there is no appropriate appellation. It is usually but not invariably accompanied by an eruption of vivid, red, pimples not larger in general than a pin's head, which spread over the breast, arms, thighs, neck and occasionally close to the hair. The eruption often disappears to a certain degree when we are sitting quiet, and the skin is cool. [48]

Temperance is required to treat this, for Henderson is of the opinion that excess bathing aggravates prickly heat (48–49). Temperance in both exercise and in bathing, then, serves as a caution against this itching.

Liver Function

Temperance, too, according to Henderson, underpins the proper maintenance of the liver. Unlike the other parts of *Shanghai Hygiene*, this part does not concern an aspect of human behavior but it concerns "the largest organ in the body." Henderson holds: "No organ is more influenced by temperature, diet, drink, perspiration, clothing and exercise" (49). The liver produces bile, and either a lack of or excess of bile is dangerous to one's constitution. To avoid such potentially fatal imbalances, Henderson advises temperance with the other non-naturals: food, drink, exercise and heat. He appeals frequently to Galenic humoralism for his analysis of the liver (50).

For Henderson, the importance of temperance is of constant emphasis. Food and drink should be simple "for if the liver is too much stimulated," this will either result in the "enlargement and chronic inflammation of the organ, or a reaction will take place, and little or no bile will be secreted" (51). Henderson cautions how too large or frequent quantities of "animal, rich and highly seasoned food" and too great a "variety of incongruous dishes, and sauces, and spices, and wines, particularly in warm countries, and seasons, are most influential causes of disease" (51).

Similarly, the excess use of "*spirituous* or other intoxicating liquors" is "productive of the diseases of this organ." Such diseases are more acute in warm climates, while in "temperate countries," the resulting diseases are "of the more chronic and structural maladies" (51–52).

Henderson cautions readers of the three dangerous conditions peculiar to the liver in hot climate: the excessive secretion of bile, the diminished secretion of bile, and the secretion of vitiated bile. In turn, he states: "Each of these conditions assumes all kinds of modifications, resulting from individual temperament, constitution, diet, drink, exercise, clothing, habits, the regulation of passions, etc." (52).

The first danger, of excessive bile secretion "irritates the stomach and bowels, producing vomiting, and a more rapid passage of substances through the intestinal tube, with severe griping pains and straining; producing in short the same effects as a large dose of an irritating purgative-medicine" (54). Henderson's solution to this is to be moderate in the consumption of food and drink.

Especially in hot weather, one should not consume too many "highly seasoned dishes," "beer and wine" and to take measures to not perspire too much, "for it will be found that the most intimate relation, and the strongest sympathy exists, between the perspiration and the secretion of the bile" (54). One can achieve the latter by avoiding "violent exercise, which will increase the perspiration, and therefore the biliary secretion" (54–55).

The second danger, of diminished bile secretion, means: "The liver will scarcely secrete a particle of bile; and thus some formidable diseases are induced, requiring powerful remedies to overcome them" (55). The solution to this problem, once again, relates to temperance and diet. That is, to not eat or drink foods that are too rich, such as "pickles, hot curries, varieties of wine, etc." (55)

The third danger is the secretion of vitiated bile. Vitiated bile has many, different symptoms, "from undefined uneasy feelings, slight nausea, headache, low spirits, to the most violent vomiting, colic, cholera and dysentery" (57). Henderson's advice is to exercise temperance in daily activity. That is, to be moderate with ordinary exercise, not to expose oneself to the heat of the sun, or drink stimulating liquids. This prevents "an increased and vitiated flow of bile" (58).

The liver, then, is central to maintaining the health of one's constitution. Henderson's advice is completely of the orthodoxy of the medicine of his day. Classical hygiene, stressing temperance, provides the medical solution that so many of his patients encounter in Shanghai, which he maintains, relate to the liver.

Sleep

Sleep, a continuation of the aforementioned topic of rest, is another requirement of hygienic medicine. The quality of sleep is of importance to Henderson, and again, moderation is advisable in all aspects of living: "The less that one perspires during sleep the better. In order to secure sound and refreshing sleep during the hot weather, late dinners and generous wines, *must* be avoided" (60–61).

Especially because of the hot weather, Henderson argues that sleep is important for one's balance. After all, "The design and end of sleep is to renew the vital energy, and to restore exhausted nature" (59). Henderson continues:

> In order to secure permanently good health, we require more sleep in a hot climate, than in a temperate one; as a general rule, if we required seven hours sleep in England, we ought to have eight in China. Sound,

> refreshing and undisturbed repose influences our health and constitution more than is generally supposed. Unfortunately when it is very hot, refreshing sleep is the exception, not the rule. Our great aim should be to *sleep cool*, and be thoroughly protected from mosquitos. [60]

In line with Henderson's opinion that more sleep is required in hot weather, he consoles his readers who cannot sleep soundly through the night that an afternoon siesta may be desirable. "Half an hour sleep after" the principal meal "may be taken as an advantage in hot weather" (61). Again, how a member of the poorer classes can afford to sleep more, Henderson does not mention.

Of great concern, then, is that the body be able to sleep cool on light stomachs and mattress-less cane beds, consistent with *Shanghai Hygiene*'s advice concerning the merits of heat restraint, the function of perspiration, early sleeping patterns, and temperance.

The Passions (Sexual Health)

Perhaps of all the non naturals, the passions best typify the integration of classical individual hygiene with the modern community-focused category of hygiene. Galenic medicine referred to the entire man as a natural balance. Morality and class influence contemporary hygiene. According to Henderson, passions have much to do with the physician, for "mind and matter are too closely combined to be studied or treated apart. To medicine alone it belongs to contemplate, and to treat the *entire man—physical, moral* and *intellectual*" (61).

Self-control is thus necessary. Henderson cautions that people must be more aware of the "great injury they sustain" if they do not control their passions. Otherwise, their health and constitution will suffer from the condition of their mind (62). Nonetheless, strong passions, with control, make the constitution and the psyche of a people great:

> England, France, and America are great, because the people have strong passions; but England is greatest because her people can command their passions. The Chinese have little passion (except those in common with the brutes, self preservation and cunning) hence every thing is stagnant, and has a low standard. [63]

Control, Henderson asserts, is essential to morality. Morality in turn dictates the happiness and balance of a person. Henderson tells of his acquaintance with various men of both classes in the East, "and for health, strength and *happiness*, the strictly moral man will contrast most favorably with one of the opposite class." By contrast, he expresses how he has "seen many suffer severely, destroy their health, happiness and life, by following the promptings of their unbridled passions; need I say, that *I have never seen a man suffer from keeping himself pure*" (65).

Morality is of particular importance because, in the periphery, many expatriates are single and bored. Henderson believes, many Europeans turn to promiscuity because of the "greater laxity of moral and religious principle" in the periphery (65–66).

A second check on passions in the tropics, writes Henderson, is to engage with refined literature. Henderson devotes a very long footnote to the importance of literature, in an elitist exposition that clearly excludes the poorer classes. He cautions how:

> The monotony of life and the apathy of mind so conspicuous in hot climates, together with the obstacles to matrimony, too often lead to vicious and immoral acts, which speedily sap the foundations of principles imbibed in early youth, and involve a train of consequences, not seldom embarrassing, if not embittering every subsequent period of life. It is here that a taste for some of the more refined, and elegant species of literature, will prove an invaluable acquisition for dispelling *ennui*—the moth of mind and body. [66]

Self-control, then, is his link between morality and health. Henderson maintains that the "influence of public and private morals on the health and welfare of communities is too little thought of, for its power is very great" (66–67). Public morality, as he sees it, is a direct determinant of public health.

Climate (Air)

Although air is, classically, a non-natural, *Shanghai Hygiene* does not explicitly treat air as a heading in itself. In Henderson's very long closing remarks, he devotes over ten pages to the topic of climate. This is in addition to his substantial and integrated sections on climate within the other non-naturals. Climate is a very important category of analysis that permeates through the entire text of *Shanghai Hygiene*.

Henderson laments at how little significance the literature on the climate of China has played, despite the substantial foreign presence over the last eighteen to twenty years. That is, little beyond the Chinese climate being "a trying climate" or "a very flat locality" or "something equally vague and indefinite: and although hosts of medical practitioners have resided at this port, professedly to treat disease, they have done nothing to prevent disease, the more important of the two" (72–73). Accordingly, he recommends: "We should study well the climate, and mold our obsequious frames to the nature of the skies under which we sojourn" (74).[35]

His concern, then, is for new residents to be aware of their own bodily constitution and to be proactive with maintaining one's hygiene, in consideration of all climate related issues, when going to a new station or posting. For, "surely a subject which so powerfully influences man's health, and consequently his happiness, demands all the attention and the most careful investigation which we can possibly give to it" (74).

Henderson understood the physical climate of a city to be dependent upon certain principal particulars: temperature, humidity, geological nature of the soil, drainage and cultivation, proximity of sea and rivers, general and local elevation, position of mountains, prevalent winds, general and local aspects, trees and vegetation (75). Besides these,

> if we wish to arrive at anything like accuracy, many other points must be observed, as perpendicular pressure of the atmosphere, electricity, the purity and transparency of the air, the quality of the water, the ozone, the moral condition of the people, their degree of intelligence, appearance, etc. and whether or not there be many aged people among them, what diseases prevail in the locality, and especially what is the type of the diseases. [75–76]

Henderson's conclusion is one of optimism, and reiterates the importance of the hygienic principle of temperance. For, if a person with a good constitution abides by temperance, strictly avoids eating "cheap Chinese fruit" as found in the streets, and also takes "care to provide against the changes of temperature, which supervene suddenly during the autumn," then with all of "*these* precautions, there is no reason to fear the climate of Shanghai" (89). Not taking a pessimistic and determinist line in relation to climate could, then, assure Britons arriving in China of their potential survival in their new posting. This is important as it ensured the European constitution's probable survival and, therefore, also survival in the colonial missions of the day.

---

35 Henderson quotes Dr. Johnson as authority.

General Remarks

Shanghai Hygiene's concluding remarks acknowledge that despite climate, Shanghai, like other foreign settlements, "may be improved to almost any extent by artificial means, if judiciously adopted and vigorously varied into operation" (89). Henderson's analysis and conclusion are more in line with modern developments in hygienic medicine, that is, he concludes in favor of a communal policy and a moral stance. In effect, Henderson makes a call for the "transformation of physical space"[36] to make China more like Britain for the foreign communities to keep healthy.

Politically, Henderson laments how "unfortunately the health, and consequently the lives of the inhabitants have occupied the smallest share of the attention of governments, legislators, political economists, and municipal authorities in most countries" (90). To him, Shanghai is no exception. Policy aside, Henderson then makes a moral complaint:

> The multifarious modes in which avarice, ignorance, low cunning, and the love of overreaching, are practiced both by natives and a certain class of foreigners, sap directly and indirectly the springs of health and life, and often frustrate the best intentions of those at the helm of affairs. [90–91]

Good public health in Shanghai requires cleanliness, drainage and street planning, which "will as surely improve the health of the Shanghai community as effect follows cause" (91–92). The provision of new hospitals, which follow the principles of classical hygienic medicine, is also necessary.

Henderson's concluding recommendations, then, are twofold. Foreign residents in Shanghai must have "a large and well arranged general hospital" and "a commodious and conveniently situated Sanatorium" (100). And so *Shanghai Hygiene* emphatically concludes, with Henderson's plea: "I am convinced, that by this simple, and eminently practical means, much disease would be averted, better health would be secured, and *many lives would be saved*" (100).

Consistency of Other Medical Reports with *Shanghai Hygiene*

Henderson was not the only British doctor in China who subscribed to hygienic medicine. The *Customs Gazette* carries reports by the doctors who served in

36 Alan Bewell, *Romanticism and Colonial Disease* (London: John Hopkins University Press, 1999), 43.

the Imperial Customs Service, and who maintained the health of the British communities in China. These reports show a high degree of consistency between the theory of *Shanghai Hygiene* and the practices of British doctors in China. Like *Shanghai Hygiene*, the concerns of these British doctors are also with motion and exercise, food and drink, retentions and evacuations, and other humoralist dichotomies. They too agree on the virtue of temperance as the morality of hygiene. And they too dismiss the Chinese just as their British-based colleagues dismiss the "great unwashed" that the working classes in Britain had become.

Dr. James Watson was one medical officer who consistently demonstrates his commitment to the principles of classical hygienic medicine. His report from Newchwang (Yingkou) in 1871, for example, shows how the principles of classical hygiene, such as air and food, inform his cure tonics. He remarks how even during the summer months, the weather was "remarkably cool."[37] He then identifies diarrhea as a common complaint of his patients, of which the cause was "the eating of unripe fruit. To these may be added indiscretions in diet generally."[38] Watson's treatment, in line with classical hygiene, is "complete rest, simple diet, a few doses of ipecacuanha and soothing injections, followed by slight astringents."[39] Watson then concludes with a caution:

> Afterwards tonics and careful living speedily restore the patient to perfect health. I find that people who during the warm weather keep out of the direct rays of the sun, wear a broad flannel belt around the bowels, and are moderately careful in diet, are seldom attacked by diarrhea.[40]

Again and again, these reports echo Henderson's views, adding particular examples and details as they do so.

British medical officers are clearly concerned with diet and make frequent references to both the Chinese and British diets. Dr. Patrick Manson and Dr. David Manson warn from Amoy (Xiamen 厦门) in 1873 that European mothers are often unable to breastfeed their children in China: the "European constitution must be altered in this respect before it could flourish here."[41] Their

37 James Watson, "Dr. James Watson's Report on the Health of Newchwang for the Half-year Ended 30th September 1871," *Customs Gazette: Medical Reports*, no. 3 (1872): 10.

38 Ibid.

39 Ibid.

40 Ibid., 10–11.

41 Patrick Manson and David Manson, "The Drs. Mansons' Report on the Health of Amoy for the Half-year Ended 30th September 1873," *Customs Gazette: Medical Reports*, no. 6 (1873): 31.

caution and solution is to improve the quality and supply of the food residents consume, in order to protect their bodies from disease.[42] In 1881, Dr. Patrick Manson warns residents who insist on eating pork to cook it in the same way that the locals do "Cooked as the natives cook it there can be little danger, but a roast leg of pork cooked in foreign style would certainly be a most dangerous dish."[43] Manson warns missionaries and those who travel much within the Chinese interior and who live on a budget to keep away from "foreign bazaars" but, "if they will have pork, they ought to have it cooked in small pieces, thoroughly, and in native fashion."[44] Dr. T. Rennie, too, at Foochow 福州 issues caution against the food and drink found there when he hypothesizes how "salad washed in unfiltered water may be the cause of the frequent occurrence of lumbrici among Europeans."[45]

Concerns about the quality of water across China remain constant in this period. During an epidemic of 1883, many members of the foreign community were immunized from cholera. Although 10,000–20,000 Chinese died, only two reported deaths among the 250–300 foreigners occurred. Both were females, "in one case the attack was traced to bad drinking water, and in the other to unsound fruit. There can be little doubt that the precautions which foreigners take with regard to drinking water account for their freedom from disease."[46] Dr. Jamieson's report from Shanghai cites academic works as authority for his suspicion that fecal matter contaminates much of the water in Shanghai.[47]

In another report, Dr. Jamieson warns against intemperance with alcohol in the hot Shanghai weather. Although he acknowledges that alcohol may sometimes assist with circulation, "the moral of course is that it is only by an abuse of terms that 'total abstinence' can be qualified as 'temperance'."[48] Dr. W.W. Myers analyzes the opinion of another medical practitioner who argues that most cases of fatal aneurism could "be traced either to intemperance in the use

42 Ibid.

43 Patrick Manson, "Trichina Spiralis in Chinese Pork by Dr. Patrick Manson," *Customs Gazette: Medical Reports*, no. 21 (1881): 26.

44 Ibid.

45 T. Rennie, "Dr. T. Rennie's Report on the Health of Foochow for the Year Ended 31st March 1881," *Customs Gazette: Medical Reports*, no. 21 (1881): 51.

46 J.J. Underwood, "Chinese Medicine: To the Editors of *The Lancet*," *The Lancet*, Oct. 20, 1888, 799.

47 Alexander Jamieson, "Dr. Alexander Jamieson's Report on the Health of Shanghai for the Half-year Ended 31st March 1873," *Customs Gazette: Medical Reports*, no. 5 (1873): 51.

48 Alexander Jamieson, "Dr. Alexander Jamieson's Report on the Health of Shanghai for the Half-year Ended 31st March 1874," *Customs Gazette: Medical Reports*, no. 7 (1874): 43.

of alcohol or to syphilis."[49] Dr. Myers' report concludes that alcohol by itself is not an evil, when taken in moderation:

> One cannot scientifically class alcohol as a food necessary to the normal man; but as a luxury, enjoyed within physiological limits, it may be taken by the majority of healthy persons, not only with impunity but according to temperament, with a certain amount of mental content. Daily experience proves how indispensable alcohol is as a medicine, whether applied to call up reserves of force, temporarily retard tissue change, or produce other beneficial chemical and physiological results.[50]

When Dr. J. Jardine diagnoses one English patient with serous, or sero-sanguineous effusion to the brain, chest and other parts of the body, he treates the patient using the principles of hygienic medicine. Dr. Jardine notes how the patient had lived almost exclusively on tea and toast—he had abstained from a fresh-meat and vegetable diet. Immediately, he "was ordered an antiscorbutic diet of a generous character, lime-juice, milk, and a tincture of per chloride of iron and quinine; but it is certain that he still continued to neglect himself."[51] Regretfully the patient died, for the patient did not sustain this diet into his lifestyle.

In order to attain balance in one's lifestyle, doctors actively encouraged their patients to exercise, temperature permitting. Dr. Jamieson praises the foreign residents in Shanghai for taking advantage of organized trips into the country to "render open air exercise on both a large and a small scale available for all sections of the community, female as well as male, children as well as adults."[52] Dr. Manson at Amoy also urges "everyone who can, especially ladies and children, to go to the hills or seaside for five weeks or two months in July and August, for when these months are tided over the great heat is past."[53] They highly recommend Kushan (within Amoy) as a sanatorium for foreigners, because foreigners could exercise and retreat here, in well-ventilated houses, to negate

---

49 W.W. Myers, "Dr. W.W. Myers's Report on the Health of Takow," *Customs Gazette: Medical Reports*, no. 28 (1884): 22.

50 Ibid.

51 J. Jardine, "Dr. J. Jardine's Report on the Health of Kiukiang for the Year Ended 31st March 1880," *Customs Gazette: Medical Reports*, no. 19 (1880): 9.

52 Jamieson, "Dr. Alexander Jamieson's Report on the Health of Shanghai for the Half-year Ended 31st March 1873," 52.

53 J.R. Somerville, "Dr. J.R. Somerville's Report on the Health of Foochow (Pagoda Anchorage) for the Half-year Ended 30th September 1875," *Customs Gazette: Medical Reports*, no. 10 (1875): 38.

the effects of the hot weather. Dr. John Kenneth Mackenzie, from Ningbo, relieves at how the health of foreign residents over the previous year "has been remarkably good, due, I have no doubt, in a great degree to the coolness of the summer, which permitted people to take more exercise than is customary among the majority of foreigners in the warm season."[54]

Clothing could sometimes moderate and assist the body's processing of hot weather. Dr. E.I. Scott warns how "intermittent fever is common among sailors who sleep on the decks of their ships with very little covering, and who swim under the hot sun." In this case, regretfully, whether or not the sailors wore a hat as protection, they would almost certainly come down with fever within 24 hours.[55] Clearly, then, a more holistic approach was required. Dr. Jamieson warns of the causes of malaria and dysentery that in his opinion, "Greater care on the part of individuals as regards diet, drink and dress has also tended to limit the number of cases, and perhaps to render those which do occur less severe."[56]

As a further precaution against cholera, Dr. E.A. Aldridge advises residents to not only boil and filter the water and be careful with diet, but also to wear appropriate clothing. A "broad thick flannel belt, even if not worn in the daytime, should always be worn at night, while the sleeping clothes should be made of flannel; … exposure to night air should be avoided, and therefore sleeping on the verandahs abandoned."[57]

British medical officers are also quick to recommend the therapeutic qualities of bathing. Dr. Myers compliments the sulfur springs at Chefoo (Yantai), as useful in "the treatment of cutaneous diseases and rheumatism consequent on constitutional taint."[58] Both the Chinese and foreigners used the springs to cure many diseases, and

> in those obstinate cases of syphilitic disease where rheumatic, ulcerative or cutaneous manifestations are unaffected by the ordinary treatment, I have in many instances found a trip to the baths either quite sufficient

54 John Kenneth Mackenzie, "Dr. Mackenzie's Report on the Health of Ningpo for the Year Ended 31st March 1877," *Customs Gazette: Medical Reports*, no. 13 (1877): 46.

55 E.I. Scott, "Dr. E.I. Scott's Report on the Health of Swatow for the Half-year Ended 30th September 1876," *Customs Gazette: Medical Reports*, no. 12 (1876): 19.

56 Alexander Jamieson, "Dr. Alexander Jamieson's Report on the Health of Shanghai for the Half-year Ended 31st March 1881," *Customs Gazette: Medical Reports*, no. 21 (1881): 84.

57 E.A. Aldridge, "Dr. E.A. Aldridge's Report on the Health of Hoihow for the Half-year Ended 30th September 1881," *Customs Gazette: Medical Reports*, no. 22 (1881): 6.

58 W.W. Myers, "Dr. W.W. Myers's Report on the Sanitary Condition of Chefoo," *Customs Gazette: Medical Reports*, no. 3 (1872): 41.

> or at least of such decided advantage as to render slight additional and subsequent treatment completely effective.[59]

Dr. J.H. Lowry thoroughly recommends the locality of Pakhoi (Beihai 北海), despite the town's dangerous miasmatic emanations. Geographically, he finds Pakhoi advantageous, for it has the benefits of both the country and the seaside, allowing for riding and exercise. In particular, "sea-bathing can be indulged in with impunity in the evenings. In the present age it is hardly necessary to speak of the advantages of the sea-bath, acting as it does very powerfully on tissue metamorphosis."[60]

Geography also determined how much one's constitution could perspire. Dr. W.A. Henderson views the northern climates as drier, and southern climates as more moist:

> From the lungs of those who drink in dry air, the dry air quaffs large draughts of water, giving rise to deliciously exhilarating feelings. Not only does dry air rob the blood of its water by the lungs, but also by the skin. Perspiration is less sensible in the dry than in the moist climate; yet we know that it is greater, the dry air rapidly carrying it off as it is formed. On the contrary, the moist climate checks evaporation from both of those organs.[61]

In relation to the air, medical missionary, Dr. Benjamin Hobson, even as early as 1848, comments on how "Lichen tropicus or prickly heat is a source of much inconvenience to foreigners." This is because towards "the close of the hot season, natives, as well as foreigners, are liable to be affected with boils."[62]

Clearly, then, the hot season was of grave concern to the balance of the British constitution. The liver was central to the functioning of the body. Dr. W.R.E. Smart studies the health of the liver according to the climatic patterns of Hong Kong and the Canton River station. His conclusions, collated by Dr. B.G. Babington as president of the Epidemiological Society, were published

---

59 Ibid.

60 J.H. Lowry, "Dr. J.H. Lowry's Report on the Health of Pakhoi for the Half-year Ended 30th September 1882," *Customs Gazette: Medical Reports*, no. 24 (1882): 27.

61 W.A. Henderson, "Dr. W.A. Henderson's Report on the Health of Ningpo for the Eighteen Months Ended 30th September 1880," *Customs Gazette: Medical Reports*, no. 20 (1880): 28.

62 Benjamin Hobson, "Brief Notice of the Hospital at Kum-Le-Fau in Canton, During the Year 1851," in *The Hobson Papers, Wellcome Manuscripts* (London: Wellcome Library, 1851), Box MS 5852/43, 25.

as a report in British Medical Journal on 1 June 1861. Dr. Smart shows a humoralist concern for climate and its effect on liver diseases. He considers that "the healthy season is the spring" and so reinforces the hygienic theme of temperance even in the seasons.[63]

The seasons also affected sleep patterns. Dr. James Watson at Newchwang is of the opinion that the "morning air is exhilarating in its charming freshness, while the cool evening soothes and refresh the weak, and sleep, which here requires no wooing, is followed by increased strength and energy."[64] Doctors also issue advice on how the quality of sleep can improve according to the dwelling one lives in. Dr. Aldridge, at Hoihow (Haikou 海口), particularly warns against living in Chinese-built houses:

> So long as foreigners here live in Chinese-built houses, and the breeze that is usually blowing is kept off by their houses being surrounded by others, they will find at the end of every summer that their constitutions have been enfeebled by excessive perspirations, sleepless nights, etc. Were they, however, to live in detached houses built on elevated ground, I feel sure that a summer's residence here would be little more trying to the constitution than in other ports in China.[65]

The climate, then, is clearly an outright concern for all British medical practitioners, and this underpins most of their advice. Heat and climate are critical considerations for the survival of the British constitution in China, and the utilization of the cautionary principles of hygienic medicine are integral to their survival. Dr. Jamieson criticizes the structure of passenger ships as having "deficient air space, and neglect of hygienic precautions in the men's quarters."[66]

Dr. Patrick Manson explicitly opposes the notion that the British should adopt the habits of the Chinese in order to adapt to the Chinese climate. His reports indicate his belief that the characters of a "race" are the results of the process of natural selection that have worked on many generations: "Appetites bred through many generations become instincts, and an Englishman must

63 W.R.E. Smart, "Reports of Societies, Epidemiological Society: On the Diseases of Hong Kong and the Canton River Station," *The British Medical Journal,* June 1, 1861, 589–90.

64 James Watson, "Dr. James Watson's Report on the Health of Newchwang for the Half-year Ended 30th September 1872," *Customs Gazette: Medical Reports*, no. 3 (1872): 15.

65 Aldridge, "Dr. E.A. Aldridge's Report on the Health of Hoihow for the Half-year Ended 30th September 1881," 6.

66 Alexander Jamieson, "Dr. Alexander Jamieson's Report on the Health of Shanghai for the Half-year Ended 30th September 1883," *Customs Gazette: Medical Reports*, no. 26 (1883): 5.

have his beef."[67] Dr. Manson also cautions that temperance and trips back to Europe or other temperate climates are important for the survival of the British constitution.

Dr. Scott, in a less antagonistic tone, is very complimentary of the air at Swatow (Shantou 汕头).

> The climate of Swatow is one of the healthiest and most delightful in the world.... Even in the hottest weather there is daily a refreshing sea-breeze which gives bloom to the cheeks and vigor to the frames of the most feeble. I have seen delicate children brought here almost dying who have got well and strong in a short time; and delicate adults who could hardly exist at home, or in other parts of China, quickly gain strength in this genial climate.[68]

Dr. McFarlane is also more conciliatory of the Chinese climate. Despite the reputation of Ichang (Yichang) as an unhealthy town, he is "decidedly of opinion that Ichang is healthy." This, he infers, is because "the hills and in the valleys on the opposite side of the river pleasant walks can be got, although the roads are bad. The air is bracing and enlivening in all the surrounding country, and only about three miles up river is the ... Yangtze."[69]

Conclusion

Using the theme of caution, this chapter analyzes the category of hygiene within the lens of British imperial medicine in early modern China because hygiene as a medical discourse seeks to prevent and caution against disease. The first section outlined the historical origins and development of Western and, in particular, British hygienic medicine and so discussed the classical origins of hygiene in Galenic medicine. Classical approaches to hygiene understood it as an individual concern and so draws on humoralism with particular reference to the principle of the non-naturals. The modern development of hygiene as a public concern coincided with the development of public health

67 Manson and Manson, "The Drs. Mansons' Report on the Health of Amoy for the Half-year Ended 30th September 1873," 32.

68 Scott, "Dr. E.I. Scott's Report on the Health of Swatow for the Half-year Ended 30th September 1876," 19.

69 E.P. McFarlane, "Dr. E.P. McFarlane's Report on the Health of Ichang," *Customs Gazette: Medical Reports*, no. 20 (1880): 19.

and with it, the introduction of racial, moral, and class prejudices into the application of the non-naturals.

The second section reviewed *Shanghai Hygiene* as a unique work that reconciles classical and modern theories of British hygienic medicine in early modern China. Henderson issues in *Shanghai Hygiene* numerous cautions to the British community in Shanghai and the rest of China in order to prevent the many diseases common to life in locations far removed from the metropolis. In doing so, Henderson mixes humoralist and public health principles with the racial, class, and moral prejudices prevalent in that period. *Shanghai Hygiene* is the only known work to have applied British hygienic medicine to the British in nineteenth-century China. As such, it is of great importance to the notion of caution that informed so many discourses of the period.

The third section selected reports from British doctors in the employ of the Imperial Customs Service in China in the period between 1861 and 1884. These records reveal that the theory of hygienic medicine that inform *Shanghai Hygiene* to be consistent with the practice of it by British doctors in China. The consistency between theory and practice further increases the importance of *Shanghai Hygiene* as an exemplar of a Chinese caution to the British constitution or, in other words, a British medical reaction to the prospect of the discourse of disease in late nineteenth-century China.

Shanghai Hygiene is a cautionary work. As such, it is part of the modern development of hygiene and it coincides with the emergence of tropical medicine as an extension of colonial rule. As medical historians point out, in order to conduct trade, "white" people needed to remain healthy amidst the "yellow," making the work of British doctors in China important for the conduct of trade and empire. Mark Harrison, Douglas Haynes, David Arnold, Michael Worboys, and Phillip Curtin all argue that colonizing various regions depende on developing immunities and understanding the diseases that the tropical world, in particular, seemed to carry.[70] Without this attention to health and hygiene,

70 Mark Harrison, "'The Tender Frame of Man': Disease, Climate, and Racial Difference in India and the West," *Bulletin of the History of Medicine* 70.1 (1996): 68–93; Mark Harrison, *Climates and Constitutions: Health, Race, Environment and British Imperialism in India, 1600–1850* (Oxford: Oxford University Press, 1999); Douglas Haynes, *Imperial Medicine: Patrick Manson and the Conquest of Tropical Medicine* (Philadelphia: University of Pennsylvania Press, 2001); Douglas Haynes, "From the Periphery to the Center: Patrick Manson and the Development of Tropical Medicine as a Medical Specialty in Britain, 1870–1900" (Ph.D. diss., University of California, Berkeley, 1992); David Arnold, *Imperial Medicine and Indigenous Societies* (Manchester: Manchester University Press, 1988); David Arnold, *Warm Climates and Western Medicine: The Emergence of Tropical Medicine, 1500–1900*, Wellcome Institute Series in the History of Medicine, vol. 35 (Amsterdam: Clio Medica,

an overseas colony, or trading post, might have easily become the site of "the white man's grave."[71]

Ruth Rogaski, in particular, argues that hygiene plays an important role in the development of Chinese modernity during the nineteenth century.[72] She writes about health and disease in Tianjin from the time of its establishment as a treaty port. Rogaski considers the adoption by expatriates and locals of *weisheng* 卫生 or "hygienic modernity" in the twofold but contradictory interest of imperialism and national sovereignty. *Hygienic Modernity* traces the evolution of *weisheng* from traditional ideas of Chinese cosmology on diet, meditation, and self-medication to modern ideas of the cleanliness of bodies and the fitness of races: qualities that the Chinese lack in the eyes of foreign observers.

At a more rhetorical level, David Armitage summarizes the ideology of the British Empire:

> The British Empire was an arena of hemispheric and international trade. Its character was therefore commercial.... Protestantism, oceanic commerce and mastery of the seas provided bastions to protect the freedom of inhabitants of the British Empire.... In sum, the British Empire was, above all and beyond all other such polities, Protestant, commercial, maritime and free.[73]

"Protestant, commercial, maritime and free" was the British imperial ideology in China. That ideology, I argue, influenced the British practice of medicine in China between 1840 and 1890. During these fifty years, China was not under British imperial government.[74] Rather, this was the period that signified the

---

1996); *Companion Encyclopedia of the History of Medicine*, s.v. "Medicine and Colonialism," by David Arnold; Philip D. Curtin, *The Image of Africa: British Ideas and Action, 1780–1850* (Madison, University of Wisconsin Press, 1964); Philip D. Curtin, *Death by Migration: Europe's Encounter with the Tropical World in the Nineteenth Century* (Cambridge: Cambridge University Press, 1989).

71 Phillip D. Curtin, "'The White Man's Grave': Image and Reality," *Journal of British Studies* 1.1 (1961): 94–110.

72 Ruth Rogaski, *Hygienic Modernity: Meanings of Health and Disease in Treaty Port China* (Berkeley and Los Angeles: University of California Press, 2004).

73 David Armitage, *The Ideological Origins of the British Empire* (Cambridge: Cambridge University Press, 2000), 8.

74 A long and well-established historiography exists on Britain's role in the economic establishment of an informal empire in China: John King Fairbank, *Trade and Diplomacy on the China Coast: The Opening of the Treaty Ports, 1842–1854* (Cambridge: Harvard University Press, 1953); D.K. Fieldhouse, *Economics and Empire, 1830–1914* (London: Weidenfeld and

height of free trade arrangements between Britain and China.[75] This was an arrangement that perfectly suited the British. Nevertheless, a pervasive ideology of domination was essential to justify their presence and rule.

Because China was never a formal realm of the British Empire, British commercial interests in China did not have the instrumentalities of the State at their disposition. They needed to find other ways to support their exploitation of China and to legitimate that exploitation in Britain itself. British imperial ideology constructed China as different in order to exploit it and at the same time cautioned Britain against China in order to legitimate that exploitation within Britain itself.[76] As a cautionary tale, *Shanghai Hygiene* was an instrument of British imperial ideology in China.

References

Armitage, David. *The Ideological Origins of the British Empire*. Cambridge: Cambridge University Press, 2000.

Arnold, David. *Imperial Medicine and Indigenous Societies*. Manchester: Manchester University Press, 1988.

———. *Colonizing the Body: State Medicine and Epidemic Disease in Nineteenth Century India*. Berkeley and Los Angeles: University of California Press, 1993.

———. *Warm Climates and Western Medicine: The Emergence of Tropical Medicine, 1500–1900*. Wellcome Institute Series in the History of Medicine, vol. 35. Amsterdam: Clio Medica, 1996.

Bewell, Alan. *Romanticism and Colonial Disease*. London: John Hopkins University Press, 1999.

Nicolson, 1973); William Roger Louis, *Imperialism: The Robinson and Gallagher Controversy* (New York: New Viewpoints, 1976). Diplomatic histories have convincingly illustrated how Britain did not establish formal rule in China due to the difficulties of funding and administering a formal imperial presence. Trade, not rule, was the ideal as seen in M.H. Wilgus' *Sir Claude MacDonald, the Open Door, and British Informal Empire in China, 1895–1900* (London: Garland Publishing, 1987), 6–36. The "Open Door" policy and other unequal treaties gave Britain a most favored nation status and, therefore, access to China's many coastal ports and permission for its companies to trade.

75 Gregory Blue and Timothy Brook, Introduction to *China and Historical Capitalism: Genealogies of Sinological Knowledge*, ed. Gregory Blue and Timothy Brook (Cambridge, Cambridge University Press, 1999), 2.

76 See Catherine Hall, *Civilising Subjects: Metropole and Colony in the English Imagination, 1830–1867* (Cambridge: Polity, 2002).

Blue, Gregory, and Timothy Brook. Introduction to *China and Historical Capitalism: Genealogies of Sinological Knowledge*, ed. Gregory Blue and Timothy Brook, 1–9. Cambridge: Cambridge University Press, 1999.

Bynum, William, and Roy Porter, eds. *Companion Encyclopaedia of the History of Medicine*. London: Routledge, 1993.

Collingham, E.M. *Imperial Bodies: The Physical Experience of the Raj, c. 1800–1947*. Cambridge: Polity Press, 2001.

Curtin, Philip D. "'The White Man's Grave': Image and Reality." *Journal of British Studies* 1.1 (1961): 94–110.

———. *The Image of Africa: British Ideas and Action, 1780–1850*. Madison: University of Wisconsin Press, 1964.

———. *Death by Migration: Europe's Encounter with the Tropical World in the Nineteenth Century*. Cambridge: Cambridge University Press, 1989.

———. *Disease and Empire: The Health of European Troops in the Conquest of Africa*. Cambridge: Cambridge University Press, 1998.

Douglas, Mary. *Purity and Danger: An Analysis of the Concepts of Pollution and Taboo*. 1966. London: Routledge, 1996.

Emch-Deriaz, Antoinette. "The Non-Naturals Made Easy." In *The Popularization of Medicine, 1650–1850*, ed. Roy Porter, 134–59. London: Routledge, 1992.

Fairbank, John King. *Trade and Diplomacy on the China Coast: The Opening of the Treaty Ports, 1842–1854*. Cambridge: Harvard University Press, 1953.

Fieldhouse, D.K. *Economics and Empire, 1830–1914*. London: Weidenfeld and Nicolson, 1973.

Hall, Catherine. *Civilising Subjects: Metropole and Colony in the English Imagination, 1830–1867*. Cambridge: Polity, 2002.

Harrison, Mark. "'The Tender Frame of Man': Disease, Climate, and Racial Difference in India and the West." *Bulletin of the History of Medicine* 70.1 (1996): 68–93.

———. *Climates and Constitutions: Health, Race, Environment and British Imperialism in India, 1600–1850*. Oxford: Oxford University Press, 1999.

Haynes, Douglas. "From the Periphery to the Center: Patrick Manson and the Development of Tropical Medicine as a Medical Specialty in Britain, 1870–1900." Ph.D. diss., University of California, Berkeley, 1992.

———. *Imperial Medicine: Patrick Manson and the Conquest of Tropical Medicine*. Philadelphia: University of Pennsylvania Press, 2001.

Henderson, James. *Shanghai Hygiene, or, Hints for the Preservation of Health in China*. Shanghai: Presbyterian Mission Press, 1863.

Hobson, Benjamin. "Brief Notice of the Hospital at Kum-Le-Fau in Canton, During the Year 1851." In *The Hobson Papers, Wellcome Manuscripts*, Box MS 5852/43, 25. London: Wellcome Library, 1851.

Inspector-General of Customs, eds. *Customs Gazette: Medical Reports*, no. 3 (1872), 5, 6 (1873), 7 (1874), 10 (1875), 11, 12 (1876), 13 (1877), 19, 20 (1880), 21, 22 (1881), 24 (1882), 26 (1883), 28 (1884).

Johnson, James, and James Ranald Martin. *The Influence of Tropical Climates on European Constitutions*. 6th ed. London: T. and C. Underwood, and Highley and Son, 1841.

Keevak, Michael. *Becoming Yellow: A Short History of Racial Thinking*. Princeton: Princeton University Press, 2011.

Louis, William Roger. *Imperialism: The Robinson and Gallagher Controversy*. New York: New Viewpoints, 1976.

Martin, James Ranald. "Review IX: The Influence of Tropical Climates on European Constitutions." *The Medico-Chirurgical Review, or, Quarterly Journal of Practical Medicine and Surgery* 18 (July–Oct. 1856): 126–35.

———. *The Influence of Tropical Climates on European Constitutions, Including Practical Observations on the Nature and Treatment of the Diseases of Europeans on Their Return from Tropical Climates*. London: John Churchill, 1861.

Morse, Edward S. "Latrines of the East." *American Architect*, Mar. 18, 1893, 1–18.

Poovey, Mary. *Making a Social Body: British Cultural Formation, 1830–64*. Chicago: University of Chicago Press, 1995.

Rogaski, Ruth. *Hygienic Modernity: Meanings of Health and Disease in Treaty Port China*. Berkeley and Los Angeles: University of California Press, 2004.

Smart, W.R.E. "Reports of Societies, Epidemiological Society: On the Diseases of Hong Kong and the Canton River Station." *The British Medical Journal*, June 1, 1861, 589–90.

Stallybrass, Peter, and Allon White. *The Politics and Poetics of Transgression*. London: Routledge, 1986.

Underwood, J.J. "Chinese Medicine: To the Editors of *The Lancet*." *The Lancet*, Oct. 20, 1888, 799.

Villalta Puig, Stephanie. "British Medical and Imperial Ideology in China: Circa 1840s–1890s." Ph.D. diss., Australian National University, 2009.

Wilgus, M.H. *Sir Claude MacDonald, the Open Door, and British Informal Empire in China, 1895–1900*. London: Garland Publishing, 1987.

CHAPTER 2

Curing Unhappiness in Revolutionary China: Optimism under Socialism and Capitalism

Wendy Larson

When Émile Coué (1857–1926) developed optimistic autosuggestion, or routine repetition, as a method of psychotherapy, touting the slogan "Tous les jours à tous points de vue je vais de mieux en mieux" (Every day in every way, I am getting better), he became a powerful proponent of a twentieth-century trend that took place in many geographical areas: the promotion of well-being, happiness, and optimism via suggestion, repetition, ritual and belief/faith rather than through a change in circumstances. Coué's ideas, which developed within the context of intense interest in the mind that the developing field of psychology engendered, motivated others, who used his ideas to transform personal relations, commerce, health, and more. Fundamentally, Coué's highly influential claim is that happiness is a state of mind, and unhappiness at best is a failure of the will; at worst, it is a psychological disease.

In socialist and revolutionary China, leadership in various fields also sought to engender and document happiness. First developed in the Soviet Union, the positive hero was avidly embraced in China, particularly in 1950s novels. This model often featured the conversion of a bystander into an enthusiastic participant in society's forward movement, and heroism on behalf of revolutionary goals in the face of terrible obstacles. The theory of the type, *dianxinglun* 典型论 "typicality" or "typical character," in literature, film, art and drama, encouraged distance from contemporary reality and an optimistic perspective. The theory of revolutionary optimism (*geming leguan zhuyi* 革命乐观主义) eventually medicalized the absence of happiness as an illness. Exhibited and encouraged in all spheres, happiness became a mandatory political goal.

The heroic model and the Maoist emphasis on a subjectivity imbued with revolutionary optimism were the Chinese socialist version of the twentieth-century tendency—in societies influenced by Enlightenment thought—to valorize happiness, and subsequently, to regard unhappiness as a serious condition or an illness that can be cured. The work of Maxim Gorky (1868–1936), whose essays, plays and novels were widely translated beginning in the 1920s, whose novel *Mother* (1932) became the founding document of socialist realism, and whose theory of typicality lay at the core of Maoist literary

 | DOI 10.1163/9789004319219_004

theories was the bridge into the literary model that embodied the revolutionary interpretation of the twentieth-century trend toward subjective enhancement of well-being. Admired and translated by Lu Xun 鲁迅 (1881–1936), Qu Qiubai 瞿秋白 (1899–1935), Feng Xuefeng 冯雪峰 (1903–1976), and others, Gorky's ideas lay at the heart of the 1935–36 debate on typicality between Zhou Yang 周扬 (1908–89) and Hu Feng 胡风 (1902–85). This debate is generally interpreted as a struggle over the meaning of realism, but it also set the stage for an expansion of typicality into a more broadly understood emphasis on happiness.

This emphasis on and promotion of happiness was not unique to socialist countries, but rather was a semi-global trend, originating in Europe, that embodied a subjective, contemporary recognition of the utopian aspects of personal, national, and world progress, or an extension of scientific rationality. In the most radical examples, utopia became not a vision of the future, but a state of mind, or happiness under present circumstances.[1] While the influence of this trend extended into many locales, in this paper I will concentrate on China and the United States, both of which, I argue, showed heightened levels of interest in producing happiness or optimism, and propelling it forward as integral aspects of their modernized culture. In this regard, we can look at the United States as an archetypical representative of rapid capitalist development, and as China as the same for socialist development; in other words, these societies are characterized by a concentration of tendencies under these regimes. Therefore, understanding the drive toward curing unhappiness in revolutionary China begins with a look at happiness in the West and more briefly in the Soviet Union, which first developed the models that became an important part of revolutionary Chinese culture. The goal of this comparative assessment is to embed Chinese socialist psycho-social practices within a global context that shows how they are part of the Enlightenment project of progress and improvement, a temporal model with far-reaching consequences.

Optimism under Capitalism: The Western Era of the Mind

During the mid to late nineteenth century, interest in mental processes flourished in many geographical areas. In Europe and the United States, "mental philosophy" was moving away from religion, and was in the process of becoming the modern field of psychology, which spread into Russia, Asia, Latin

1 Lisa Garforth, "No Intentions? Utopian Theory After the Future," *Journal for Cultural Research* 13.1 (Jan. 2009): 5–27.

America and other locales. As a research field, psychology was conceptualized as working within the realm of science rather than as part of metaphysics or religion.[2] However, not only in terms of research and eventually clinical treatment, but also from the perspective of models and ways of thinking about the mind, psychology forged new roads for the professional and the commoner. Joseph Haven's influential 1857 *Mental Philosophy: Including the Intellect, Sensibilities, and Will*, translated and used as a textbook in Japan in 1875 and China in 1889, valorized introspection, which he viewed as a scientific methodology that could lead to an understanding of not only the mind, but also of the self.[3] Interest in the self and in a subjective understanding of one's life, thoughts, and emotions exploded in the twentieth century as psychology, with its many branches and approaches, developed into a full-fledged discipline with influence well beyond the professional and academic realms, into business, politics, human relationships, and most aspects of daily life.[4]

The discipline's emergence as part of scientific discourse was fraught with danger, not only from metaphysics and religion, but also from related fields that spun into long-lasting and popular trajectories. The question of what could influence minds and bodies was a central concern of Franz Anton Mesmer's (1734–1815) theory of animal magnetism, which held that a life energy or magnetic fluid resided in animate beings. Early proponents of mesmerism followed up on Mesmer's work and contributed to the theory in a way that eventually was significant for the development of psychotherapy and patient agency. One of Mesmer's most important disciples was Armand-Marie-Jacques de Chastenet, Marquis de Puységur (1751–1825). Working in Soissons, Puységur put forward the idea that magnetic effects were related to the patient's belief in the efficacy of the cure. At the heart of this belief was the relationship between

2 Joseph Haven, *Mental Philosophy: Including the Intellect, Sensibilities, and Will* (Boston: Gould and Lincoln, 1862), 16.

3 Ibid., 342–76.

4 For an early discussion of the effects of the discipline of psychology as it was developing, see Arthur G. Tansley, *The New Psychology and Its Relation to Life* (London: G. Allen & Unwin, 1920). For a discussion of psychology's role in medicalizing common human conditions, see Thomas S. Szasz, "The Myth of Mental Illness: Foundations of a Theory of Personal Conduct," *American Psychologist* 15 (1960): 113–18; and his *The Myth of Psychotherapy: Mental Healing as Religion, Rhetoric, and Repression* (Cambridge: Oxford University Press, 1978). For a discussion of the influence of Freudian theory in American culture, see E. Fuller Torrey, *Freudian Fraud: The Malignant Effect of Freud's Theory on American Thought and Culture* (New York: Harper Collins, 1992). A good source for an historical approach to the modern self is Charles Taylor, *Sources of the Self: The Making of the Modern Identity* (Cambridge: Harvard University Press, 1989).

the magnetizer and the patient, a focus that became apparent in psychoanalysis, where a certain relationship between the analyst and the analysand was crucial for success. Abbé José Custodio de Faria (1746–1819), also a disciple of Mesmer, conducted experiments to prove that mesmeric trances were the product of suggestion, and no external cause was necessary. His 1819 *De la cause du sommeil lucide* emphasized the will of the subject and the availability of suggestion as a means to change behavior and physical reality not only in trance, but also in the waking state. In 1843, James Braid (1795–1860) published *Neuryphology; or, the Rationale of Nervous Sleep, Considered in Relation with Animal Magnetism*, arguing that the physical effects of mesmerism came about through an abstract attention to sleep, which resulted in a state of nervous sleep that he called "hypnotism." He linked this state to brain physiology and developed a set of terms that were acceptable to the medical community. August Amboise Liébeault (1823–1904) also focused on the power of suggestion.

A well-known debate on the nature of hypnotic suggestion was raging when Sigmund Freud (1856–1939) visited first Paris and then Nancy. In the work of Pierre-Marie-Fêlix Janet (1859–1947), Josef Breuer (1842–1925), and Sigmund Freud, the trajectory of mesmerism and hypnosis led to an emphasis on the subconscious, and on accessing the subconscious for healing, which is characteristic of the modern field of psychoanalysis.[5] It also led to a focus on the way in which desires that are not totally conscious can be accessed or created in the average healthy person.[6] The immensely fashionable ideas of and practices promoted by Émile Coué, who studied hypnosis with Liébeault and others, expanded theories of the importance of the mind into the popular realm. Coué moved away from suggestion under trance or sleep (hypnotism) towards conscious suggestion that accessed the "imagination"

5 Unless otherwise noted, the information on the history of mesmerism, hypnotism, suggestion, and psychology in these paragraphs was taken from Robert H. Wozniak, "Mind and Body: Réne Descartes to William James," *Serendip*, 1995, http://serendip.brynmawr.edu/Mind/(accessed Jan. 5, 2014); originally published in 1992 at Bethesda, MD & Washington, DC by the National Library of Medicine and the American Psychological Association.

6 Commenting on the general atmosphere of "meta-physical novelties," M.M. Mangasarian puts "Mysticism, Spiritualism, Eddyism, Couéism, Freudism, Revivalism, Blavatskyism" together as movements motivated by irrationality and propelled forward mainly by women. Although compared with Freud, "Couéism is a little simpler as it does not over-emphasize the sub-conscious," the Coué "daily prayer" as well as the group dynamics and psychology, and "sing-song, soothing, lullaby style of voice" that Coué uses when treating patients "helps to bring about an atmosphere conducive to hypnotic operations." See Mangasarian, *Psychoanalysis and Autosuggestion: Sigmund Freud and Emile Coue* (Chicago: Independent Religious Society, n.d.), 5, 17.

via simple techniques.[7] Proposing a method that anyone could deploy—with some practice and without the costly intervention of experts—Coué harnessed the 300-year fascination with suggestibility and transformed it into a popular methodology that focused on producing individual well-being. He established a framework for both recognizing that happiness was a state of mind, and for accepting as fact the idea that personal well-being was within the bounds of individual mind control. Although Coué dealt in medical cures, his focus, as C. Harry Brooks explains, was on state of mind and lifestyle:

> But as long as we look on autosuggestion as a remedy we miss its true significance. Primarily it is a means of self-culture, and one far more potent than any we have hitherto possessed.... It is essentially an individual practice, an individual attitude of mind.... It touches our being in its wholeness.... It teaches us that the burdens of life are, at least in large measure, of our own creating.... If fear and disease were banned from the individual life, could they persist in the life of the nation?[8]

Although in 1922 Brooks imagined social transformation from Couéism, especially in the treatment of criminals and the resolution of human greed, as we will see, Coué's methods were quickly picked up by business, which used them as a force to make profit rather than a "force making for goodness."[9]

After studying hypnosis, Coué published *Self-Mastery through Conscious Autosuggestion*, first in England (1920) and two years later in the United States. In France, Coué set up his clinic at Nancy, where he treated thousands free of charge, almost always in large groups at his home.[10] His theory of self-improvement through optimistic autosuggestion proposed that through

---

7 For a discussion of Coué's relationship with Liébeault, see Charles Baudouin, *Emile Coué and His Life Work* (New York: American Library Service, 1923).

8 C. Harry Brooks, *The Practice of Autosuggestion by the Method of Emile Coué* (New York: Dodd, Mead, 1922), 116–17.

9 Ibid., 118.

10 As Ella Boyce Kirk (b. 1842) noted in her *My Pilgrimage to Coué* (New York: American Library Service, 1922), 78–79, although for "the more sophisticated mind" it may take time to benefit from Coué's treatment, "simple people, however, children, and the peasants, who flock in such numbers to the clinic, and persons of marked religious tendencies are likely to be benefited at once," mostly because they are "prepared to believe." A well-educated woman with a negative opinion of "faith healers," Kirk nonetheless went from New York to Nancy to be treated for various physical pains resulting from her weight. Her "pilgrimage" gained such spectacular results that she wrote an engaging account of it and became an accredited teacher of Couéism. Kirk was superintendent in a Pennsylvania school, where

repetition of phrases that affirmed one was happy, cured, or otherwise altered, such a situation would become reality. As Coué explained:

> I know that one generally passes for mad in the eyes of the world if one dares to put forward ideas which it is not accustomed to hear. Well, at the risk of being thought so, I say that if certain people are ill mentally and physically, it is that they *imagine* themselves to be ill mentally or physically. If certain others are paralytic without having any lesion to account for it, it is that they *imagine* themselves to be paralyzed, and it is among such persons that the most extraordinary cures are produced. Or others again are happy or unhappy, it is that they *imagine* themselves to be so, for it is possible for two people in exactly the same circumstances to be, the one *perfectly happy*, the other *absolutely wretched*.[11]

Contrasting imagination and will, Coué advised his patients to prevent the will—which tended to recognize and emphasize limitation—from controlling agency.[12] Instead, the patient should invoke and give free rein to the more powerful imagination by repeating phrases such as "Every day in every way, I am getting better" and "It passes," which altered the subjective sense of well-being and, supposedly, even cured physical illness. Coué's writing is full of testimony about miracle cures.[13] His supporters and critics recognized the

---

she edited a school-version of Charles Dickens' *A Tale of Two Cities* (New York: American Book, 1899).

11 Émile Coué, *Self-Mastery through Conscious Autosuggestion* (New York: American Library Service, 1922), 12–13.

12 Ibid., 7–10.

13 Criticism directed at Coué includes the fact that he is not a "member of the medical profession," and that his methods risk that "persons with organic disease susceptible of the cure by operation or otherwise may go on assuring their 'unconscious' that 'it's going' or 'I'm getting better' until the condition becomes incurable" (*The British Medical Journal*, Apr. 8, 1922, 575). Editorial write-ups in *The British Medical Journal*, Nov. 29, 1924, 1010, also criticize a spin-off by Coué disciple R.C. Waters, *Auto-Suggestion for Mothers*, in which the author argues that "it should be theoretically possible to determine the sex of a child by auto-suggestion practised by the prospective parents before and after conception," as "somewhat fantastic." And, after going through a history of hypnotism that ends with a long quote from Coué, Clark L. Hull notes in his "Hypnotism in Scientific Perspective," *Scientific Monthly* 2 (1929): 160: "All sciences alike have descended from magic and superstition, but none has been so slow as hypnosis in shaking off the evil associations of its origins." Originally a skeptic but after a visit to Coué in Nancy becoming a supporter, Hugh Macnaghten, Vice-Provost of Eton College, noted in his *Émile Coué: The Man and His Work* (New York: Dodd, Mead, 1922), 4, that he did not see any miracle cures at Nancy, and that Coué sent people with broken legs to surgeons, stating that "he works no miracles." The

intellectual field of psychology and particularly Freudian psychoanalysis, with its interest in the unconscious, subconscious, and conscious, as the environment within which Coué worked. As J. Herbert Duckworth explains, "Autosuggestion, as taught at the new Nancy School, is a science by which is put to practical purposes logical lessons learned from the study of the *subconscious mind*—that great, and, until comparatively recently, uncharted ocean whose fascinating mysteries have been so thoroughly explored by Freud, Jung and other psychoanalysts."[14]

In the following discussion, I will consider the American tendency to valorize self-help as a cure for unhappiness as a powerful and influential trend in twentieth-century optimism. Psychotherapy became extremely popular throughout the American twentieth century and into the twenty-first, with different trajectories developing in medicine, mental health, self-help/popu lar culture, religion, and commerce. Within this context, the trajectory of the nineteenth-century concern with mental processes in America produced the therapeutic society in which the dynamic, changeable, and affirmative nature of the self is assumed, in which self-esteem, self-expression, and the development of personality have become the most important values, and in which the self can grow and improve.[15] Compared with Europeans, Americans are often found by non-Americans to be optimistic and even overly happy.[16] And finally, although the influence of Coué's work in America is generally recognized,

---

apparent miracle cures that Coué achieved are not cures of those with physical problems, Macnaghten argues, but are cases of people who only believe they have physical problems (4–6). In *The Realm of Delight* (London: Adlard & Son & West Newman, 1923), Alice Baird argues against the idea that Coué is a magician, while beginning her book with a drawing of Coué in a magician's hat and gown, holding a wand and with a cat next to him. Henry Amos Purcell, in the penname of Another Gentleman with a Duster, argues in his *Is Coué a Foe to Christianity?* (New York: Frederick Moore, 1923), 78–79, that Coué and Freud "supplement each other—like the two halves of an apple!" and describes Couéism as an enemy of Christianity that could be part of a "world-wide religious class" pitting the anti-Christian people of the Orient with Russia and Islamic culture against Christians. The author also notes that although Coué does not think religion is necessary, he "*plays upon the religious emotions*" and appeals more to Protestants than to Catholics, who generally ignored him (25). For a detailed description of Coué's on-the-ground practice, see Charles Baudouin's preface to *How to Practice Suggestion and Autosuggestion*, by Émile Coué (New York: American Library Service, 1923), 9–25; and Kirk, *My Pilgrimage to Coué*.

14 J. Herbert Duckworth, *Autosuggestion and Its Personal Application* (New York: James A. McCann, 1925), viii.

15 Philip Cushman, *Constructing the Self, Constructing America: A Cultural History of Psychotherapy* (Reading, Mass.: Addison-Wesley, 1990).

16 Christina Kotchemidova, "From Good Cheer to 'Drive-By Smiling': A Social History of Cheerfulness," *Journal of Social History* 39.1 (2005): 5–37.

Baudouin notes that the impetus for his theories to some extent may have come from the United States:

> Meanwhile, the ideas of the Nancy school had spread. In America they were being exploited and popularized with all the claptrap and noise that accompanies bluff. In that mass of very uninteresting literature, Mr. Coué thought there was perhaps something to be found, and his merit lies in having been able to extract the strong, vital principle from all that trash. In one of those American pamphlets which he describes as "very indigestible," he at least found indications of experiments which he had the patience to try out, and in which he believed he saw the necessary basis for the "method" he had been seeking ever since his meeting with Liébeault. This brings us to 1901.[17]

While his work never assumed a historical significance as great as that of Freud or Jung, Coué is important because his method of optimistic autosuggestion became a route to success in business that associated the curing of unhappiness with economic prosperity. After his lecture tour in the U.S. in 1923, Coué's influence in American expanded rapidly. He spoke to large crowds, including 3,000 at the Orchestra Hall in Chicago.[18] Very rapidly, Coué's ideas stimulated interest in using autosuggestion to enhance sales, and it was in the developing capitalist economy that his work found many followers.[19] Frank Lincoln Scott's *Autosuggestion and Salesmanship, or Imagination in Business* was published in 1923, the same year Coué lectured in the U.S. and only a year after his book was published in English. Dedicating the book to a friend who introduced him to Coué's writing, Scott quotes Coué throughout and writes about his influence in the world of sales, crediting him for making "one discovery that marks the beginning of an exact science of salesmanship," which is the conflict between will and imagination.[20] Scott addresses criticism of selling by hypnosis by noting that according to Coué, "suggestion can be used successfully only when

17 Baudouin, *Emile Coué and His Life Work*, 17–18.

18 John R. Schmidt, "Emile Coué: Chicago's Miracle Man," *Chicago History Today*, 2012, http://www.wbez.org/blog/john-r-schmidt/2012-02-06/emile-coue-chicagos-miracle-man-95980 (accessed May 17, 2012, no longer available).

19 Coué became aware of this possibility when he was asked about using autosuggestion in business while speaking to a group of businessmen in Cleveland, and responded in the affirmative. See Émile Coué, *My Method: Including American Impressions* (Garden City: Doubleday, Page, 1923), 143.

20 Frank Lincoln Scott, *Autosuggestions and Salesmanship, or Imagination in Business* (New York: American Library Service, 1923), 24.

the suggestion made squares with the desire of the patient, or in this case, the prospective customer."[21]

Coué's theories were an important source for Dale Carnegie (1888–1955), who in 1936 published the global blockbuster *How to Win Friends and Influence People* (updated in 2011 as *How to Win Friends and Influence People in the Digital Age*), as well as other self-help books. Carnegie also developed the Dale Carnegie Course, a series of lessons derived from his experience in marketing, salesmanship, and public speaking. Carnegie's books and courses were part of the developing fields of popular psychology, human potential, and self-help, which continues as a robust area in the United States today. One of his favorite quotes was "Act enthusiastic and you will be enthusiastic!"[22] Carnegie translated the mutability of the mind and the power of the individual to self-cure that motivated Coué into a business context and a recipe for success, both in business and in personal relationships. He argued that salesmen should always wear a smile and train themselves in cheerfulness, no matter how rude their customers may be.[23]

A second major American figure influenced by Coué was Norman Vincent Peale (1898–1993), founder of the long-lived radio show "The Art of Living" in 1935, a founding editor of *Guideposts* in 1945, and the author of the blockbuster *The Power of Positive Thinking* (1952) as well as many other books. While living in Boston, Peale made a special effort to hear Coué speak, and was intrigued by his ideas.[24] Like Coué, Peale emphasized the repetition of phrases and other

21 Ibid., 61.

22 The Dale Carnegie Course is still available, and has expanded to include online training. Carnegie's book has been adapted as *How to Win Friends and Influence People in the Digital Age*, and the official website bears the name Dale Carnegie Training, http://www.dalecarnegie.com (accessed Jan. 7, 2014).

23 Kotchemidova, "From Good Cheer to 'Drive-By Smiling'," 13.

24 Carol V.R. George, *God's Salesman: Normal Vincent Peale & the Power of Positive Thinking* (New York: Oxford University Press, 1993), 48–49. Coué argued that his theories were unrelated to religion, and that his methods could be used effectively by anyone "be Protestants or Catholics, be Bhuddists [sic] or Mohammedans, be what you will: it does not concern me whether you are zealots or Freethinkers: I only desire that all of you, from every point of view, Catholic, Nonconformist, or Agnostic, may grow daily better and better." Quoted in Macnaghten, *Émile Coué*, 38; see also Chap. 7, "M. Coué in His Relation to Christianity," 43–44, in which Macnaghten suggests that miracles performed by Christ may be similar to those performed by Coué: "And some future day some disciple of M. Coué, less wise, less busy, and rasher, may rush in and answer [the question of whether Christ performed miracles] that the miracles of Christ are no miracles: they can all be explained away quite naturally." Coué's American followers found no contradiction between his work and their Christian beliefs.

mechanical devices to push the mind toward a more positive state. Although crediting God, Peale put his attention on the ability of the individual, "grasping themes that were alive in the culture and then offering them in a practical, entertaining form that helped people achieve results *for themselves*."[25] Peale viewed the mind as dynamic, self-healing, and creative, a channel for divine energy that could be activated via the three-step approach of picturizing, prayerizing, and actualizing.[26] Appealing to business leaders such as J.C. Penney, Howard Pew, Stanley S. Kresge and many others, Peale built on the relationship between religion and business that Max Weber identified as uniquely American.[27] This "Practical Christianity" used optimism to celebrate social mobility and individual success, enhance personal autonomy, celebrate individual success, and build satisfaction. Despite his popularity, Peale's work was criticized from many angles, and labeled a cult of reassurance, positive thinking, easy religion, and happiness.[28]

As Alfred E. Johns noted in 1950, although Couéism had faded after the high point of 1923, when Coué gave clinics all of the United States, and particularly after Coué's death in 1926, much of "Coué's theory, however, had been incorporated in to the psychiatric and mental healing field."[29] The notion that optimism is not the result of better circumstances but rather an internal process that can be willed into existence by the self has become commonplace in American life. Furthermore, the idea that optimism can influence one's physical health

25 Sarah Forbes Orwig, "Business Ethics and the Protestant Spirit: How Norman Vincent Peale Shaped the Religious Values of American Business Leaders," *Journal of Business Ethics* 38.1/2 (June 2002): 82.

26 George, *God's Salesman*, 139.

27 Orwig, "Business Ethics and the Protestant Spirit," 83.

28 George, *God's Salesman*, 142–43. One of the criticisms directed at Peale in *God's Salesman*, 128, was that his approach was "Couéism with organ music." Others who worked in the public sphere to bring autosuggestion, positive thinking, or optimism together with religion, happiness, mental health, and success in life and business include Alfred E. Johns (*Scientific Autosuggestion for Personality Adjustment and Development*, 1952); Napoleon Hill (1883–1970; *Think and Grow Rich*, 1937); Frederick Eikerenkoetter (1935–2009), known as "the Success and Prosperity Preacher"; Robert H. Schuller (1926–), founder of Crystal Cathedral Ministries, televangelist on *Hour of Power* from 1970 to 2006, and author of some thirty-seven books, including *The Eight Proven Principles of Possibility Thinking* (1998); Joel Osteen (1963-; *Become a Better You: 7 Keys to Improving Your Life Every Day*); and Steven Covey (1932–; *7 Habits of Highly-Effective People*). Coué's popularity is testified to by the seven printings, all in 1922, of Cyrus Harry Brooks' book *The Practice of Autosuggestion by the Method of Emile Coué*.

29 Anonymous, "Ancient Fads Still Rolling," *Spokane: The Spokesman-Review*, Mar. 27, 1950, 14.

has gained currency within medical circles, and researchers have studied it as a form of therapy. One study concludes: "An optimistic explanatory style may protect against risk of coronary heart disease in older men."[30] Other studies have concluded that optimistic patients are less likely to be bothered by symptoms.[31] Optimism has been studied in relation to prostate cancer, adiposity, multiple sclerosis, infectious diseases, placebo effects, stress and immunity, oral cavity cancer, and of course mental illnesses such as depression and mood disorder.[32] The Program in Placebo Studies and Therapeutic Encounter at Beth Israel Deaconess Medical Center at Harvard supports studies into the way in which placebos—suggestion in the form of a pill or injection—as well as simple physician empathy (verbal suggestion) can produce chemical changes in the body that lead to patient improvement. Rather than comparing placebos to drugs, the researchers there, led by Ted Kaptchuk, try to understand what makes a placebo—or suggestion—powerful.[33]

The creation of optimism via positive thinking emerged from an early form of hypnotism, in which hypnotic trance was believed to be based on transfer of magnetic fluid from hypnotist to patient. The trajectory progressed through abandonment of the idea of fluid and focus on the trance, induced sleep, or

---

30 Laura D. Kubzansky et al., "Is the Glass Half Empty or Half Full? A Prospective Study of Optimism and Coronary Heart Disease in the Normative Aging Study," *Psychosomatic Medicine* 63 (2001): 910.

31 Michael F. Scheier and Charles S. Carver, "Optimism, Coping, and Health: Assessment and Implications of Generalized Outcome," *Health Psychology* 4.3 (1985): 219–47.

32 Suzanne K. Steginga and Stefano Occhipinti, "Dispositional Optimism as a Predictor of Men's Decision-Related Distress after Localized Prostate Cancer," *Health Psychology* 25.2 (Mar. 2006): 135–43; D. Khullar et al., "Optimism and the Socioeconomic Status Gradient in Adolescent Adiposity," *Journal of Adolescent Health* 49.5 (2011): 553–55; Marijda Fournier, Denise de Ridder, and Jozien Bensing, "Optimism and Adaptation to Multiple Sclerosis: What Does Optimism Mean?" *Journal of Behavioral Medicine* 22.4 (1999): 303–26; W. Lang, "Infectiology and Optimism in Medicine," *Munchener Medizinische Wochenschrift* 127.9 (1985): 191–92; Debbie Morton et al., "Reproducibility of Placebo Analgesia: Effect of Dispositional Optimism," *Pain* 146.1/2 (2009): 194–98; Lena Brydon et al., "Dispositional Optimism and Stress-induced Changes in Immunity and Negative Mood," *Brain, Behavior & Immunity* 23.6 (2009): 810–16; Samuel Ho et al., "The Roles of Hope and Optimism on Posttraumatic Growth in Oral Cavity Cancer Patients," *Oral Oncology* 47.2 (2011): 121–24; and Kim Kronstrom et al., "Optimism and Pessimism as Predictors of Work Disability with a Diagnosis of Depression: A Prospective Cohort Study of Onset and Recovery," *Journal of Affective Disorders* 130.1/2 (2011): 294–99.

33 Beth Israel Deaconess Medical Center, "Program in Placebo Studies & Therapeutic Encounter (PiPS)," Harvard Medical School, http://programinplacebostudies.org/(accessed Jan. 9, 2014).

mental state, to a recognition that one could self-hypnotize by means of repetition and ritual, and finally, to the value of positive thinking in general. In the United States, Coué's attempt to use conscious desire to suppress the will and invoke the imagination became intertwined with many fields, but especially with business and advertising, the latter of which relies on what can be extremely indirect suggestion to sell goods or services. Promoting life-styles, attitudes, image, and group inclusion, advertisements make symbolic or abstract connections that appeal to the viewer's imagination. Variously called "capital realism" or "commercial realism," advertising that distances itself from the qualities of goods or services—or information about products—and focuses instead on creating ambiance or association—or manipulation, or the creation of new desires, aspirations, and values—is part of the overall deployment of suggestion and autosuggestion within commerce.[34]

When advertising moved from the "warning" ad, which testified to dire consequences if the product was not used (Listerine linking bad breath to spinsterhood), to the "product satisfaction" ad, which promised happiness (security and health), the link between Coué's methodology and optimism was complete. Smiling, cheerfulness, and enjoyment were important emotional aspects of consumer culture, expressed in comics and cartoons (the "funnies"), music (crooning), television (the "maddening jingle" and the laugh track, an American invention), and beginning in 1971, the ubiquitous smiley face.[35] Earlier somber rituals, such as the funeral, were replaced by the celebration of life, with sadness replaced by joy, and other social practices also have slowly changed in the direction of encouraging optimism and the curing of unhappiness.

In fact, the trajectory of advertising, which moved from creating fear to suggesting pleasure, was only one aspect of a broader transformation that centered cheerfulness and optimism as important public and personal values. In Europe and the United States, sentimental sadness was "the badge of a way of

---

34 See John Kenneth Galbraith, *The Affluent Society* (Boston: Houghton Mifflin, 1958); Erving Goffman, *Gender Advertisements* (New York: Harper and Row, 1976); Raymond Williams, "Advertising: The Magic System," in *Problems in Materialism and Culture* (London: Verso, 1980), 170–95; Michael Schudson, "Advertising as Capitalist Realism," in *Advertising, the Uneasy Persuasion: Its Dubious Impact on American Society* (New York: Basic Books, 1984), 209–33; Roland Marchand, *Advertising the American Dream* (Berkeley and Los Angeles: University of California Press, 1985); and Sal Randazzo, *Mythmaking on Madison Avenue* (Chicago: Probus, 1993).

35 The smiley face sold over 50 million buttons at its peak, and developed into the World Smile Corporation and the Smiley Store. See Kotchemidova, "From Good Cheer to 'Drive-By Smiling,'" 20.

life" until the eighteenth century, when in the United States, the public's embrace of melancholy began to shift.[36] The result was an ever-increasing emphasis on optimism and happiness, culminating in a demand for cheerfulness in almost all contexts, including those previously marked by a publicly expressed sadness. Before and even into the twentieth century, crying in public was common for both sexes in Europe, as "tears implied a noble soul and a sad face" (both signs of sensibility), Christian suffering, compassion, and self-sacrifice.[37] What impacted the "culture of sadness" was the increase in human agency, which demanded that people not be resigned to their situations but rather, believe that they can put changes into effect, and the emphasis on individualism, which promoted self-love. Both changes in focus were part of modernization, which developed under a burgeoning capitalist expansion that needed a large corps of productive workers and an expanding middle class. Cheerfulness for both sexes, which had to be deeply felt rather than simply enacted, eventually made its way into national character and the American myth, melding with the de-intensification of emotions that began in the mid-1800s.[38]

American optimism, as it came to be known, provided a perfect environment for the explosion of Couéism in the twentieth century. The exceptional good humor of Americans under many situations, especially labor, was noted well before this time by European commentators.[39] As the importance of cheerfulness continually expanded, the quality turned into a desired personality characteristic for employers. Expressed happiness was publicly proclaimed in the guidelines of developing community organizations such as the Boy Scouts, which listed cheerfulness as one of the twelve characteristics of a Scout.[40] By the twenty-first century, America had become so enamored of happiness that people holding signs felt it was fine to aggressively demand that passersby smile, and the website www.about.com, under the category of "longevity," listed ten reasons why smiling was important for health and well-being: making us attractive, changing our mood and that of others, relieving stress, boosting the immune system, lowering blood pressure, releasing natural pain killers, making us look younger, making us seem successful, and helping

36 Anne Amend, "Melancholy," in *Encyclopedia of the Enlightenment*, ed. Michel Delon (Chicago: University of Chicago Press, 2001), 822–26; quoted in Kotchemidova, "From Good Cheer to 'Drive-By Smiling'," 7.

37 Kotchemidova, "From Good Cheer to 'Drive-By Smiling'," 7.

38 Ibid., 12–13.

39 Ibid., 9–11. British journalist William Corbett, British traveler Joseph Grund, British barrister Alexander Mackay, German emigrant and eventual Harvard psychology professor Hugo Münsterberg are a few examples.

40 Ibid., 17.

us stay positive.[41] Within the psyche and in public contexts, optimism had become the norm, expected of all and admired in those who embraced it thoroughly. Within a scant hundred years, the United States seems to have become the happiest nation on earth.

Optimism under Socialism: Gorky and the USSR

While individualism was an important factor in the development of optimism in the United States, in both China and the USSR, where many models of revolutionary socialist culture were developed, although individualism was criticized, optimism was widely encouraged.[42] In nineteenth-century Russia, interest in the mind developed rapidly, with strong attention to a variety of practices, from mesmerism and hypnosis to psychoanalysis. Early Russian philosophers developed several strands of thought that expressed ideas about the function of the unconscious.[43] Hypnotism was regulated by the law, which also protected the population against unlicensed medical practices since 1788, when the Russian Medical College determined that practitioners must be validated by medical experts.[44] Although the Tsar's family was treated by Jean-Martin Charcot (1825–93), hypnotism as both a window into how the mind worked and as a therapy that could direct and change behavior through access to the unconscious was superseded among intellectuals by Freudian psychoanalysis, which from the beginning had strong roots in Russia. Not only did

41 Mark Stibich, "Top 10 Reasons to Smile," Feb. 4, 2010, http://longevity.about.com/od/lifelongbeauty/tp/smiling.htm (accessed Jan. 9, 2014).

42 Kotchemidova, "From Good Cheer to 'Drive-By Smiling'," 14, argues: "The philosophy of individualism defined cheerfulness as the most beneficial of emotions since it served the self. (In contrast, group cultures, such as traditional nationalism or pre-Reformational Christianity, tend to promote sadness as part of the ethic of compassion or self-sacrifice. A recent example was Milosevic's political metaphor of Mother Serbia as a martyr, which drew on Eastern Orthodoxy and evoked sorrow)." Socialism may be the exception to this general tendency, a fact that supports the interpretation of socialist culture as one trajectory of modernity.

43 Alberto Angelini, "History of the Unconscious in Soviet Russia: From Its Origins to the Fall of the Soviet Union," *Institute of Psychoanalysis* 89 (2008): 369.

44 In 1912, the *British Medical Journal* noted that not only were regulations in effect in Russia in the eighteenth century, but by 1845, penalties were set by the government—whereas Germany had significantly lesser protection against quackery ("Quackery in Russia and Germany," 1087–88). In 1895, the same journal noted that the "practice of hypnotism is strictly regulated by law in Belgium, Hungary, and Russia" ("Hypnotism and the Law," 437).

many of Freud's patients in his early practice come from East Europe and Russia, but also, the cultural space of Eastern Europe, divided into the Russian and Austro-Hungarian empires, was shared by Russian-Jewish intellectuals and Freud's circle. Major figures within psychoanalysis were of Russian origin, including Sabina Spielrein, Lou Andreas-Salome, and Max Eitingon. Freud, whose mother was from Odessa and who was long interested in the Russian psyche or national character, believed that "Russians are closer to the unconscious than Western people," which to him was supported by the early reception of psychoanalysis in Russia.[45] His affinity with Russia contrasted strongly with his opinions of America, which he visited in 1909 and professed to hate. Freud believed that Americans had created the ultimate material society and had lost their respect for authority, undermining the basis of civilization.[46]

In Russia, Freud's theories spread rapidly, not only dominating the various fields of mental health, from where it attacked the influential field of hypnosis, but also extending into literature, arts, sociology, pedagogy, ethics, and aesthetics.[47] Two pioneers of Russian psychoanalysis, Nicolai Osipov (1877–1934) and Tatiana Rosenthal (1885–1921), were also political activists, and psychoanalysis found many adherents among those who wanted to completely remake society and construct a new kind of person in a new kind of society. The most radical initiative in this direction was the Psychoanalytic School of Moscow, founded in 1921 by Vera Schmidt (1998–1935), where educators "would try to understand and interpret the unconscious derivatives of the infantile unconscious and separate them from conscious manifestations."[48] When the State Psychoanalytic Institute was founded in 1923, the problems of freedom, submission, and power were central for Russian psychoanalysts, forming directions that seemed to promote the "newest, most 'progressive' developments of radical social thought…being able to change history, society and human nature."[49] In 1925, Alexander Luria and Lev Semenovic Vygotski wrote glowingly about the "new and original direction in psychoanalysis" that "creates a synthesis of

---

45 Alexander M. Etkind, "How Psychoanalysis Was Received in Russia, 1906–1936," *Journal of Analytical Psychology* 39 (1994): 191–92; James L. Rice, *Freud's Russia: National Identity in the Evolution of Psychoanalysis* (New Brunswick: Transaction, 1993). Rice has studied Freud's Russian background and connections in detail, focusing on Freud's reception of Dostoevsky.

46 Herbert Kaye, "Why Freud Hated America," *The Wilson Quarterly* 17.2 (Spring 1993): 118–25.

47 Etkind, "How Psychoanalysis Was Received in Russia, 1906–1936," 194–97; Arthur Petrovsky, *Psychology in the Soviet Union: A Historical Outline*, trans. Lilia Nakhapetyan (Moscow: Progress, 1990), 153.

48 Angelini, "History of the Unconscious in Soviet Russia," 371.

49 Etkind, "How Psychoanalysis Was Received in Russia," 200.

Freud's teachings and of Marxism on the basis of the Pavolvian theory of conditional reflexes."[50]

In the mid-1920s a debate about the concept of consciousness also took place, with one side branding it a "mentalistic superstition" and proposing in its place the study of behavior, and another group supporting the concept as valid.[51] By the mid-1930s, the unconscious was disavowed in favor of the conscious mind, and along with it went psychoanalysis, which was banned.[52] From that point on, psychoanalysis was regarded as anti-Soviet and bourgeois and the Stalinization of the discipline was underway.[53] Although for several years hypnosis had been the major enemy of Russian psychoanalysis—with Rasputin having taken lessons from a "magnetizer"—it was the only type of psychotherapy to survive in the Soviet period.[54] The idea of the New Mass Man, the New Socialist Man, or just the New Man, and the importance of the conscious mind did survive, however, becoming the backbone of the Soviet model of the human being. This complex construction involved many spheres, but in literary culture, Maxim Gorky's role was crucial. Credited with founding socialist realism even though the directive many not have come from him, Gorky helped create the New Man through his fiction and essays.[55] The Central Park of Culture and Leisure in Moscow, which was engineered to promote soviet collectivist values and the building of the New Man, was renamed Gorky Park in 1932, and the search for proletarian heroes began, led by Gorky's novel *The Mother*.[56] Stalin's famous 1935 comment, "Life has become more joyous,

---

50 Ibid., 197. The development of psychoanalysis in the USSR resulted in strong resistance from liberal Russian intellectuals, including the poet Anna Akhmatova, who professed to hate Freud; also Vladimir Nbokov, and Mikhail Bakhtin, who called psychologists "spies." Ibid.,202.

51 Angelini, "History of the Unconscious in Soviet Russia," 377.

52 For a detailed history of psychiatry and psychoanalysis in Russia and Soviet Russia, see Miller, *Freud and the Bolsheviks*.

53 Ibid., 103–13. See also V.N. Buzin, "Psychoanalysis in the Soviet Union: On the History of a Defeat," *Russian Social Science Review* 36.61 (Nov.–Dec. 1995): 65–73.

54 Etkind, "How Psychoanalysis Was Received in Russia," 194.

55 As Lidiia Siridonova states, the "stormy waves of time are slowly washing away the image of Maxim Gorky, Lenin's enthusiastic friend and Stalin's accomplice and comrade-in-arts, as the 'founder of Socialist Realism'.... [I]t has become clear that Gorky was neither an orthodox Marxist nor a devout Bolshevik.... [I]n the 1930s he was almost the only one who dared to protest the politicization of literature and the creation of the 'cult of personality', refusing to work with the functionaries on the board of the Writers' Union." Lidiia Siridonova, "Gorky and Stalin (According to New Materials from A.M. Gorky's Archive)," *The Russian Review* v.54 (July 1995): 413.

56 Claire Shaw, "A Fairground for 'Building the New Man': Gorky Park As a Site of Soviet Acculturation," *Urban History* 38.2 (2011): 325–37.

comrades!" took form in an annual carnival, a "riot of song, dance, food and drink" orchestrated within the park.[57] The old misery was replaced by a new happiness oriented toward modern attitudes and the joyous new society that had transformed the miserable past: "Remember the dust, the crush, the bad language of the cops forcing back the tired and embittered crowd."[58] Progress and the future were the hallmarks of this celebration, and carnivals in Nice and Paris could not compete because the future of their citizens was "shrouded in gloom," completely unlike a Soviet citizen who "felt himself master of his life and country."[59]

As a well-respected writer who, like Lu Xun, had emerged out of the pre-socialist era, Gorky's evolution toward a proletarian perspective seemed to embody a natural progress:

> Gorky's aesthetic itself possessed an enormous inner integrity, since it was the fruit of his own biography. It was not an acquired aesthetic, not developed by someone else, not a received aesthetic, but rather one attained to by Gorky during the course of his entire life.... It was for this reason that with such passion Gorky stamped his own aesthetic code onto the new Socialist Realist aesthetics that he created.[60]

Crucial to Gorky's aesthetic was knowledge of life, exactness of portrayal, truth, verisimilitude, and realism. Writers needed a courageous spirit—the "spirit of heroism"—which could be accessed as long as the writer was in tune with reality, since "reality is already heroic."[61] The utopian, future-directed aspect of

---

57 Ibid., 338.

58 L. Nikulin, "Karnaval molodosti," *Pravda*, July 13, 1936; quoted in Shaw, "A Fairground for 'Building the New Man'," 339.

59 Ibid.

60 Dobrenko, *The Making of the State Writer* (Stanford: Stanford University Press, 2001), 358–59.

61 Ibid., 359, 362. In 1900 Gorky had recognized a social need for "the heroic" in a letter to Chekhov, and his quest for moral purity was in part a quest for heroes within all classes and groups. See Rufus W. Mathewson, Jr., *The Positive Hero in Russian Literature* (Stanford: Stanford University Press, 1975), 166. Although he became established as the voice of Soviet socialist realism, only a decade earlier Gorky had doubts that the Russian people could successfully undertake any revolution. In essays later called by the authorities "mistakes," he complained of their laziness, passivity, spinelessness, cruelty, lack of initiative, and so on, and Lenin, and more generally the Bolsheviks, as cold-blooded and immoral. See Maksim Gorky, *Untimely Thoughts: Essays on Revolution, Culture, and the Bolsheviks, 1917–1918*, trans. Herman Ermolaev (New York: Paul S. Eriksson, 1968). In general, for the massive construction of the Soviet writer and reader, see Dobrenko, *The*

socialist realism (and of scientific rationalism) was embedded in the project, as Gorky spoke out against the "poisonous unbearable nastiness of the past" in favor of "the height of the accomplishments of the present, from the height of the great goals of the future."[62] *Mother*, published in 1907, followed Lenin's 1905 article "Party Organization and Party Literature" in substituting "a programmatic, declamatory optimism" for the search into the many experiences of life, especially suffering, which had been the basis of classical fiction.[63] Two motifs of *Mother* became common in socialist realism: the "conversion of the innocent, the ignorant, or the misled to a richer life of participation in the forward movement of society," and "emblematic political heroism in the face of terrible obstacles."[64] Moral qualities animate the behavior of the hero, who as does Pavel to his mother, proclaims that engaging in dangerous behavior is his "happiness," and asks that she rejoice in sending her children to death.[65] The revolutionary characters' passion suggests their dedication to a powerful vision of the future, which speaks to their amazing and profound optimism.[66]

Clearly, as in the United States, happiness was a mandatory value in the Soviet Union, which similarly expanded the public space within which happiness could and should be expressed. *Petrified Utopian: Happiness Soviet Style* (2011), a collection of academic articles about the various realms where happiness was promoted, speaks to the breadth of the movement. Joy was expected of children (even orphans) and more generally, within and on behalf of childhood. Painting, posters, advertisements, and other visual representations displayed happy workers, peasants, and others. Happiness was associated with cuisine, sewing, poetry and literature, house and home, and holidays. It was projected through architecture, in films, and by means of self-construction, which was guided in a number of ways. Evaluating the many spaces and times of happiness in the Soviet Union makes it obvious that socialist happiness could rival capitalist happiness, both in its intensity and in the social strategies that sustained it.

Making of the State Reader: Social and Aesthetic Contexts of the Reception of Soviet Literature, trans. Jesse Savage (Stanford: Stanford University Press, 1997) and *The Making of the State Writer*; also Dobrenko, *Aesthetics of Alienation: Reassessment of Early Soviet Cultural Theories* (Evanston: Northwestern University Press, 2005) for the relationship between Soviet realism and the economy.

62 Dobrenko, *The Making of the State Writer*, 363.

63 Mathewson, *The Positive Hero in Russian Literature*, 167, 156–76.

64 Ibid., 176.

65 Ibid., 169.

66 Ibid., 173.

Optimism under Chinese Socialism: Curing Unhappiness

In 1973, after she returned from two visits to China, Ruth Sidel presented a talk to the American Orthopsychiatric Association in New York. Entitled "The Role of Revolutionary Optimism in the Treatment of Mental Illness in the People's Republic of China," the article detailed the way in which revolutionary optimism was used as a psychological cure at the Third Beijing Hospital (90 beds) and the Shanghai Mental Hospital (916 beds).[67] She also met with professors at the Beijing Medical College. Sidel emphasized that training in revolutionary optimism was not the only therapy, but was used in combination with drugs, acupuncture, physical therapy, and talk therapy. The root of psychological optimism lies in the old Yan'an idea of "regeneration through one's own efforts," Sidel argued, and the notion that "a man has infinite power to remold his environment given sufficient will" is evident in many aspects of socialist culture.[68] Viewed as an enemy, mental illness must be fought via a correct relationship between the doctor and the patient that works toward a victorious resolution, with patients organized into "fighting groups."[69] Self-sacrifice, changing sorrow into strength and low spirits into high spirits are all aspects of revolutionary optimism.[70] The four beliefs that underlie the theory are subordinating individual needs to those of the group, understanding that the individual is part of the larger revolution, believing that participating in the successful revolution generates happiness and meaning in life, and accepting that human beings have an infinite capacity to learn and change.[71] Mental illness was a "paper tiger" that, once it was understood by the patient, could be conquered.[72]

---

67 Ruth Sidel, "The Role of Revolutionary Optimism in the Treatment of Mental Illness in the People's Republic of China," *American Journal of Orthopsychiatry* 43.5 (Oct. 1973), 732–36.

68 Ibid., 734.

69 Ibid.; Kam-Shing Yip, "An Historical Review of the Mental Health Services in the People's Republic of China," *International Journal of Social Psychiatry* 51.106 (2005): 109.

70 Sidel, "The Role of Revolutionary Optimism in the Treatment of Mental Illness in the People's Republic of China," 735.

71 Ibid., 736.

72 Ibid., 734; Yip, "An Historical Review of the Mental Health Services in the People's Republic of China," 109. For a detailed discussion of the medicalization of revolutionary optimism, see Wendy Larson, *From Ah Q to Lei Feng: Freud and Revolutionary Spirit in 20th Century China* (Stanford: Stanford University Press, 2009), 96–109. See also Robert Chin and Ai-li S. Chin, *Psychological Research in Communist China, 1949–1966* (Cambridge: MIT Press, 1969).

The texts that were used to train patients in revolutionary optimism are the classic Maoist texts that emphasize will over material constraint: "On Practice" ("Shijian lun" 实践论), "On Contradiction" ("Maodun lun" 矛盾论), "Serve the People" ("Wei renmin fuwu" 为人民服务), "The Foolish Old Man Who Moved the Mountain" ("Yugong yi shan" 愚公移山), and "Where Do Correct Ideas Come From?" ("Ren de zhengque sixiang shi nali lai de?" 人的正确思想是哪里来的?).[73] These texts were the basis of Maoism-in-practice in many aspects of life, far exceeding the medical sphere, influencing art, literature, and daily life. Maoism emphasized voluntarism and change, romanticizing the rural as a physical site of transformation and an inspirational ideal. According to Maurice Meisner's well-known study, Maoism "replaces the Marxist belief in objective laws of history with a voluntaristic faith in the consciousness and the moral potentialities of men as the decisive factor in sociohistorical development."[74] Maoist emphasis on will, subjectivity, and personal or cultural transformation through individual and group efforts was expressed through a consistent discourse of spiritual development that aligns well with Coué's "Every day in every way, I am getting better." Self-criticism, personal sacrifice, and a fine sense of one's positive role in social hierarchy all were part of this comprehensive spiritual discourse.[75] And mandatory for the revolutionary subject was happiness and joy, which increased along with the development of production or anticipation of the same.[76]

In literature, revolutionary optimism developed in the styles of socialist realism and revolutionary romanticism, which required certain kinds of conflicts and characters. The expression of emotion, dialogue, narrative, and other literary concerns all were influenced by revolutionary optimism. Maxim Gorky was extraordinarily influential in China over the twentieth century. Gorky's ideas, among others, motivated the tremendous rethinking of literature—its

---

73 Sidel, "The Role of Revolutionary Optimism in the Treatment of Mental Illness in the People's Republic of China," 733; Yip, "An Historical Review of the Mental Health Services in the People's Republic of China," 109.

74 Maurice Meisner, *Marxism, Maoism, and Utopianism: Eight Essays* (Madison: Wisconsin University Press, 1982), 61. Actually, a strain of idealism long existed in Marxism in the idea of permanent revolution, or the possibility of skipping over the stage of capitalism and going directly into socialism.

75 Larson, *From Ah Q to Lei Feng*, 90–96.

76 Liu Chengjie 刘成杰, Wang Tianhou 王天厚, and Zhang Mingjuan 章明娟, "Xianjin shengchanzhe de xinli tedian: Lun gongchan zhuyi laodong taidu 先进生产者的心理特点：论共产主义劳动态度 [The Psychological Characteristics of Progressive Producers: On the Work Attitude of Communism]," *Beijing daxue xuebao* 北京大学学报(哲學社會科學版) (Journal of Peking University [Philosophy and Social Sciences]), 1958, no. 4:47.

role and social function, its goals, and its techniques—that recreated the entire enterprise of Chinese literature from the teens through the revolutionary period.

Although some of Gorky's fiction came was translated and published in 1907, his essays—which ultimately transcended his fiction in terms of influence—did not come out in China until 1920, when the May Fourth Movement was well underway. At that time, *New Youth* (*Xin qingnian* 新青年) published "Literature and Modern Russia," translated by Zheng Zhenduo 郑振铎. In Russia, the article was originally published as an introduction to a world literature anthology project that planned to produce 1,500 volumes at 320 pages each, and 3,000 to 5,000 smaller volumes of 32–64 pages. Emphasizing the important role of literature in society—a sentiment that strongly supported May Fourth tendencies to valorize the ability of literature to transform thinking and thus society—Gorky proclaimed that "literature is the heart of the world" and the "mirror of human movement."[77] As Liu Qingfu explains, the essay "expresses complex human emotions and thought, and reflects the rich inner world. It deeply grasps our intent, connecting with the thoughts of people in many countries, instigating the awakening of slaves, shining light on the way for people to attain their goals."[78]

As the leftist literary movement progressed, Gorky was increasingly translated, often via English translations. Although the next translation (by Yu Dafu 郁达夫) did not come out until seven years later, throughout the 1930s, 1940s, 1950s, 1960s and later, Gorky's essays were regularly published. His essays from his later years were almost all translated and published, and he became the most influential foreign literary theorist in China, proclaimed by Lu Xun and Guo Moruo 郭沫若 (1892–1978) as "unsurpassable."[79] In the 1950s, as revolutionary culture stabilized, Gorky's work continued to be extremely important. In two collections used in colleges and universities, *Introduction to Literature* (*Wenxue gailun* 文学概论) and *The Basic Principles of Literature* (*Wenxue de jiben yuanli* 文学的基本原理), Gorky's work was referred to more often than any single author other than Marx, Lenin, and other foundational revolutionary thinkers.[80]

Gorky's influence in the 1920s and early 1930s was primarily among literary intellectuals and students, and he was an inspiration for May Fourth stand-outs

77 Liu Qingfu 刘庆福, "Gao Erji wenlun zai Zhongguo 高尔基文论在中国 [Gorky's Literary Theories in China]," *Sulian wenxue* 苏联文学 (Soviet Literature), 1988, no. 4:88.

78 Ibid.

79 Ibid., 92.

80 Ibid., 96.

such as Ding Ling 丁玲 (1904–86) and Shen Congwen 沈从文 (1902–88).[81] At the same time, however, his attention to those who were oppressed but struggling to fight against their oppressors endowed his work with a deeply realistic yet simultaneously heroic quality that only enhanced his reputation, allowing him a smooth transition from early romanticism into later socialist realism.[82] But by the mid-1930s, Gorky's writings were dragged into a formative literary debate, becoming important sources in the argument between Zhou Yang and Hu Feng on typicality in literature. As Qiu Yunhua 邱运华 argues, what is crucial to recognize is that in China, the debate about typicality is what transformed Gorky—formerly a multi-faceted writer/theorist whose ideas spanned the literary logics of different periods including theories of individual expression, pure literature, the spirit of the era—into a revolutionary tool to be used to move literature in front of rather than behind reality, as Zhou Yang put it.[83] In this metamorphosis, Gorky's work on the instrumental nature of literature as the eyes, ears, throat and tongue of class became paramount.[84] The crisis of the Japanese invasion propelled Zhou Yang and the Chinese Gorky to this radical instrumentalization of literature, which ultimately pushed aside earlier concerns, including questions of individuality and what makes humans human. The creative misreading of Gorky's theory of typicality in China, influenced by a 1955 literary policy in the Soviet Union that stipulated that typicality was always a political issue related to the nature of the party, threw aside

---

81 Jeffrey Kinkley, "Echoes of Maxim Gorky in the Works of Ding Ling and Shen Congwen," in *Interliterary and Intraliterary Aspects of the May Fourth Movement 1919 in China*, ed. Marian Galik (Bratislava: Veda, 1990), 179–88.

82 For the influence of Gorky's "political study romanticism" on Yu Dafu and in general, see Yu Zhaoping 俞兆平, *Langman zhuyi zai Zhongguo de si zhong fanshi—Lu Xun, Shen Congwen, Guo Moruo, Lin Yutang* 浪漫主义在中国的四种范式——鲁迅、沈从文、郭沫若、林语堂 [Four Types of Romanticism in China: Lu Xun, Shen Congwen, Guo Moruo, and Lin Yutang] (Guilin: Guangxi shifan daxue chubanshe, 2011), esp. 150–66 on Gorky's so-called "political study romanticism" (*zhengzhixue langman zhuyi* 政治学浪漫主义).

83 Qiu Yunhua, "Xiandai Zhongguo wenlun jianshe guocheng zhong de Gao Erji dianxinglun—sanshi niandai Zhou Yang, Hu Feng yu dianxingshuo lunbian 现代中国文论建设过程中的高尔基典型论—三十年代周扬、胡风与典型说论辩 [Gorky's Theory of Typicality in the Development of Modern Chinese Literary Theory: The 1930s Debate on the Theory of Typicality by Zhou Yang and Hu Feng]," *Xiangtan daxue xuebao* 湘潭大学学报(哲学社会科学版) (Journal of Xiangtan University [Philosophy and Social Sciences]), 1997, no. 6:76. The literary and artistic theory of typicality was established as part of socialist realism in the Soviet Union in the 1930s.

84 Ibid.

earlier interest in the social role of literature. Under first Lenin and then Stalin, Gorky became a political pawn, and China followed suit.[85]

The relevance of this debate and transformation of Gorky into a beacon of revolutionary optimism has to do with the insertion of a pronounced temporal aspect, the wonderful future, into literary form and into general expectations toward humanistic intellectuals, with their "vanguard" function. Rather than focusing on the social role of literature, Gorky's apologists used him as a tool to mold the correct utopian perspective:

> Gorky believed that literature was the "textbook of life," and writers were then the teachers of life. Because of this, he hoped that writers would write works that were truthful and that helped the working people become educated. In order to meet the educational goals of literature, Gorky often emphasized the function of thought in literary creation. He tirelessly struggled on behalf of elevating thought in Soviet literature, and he always opposed the cool attitude toward reality that paid no heed to political trends. Gorky emphasized a writer's world view and social position. He felt that working in literature was simply a method of serving the vast majority of people, not a job that meant searching for individual fame.[86]

Gorky, who once lambasted Lenin and the Bolsheviks for restricting free speech and betraying the ideals of the reformers, in the Soviet Union and in China came to stand for a narrow vision that zeroed in on the writer's role in developing, representing, and projecting the utopian vision inherent in present policies. Gorky's socialist hero, struggling throughout his life on behalf of the people, was transformed into an embodiment of the future in the present who, in his or her optimistic attitude and personality, internalized the glorious future predicted by the regimes' success, in literature via the theory of

85 Although Gorky's writing over decades was too complex to be branded as naïve class propaganda, by the 1930s, he became known for his support for socialist realism and his relationship with Stalin. See Siridonova, "Gorky and Stalin," 413–23. In this way as well as in his more classical background, he may be similar to Lu Xun, whose late-in-life immersion into Marxist literary theories opened the door for Mao's deployment of Lu Xun as a symbol of his political goals.

86 Zhang Tiexian 张铁弦, "Gao Erji yu wenxue sixiang douzheng 高尔基与文学思想斗争 [Gorky and the Debate on Literary Thought]," *Renmin wenxue* 人民文学 (The People's Literature), 1958, no. 3:7–8.

revolutionary romanticism.[87] One famous example of this process in film is the transformation of Lin Daojing 林道静 in Cui Wei's 崔嵬 film *Song of Youth* (*Qingchun zhi ge* 青春之歌, 1959), the journey from self-centered bourgeois subjectivity to revolutionary ardor produces a cathartic moment of pleasure which, formalized in the model operas of the Cultural Revolution, becomes in the most revolutionary heroes a rapture through which the hidden truth of reality is revealed.[88]

Unsurprisingly, it is during the 1950s and 1960s that happiness and optimism reached their heights, riding on the expectation of an imminent realization of socialist paradise. It was "an age of great passion and expectations, an age in which the boldest dreams about human happiness were collectively dreamed, and the most ordinary moments in life gloriously poeticized."[89] The combination of revolutionary realism and revolutionary romanticism, proclaimed by Mao as the only suitable literary theory, produced an exuberant lyricism that pushed out unhappy thoughts and expressions, becoming "a technical solution, a strategy of mobilization that serves to engage and coordinate the young population."[90] In 1963, *China Youth Magazine* (*Zhongguo qingnian* 中国青年) began a discussion on the correct understanding of happiness, repeating the old binaries of "self and collective, bourgeois hedonism and proletarian asceticism, material satisfaction and revolutionary determination" while nonetheless focusing on convincing the reader: "You are actually happy"; "Young comrades, we now live in a happy country," the article proclaimed, echoing Stalin, "We must not live in happiness without knowing what it is."[91] In revolutionary culture, the disease of unhappiness, which had plagued May Fourth writers and was wiped out only by decades of harsh training, was on the verge of disappearing. Because unhappiness indicated that one did not grasp a future which already existed in the present or, in other words, that one did not grasp the direction of history and its meaning, it signaled personal dysfunction. And

87 Lan Yang, "'Socialist Realism' versus 'Revolutionary Realism plus Revolutionary Romanticism'," in *In the Party Spirit: Socialist Realism and Literary Practice in the Soviet Union, East Germany and China*, ed. Hilary Chung with Michael Falchikov, Bonnie S. McDougall, and Karin McPherson (Amsterdam: Rodopi, 1996), 88–105.

88 Jason McGrath, "Cultural Revolution Model Opera Films and the Realist Tradition in Chinese Cinema," *The Opera Quarterly* 26.2–3 (2010): 343–76.

89 Xiaobing Tang, *Chinese Modern: The Heroic and the Quotidian* (Durham: Duke University Press, 2000), 165.

90 Ibid., 171.

91 "Zenyang peiyang he baochi wangsheng de geming reqing 怎样培养和保持旺盛的革命热情 [How to Train and Maintain Vigorous Revolutionary Ardor]," quoted in Tang, *Chinese Modern*, 175.

as happiness became the norm, unhappiness became a convenient indication of who was mentally ill, which pointed toward therapy that could range from help and encouragement to punishment.[92] The unhappiness of many people presented the dangerous possibility that it was not caused by mental illness, but rather by social dysfunction, which was impossible. Therefore, by the Cultural Revolution, unhappiness was virtually wiped away, replaced by a willing corps of youth surging into the future, pleasantly cooperative workers ready to do their part, dancing and singing minorities, and smiling, hard-working peasants. With the perfect society on the cusp of its emergence, the disease of unhappiness was almost completely cured.

It was also during the Cultural Revolution that the idea of "remembering (past) bitterness to savor (present) sweetness, pondering the old to understand the new" (*yiku sitian, wengu zhixin* 忆苦思甜，温故知新), a Land Reform phrase that elegantly encompassed and projected a tight temporal narrative, became formalized as a cliché. The past, only implied in the Chinese phrase, was society before 1949, after which the present began:

> In 1949, the entire country was liberated, and I, who had lived such a long time in hell, saw the light and began a new life. In 1952 in the countryside we started land reform and I spoke out against the cruelty of my landlord's evil control, spitting out the bitter fluid in my heart, overturning the landlord and returning land we once had for thousands of years to our family. The following year, I enthusiastically responded to the government's call and took leadership in establishing a cooperative, and was chosen as head of the cooperative. Through this organization we became strong and harvest was good; from this point on, bitterness was over and sweetness arrived, and our days became happier and happier.[93]

92 For a full history of the abuses of psychiatry and mental health treatment in China, see Robin Munro, *Dangerous Minds: Political Psychiatry in China Today and Its Origins in the Mao Era* (New York: Human Rights Watch; Hilversum, Netherlands: Geneva Initiative on Psychiatry, 2002). For the fine line between victimization, which could be treated with therapy, and counterrevolutionary intent, which had to be stamped out, as well as a discussion of the various forms of resistance and accommodation in revolutionary China, see Aminda M. Smith, "Thought Reform and the Unreformable: Reeducation Centers and the Rhetoric of Opposition in the Early People's Republic of China," *The Journal of Asian Studies* 72.4 (Nov. 2013): 937–58.

93 Chen Wangya 陈望伢, "Yiku sitian yong bu wangben 忆苦思甜永不忘本 [In Remembering Bitterness and Savoring Sweetness Never Forget What Happened]," *Zhongguo nongken* 中国农垦 [Chinese Agriculture], 1965, no. 4:28. See also Liu Deyi 刘德一, "Yiku sitian, wengu zhixin: Du *Chuangguan de renmen* 忆苦思甜，温故知新：读《闯关的人们》

The old/new, past/present dichotomies do not include a clear gesture toward the future which, as Chen Wangya's final lines indicate, has been absorbed into the present.[94]

The Global Spread of Scientific Rationalism: Be of Good Cheer

The usefulness of optimism and good cheer, whether under capitalist or socialist conditions, led to its encouragement through models, images, and narrative in self-help manuals, literature, essays, advertising, and media, even though other emotions may have been relatively acceptable in some of these cultural arenas. In the United States, the culture of commerce—with its organization of life through spatial compartmentalization and efficient time-keeping—emerged out of scientific rationality, which attempted to understand, categorize, and define all aspects of material and spiritual life for the purpose of deploying them on behalf of progress. Cheerfulness became the "most useful of emotions in an increasingly rational culture," and other emotions were "carefully directed to special niches, such as the theater, the pub, the dance club, film and fiction, various types of TV programming, the sensationalist press, and so on."[95] Thus although non-optimistic emotions were still a valid part of experience, in certain environments, or "time-space-consumer group cells," cheerfulness was still the "only emotion that is almost always appropriate in

---

[Remembering Bitterness and Savoring Sweetness, Pondering the Old to Understand the New: On Reading *Those Who Stormed the Gate*]," *Shanhua* 山花 [Mountain Flowers], 1963, no. 10:47. Liu describes the writing of *Those Who Stormed the Gate*, a history of the Guizhou Automobile Factory (Guizhou qiche zhizaochang 贵州汽车制造厂), which includes self-told stories by older workers about the hardships (bitterness) of their former lives, oppression under the Nationalists, and their new existence in which "life could not be happier." In conclusion, Liu repeats the temporal phrases: "Remember bitterness to savor sweetness, ponder the old to understand the new, compare the old and the new, and you will deeply hate the old society and fervently love the new society."

94 The visual metaphor was darkness vs. lightness, with darkness not only assigned to the past, but also to the capitalist representative the United States. In a study of textbooks from 1949 to 1966, Miin-ling Yu 余敏玲 describes a lesson entitled "In the USA, a Kid Was Killed," which ends "describing how Chinese Young Pioneers were bathed under a golden sun and joyfully played in the green river and pine woods. The contrast between light and darkness illuminates China's progress and people's happiness." See Miin-ling Yu, "From Two Camps to Three Worlds: The Party Worldview in PRC Textbooks (1949–1966)," *The China Quarterly* 215 (Sept. 2013): 682–702.

95 Kotchemidova, "From Good Cheer to 'Drive-By Smiling'," 17.

the vast public space."[96] Under this model, efficiency of production drove the ethos of mandatory happiness and modulated the intensity of emotions and their context of expression.

It is not difficult to recognize similarities in the century-long molding of happiness and optimism under capitalism and under socialism, and in the development of disincentives or cures for unhappiness and gloom. However, the struggling yet joyful heroes of revolutionary China—the aspiring Lei Fengs 雷锋 who conquer any difficulty with a smile, and the multitude of positive heroes in fiction and film—give testimony to the "increasing distance between ideological formalization and reality" that may have contributed to the end of the Maoist regime.[97] Formalism, or the stock gestures, tones, and gazes of an inspired revolutionary, went so far that by the end of the Cultural Revolution, irony had set in and revolutionary morés were actively parodied.[98] In the United States, the increasingly valued ability to seem happy even under bad conditions, and to "always wear a smile" also demanded some distance between reality and expression. And as in China, not only did resistance to mandated happiness appear, but the culture of "cool" also expanded, becoming not only an aspect of the diminishment of emotional investment and the increase in nonchalance and disengagement after WWII, but also a site where irony could grow.[99]

Coué's mantra aimed to enhance lived reality through the exercise of optimism. Optimism is clearly an emotional value that can boost efficiency and

---

96 Ibid., 18.

97 McGrath, "Cultural Revolution Model Opera Films and the Realist Tradition in Chinese Cinema," 372.

98 Paul Clark, *The Chinese Cultural Revolution: A History* (Cambridge: Cambridge University Press, 2008), quoted in McGrath "Cultural Revolution Model Opera Films and the Realist Tradition in Chinese Cinema," 373.

99 Peter N. Stearns, *American Cool: Constructing a Twentieth-Century Emotional Style* (New York: New York University Press, 1994), analyzes American cool mostly as part of the deintensification of emotions beginning in the early twentieth century and becoming the predominant model by mid century. In seeing it as the precursor of an ironical opposition to mandated happiness, I find in it some similarity to the mocking of Soviet ideological expressions that occurred in the early 1970s in the Soviet Union and the mid-1970s in China. For the Soviet "sots-art," see Nancy Condee, "Postmodernism, Communism, and Sots-Arts," in *Endquote: Sots-Arts Literature and Soviet Grand Style*, ed. Marina Balina, Nancy Condee, and Evgeny Dobrenko (Evanston: Northwestern University Press, 2000), 3–31. In China, the struggle between those who insist on understanding the revolutionary icons as expressing something real, good, and true and those who mock them as either outdated relics or as symbols of brainwashing continues in the various uses of these icons in art and other contexts.

the smooth functioning of society, whether under socialism or capitalism. My study of optimism under two major twentieth-century political, economic and cultural movements suggests that both have inherited the mandates of scientific rationality—or, in other words, both directions are modern developments of Enlightenment thought or trajectories of modernity. In particular, the ideals of progress and improvement directed the gaze of all post-Enlightenment societies toward the future and organized the present to get there quickly and efficiently, effectively incorporating the future into the present. This utopian undercurrent gave meaning to the present in China, the Soviet Union, and the United States, subtly or obviously, motivating institutions and individuals, driving production, and encouraging expansion.

Perhaps, then, the gap between the socialist and the capitalist need to cure or eliminate unhappiness is not as great as we might imagine. Yet we have to suspect that capitalism, with its greater emphasis on efficiency and the conquering and utilization of nature, grasped the logic of scientific rationality somewhat better than did socialism, with its egalitarian focus and rapid, intense reconstruction of the mentality of its subjects. The movement toward increased happiness—originally a spiritual or religious movement that was quickly picked up by the business community—over the American twentieth century lubricated the transactions of production and all aspects of work, which enabled more efficient transformation of human and natural resources into progress. Under socialism in the Soviet Union and China, the connection between productive efficiency and optimism, while touted in psychological therapy and in the "model workers" who were recognized as the ideal, was unable to match the rapid industrialization of the capitalist world, with its emphasis on development and expansion. In China, Maoism social practices such as self-criticism and mass criticism, institutionalized within schools and work places, pulled attention away from production and progress toward enhancing qualities of the mind. This intense enrichment of socialist mentality was supposed to allow the subject to maintain happiness, a cooperative attitude, and a focus on labor even when the great society was a bit delayed. As new research on the Great Leap Forward has shown, it also required an active refusal to recognize stark disparities between the realities of material life—in this case, widespread famine—and the discourse through which they are understood.[100]

---

100 Kimberley Ens Manning and Felix Wemheuer, eds., *Eating Bitterness: New Perspectives on China's Great Leap Forward and Famine* (Vancouver: University of British Columbia Press, 2011).

The spiritual-material contradiction was always a conundrum in socialist China. On one hand, as the 1963 discussion of happiness and youth in the journal *China Youth Magazine* illustrated, communism seemed to promise increased material comfort for the greatest number of people while simultaneously avoiding the capitalist problems of wealth accumulation in a small minority, exploitation of the poor, and the emotional emptiness that could result from excessive focus on money. The discussion and student letters focus on one problem: is the greatest happiness in eating well, having nice clothes to wear, and living in a nice place—as the 1949 "rescue from the sea of bitterness" seemed to imply for the mass of impoverished, suffering, and exploited peasants—or is it in serving the people and promoting communism?[101] The implication of material improvement for the masses but mandatory and continual misery for the revolutionary, who must constantly struggle and take on the most arduous tasks, was a difficult contradiction to solve. Not only did it elevate the revolutionary to an elite status and distance him or her from the commoner, but it also suggested that only in constant turmoil could the true revolutionary find happiness.[102] The cure for unhappiness, therefore, may be better living conditions for peasants and workers, but for the revolutionaries themselves, it was divorced from any material gain, existing completely within the realm of mental discipline and self-sacrifice.

Today, China and Russia do not rank high on the "happiness scale," with the former at #93 and the latter at #68, whereas the United States comes in at #17.[103] The Chinese leadership regularly encourages moral values that include hard work and support of the existing social system, implying a constant attitude adjustment that will promote satisfaction and happiness. At the same time, the much-discussed "Chinese dream" (*Zhongguo meng* 中国梦), put forward by President Xi Jinping 习近平 at the National People's Congress in 2013, embraces national strength and prosperity, with a promise to double per capita GDP by 2020.[104] Ever since Mao's death in 1976, China has relentlessly

101 Hu Dongyuan 胡东渊, "Qingnian yinggai you shenmayang de xingfuguan?—Xiang Lei Feng tongzhi xuexi ying jiejue de yi ge zhongyao wenti 青年应该有什么样的幸福观?—向雷锋同志学习应解决的一个重要问题 [What Perspective Should Youth Have on Happiness?—An Important Problem That Study of Lei Feng Should Solve]," *Zhongguo qingnian* 中国青年 (China Youth Magazine), 1963, no. 7:15.

102 Ibid., 1963, no. 9:20.

103 John Helliwell, Richard Layard, and Jeffrey Sachs, eds., *World Happiness Report 2013* (New York: UN Sustainable Development Solutions Network, 2013), http://unsdsn.org/files/2013/09/WorldHappinessReport2013_online.pdf (accessed Feb. 6, 2014).

104 Ding Yi and Sun Mei, "Commentary: 'Chinese Dream' Carries Global Significance," *Xinhuanet*, Mar. 17, 2013, http://news.xinhuanet.com/english/indepth/2013-03/17/c_132240767.htm (accessed Feb. 6, 2014).

focused on economic development. Clearly, the American tendency to enhance capitalist innovation and production in order to bring about changes in material conditions is a powerful model for developing nations.[105] Recently, however, this fiscal leap into the future has engendered middle-and-lower-class protests about air pollution, food safety, land grabbing, corruption and other social problems. Another contradiction, therefore, has emerged: if the speed is too great and regulatory agencies are not functional, economic development opens the door to another kind of unhappiness, which also must be addressed.

References

Amend, Anne. "Melancholy." In *Encyclopedia of the Enlightenment*, ed. Michel Delon, 822–26. Chicago: University of Chicago Press, 2001.

Angelini, Alberto. "History of the Unconscious in Soviet Russia: From Its Origins to the Fall of the Soviet Union." *Institute of Psychoanalysis* 89 (2008): 369–88.

Anonymous. "Hypnotism and the Law." *British Medical Journal*, Feb. 23, 1895, 437–38.

———. "Quackery in Russia and Germany." *British Medical Journal*, May 11, 1912, 1087–88.

———. "Ancient Fads Still Rolling." *Spokane: The Spokesman-Review*, Mar. 27, 1950, 14.

Another Gentleman with a Duster [Henry Amos Purcell]. *Is Coué a Foe to Christianity?* New York: Frederick Moore, 1923.

Baird, Alice. *The Realm of Delight*. London: Adlard & Son & West Newman, 1923.

Balina, Marina, and Evgeny Dobrenko. *Petrified Utopian: Happiness Soviet Style*. London: Anthem Press, 2011.

Baudouin, Charles. *Emile Coué and His Life Work*. New York: American Library Service, 1923.

———. Preface to *How to Practice Suggestion and Autosuggestion*, by Émile Coué, 9–25. New York: American Library Service, 1923.

Beth Israel Deaconess Medical Center. "Program in Placebo Studies & Therapeutic Encounter (PiPS)." Harvard Medical School. http://programinplacebostudies.org/ (accessed Jan. 9, 2014).

105 Even in Bhutan, where the idea of "gross national happiness" was first developed in 1972 by King Jigme Singye Wangchuck as an alternative to gross national product, newly elected Prime Minister Tshering Tobgay has downplayed the idea, instead focusing on national debt, high unemployment, inadequate infrastructure, and rule of law. See Gardiner Harris, "Index of Happiness? Bhutan's New Leader Prefers More Concrete Goals," *The New York Times*, Oct. 4, 2013, http://www.nytimes.com/2013/10/05/world/asia/index-of-happiness-bhutans-new-leader-prefers-more-concrete-goals.html?_r=0 (accessed Feb. 6, 2014).

Brooks, C. Harry. *The Practice of Autosuggestion by the Method of Emile Coué*. New York: Dodd, Mead, 1922.

Brydon, Lena, et al. "Dispositional Optimism and Stress-induced Changes in Immunity and Negative Mood." *Brain, Behavior & Immunity* 23.6 (2009): 810–16.

Buzin, V.N. "Psychoanalysis in the Soviet Union: On the History of a Defeat." *Russian Social Science Review* 36.61 (Nov.–Dec. 1995): 65–73.

Chen Wangya 陈望伢. "Yiku sitian yong bu wangben 忆苦思甜永不忘本 [In Remembering Bitterness and Savoring Sweetness Never Forget What Happened]." *Zhongguo nongken* 中国农垦 [Chinese Agriculture], 1965, no. 4:28.

Chin, Robert, and Ai-li S. Chin. *Psychological Research in Communist China, 1949–1966*. Cambridge: MIT Press, 1969.

Clark, Paul. *The Chinese Cultural Revolution: A History*. Cambridge: Cambridge University Press, 2008.

Condee, Nancy. "Postmodernism, Communism, and Sots-Arts." In *Endquote: Sots-Arts Literature and Soviet Grand Style*, ed. Marina Balina, Nancy Condee, and Evgeny Dobrenko, 3–31. Evanston: Northwestern University Press, 2000.

Coué, Émile. *Self-Mastery through Conscious Autosuggestion*. New York: American Library Service, 1922.

———. *My Method: Including American Impressions*. Garden City: Doubleday, Page, 1923.

Cushman, Philip. *Constructing the Self, Constructing America: A Cultural History of Psychotherapy*. Reading, Mass.: Addison-Wesley, 1990.

Ding, Yi, and Sun Mei. "Commentary: 'Chinese Dream' Carries Global Significance." *Xinhuanet*, Mar. 17, 2013. http://news.xinhuanet.com/english/indepth/2013-03/17/c_132240767.htm (accessed Feb. 6, 2014).

Dobrenko, Evgeny. *The Making of the State Reader: Social and Aesthetic Contexts of the Reception of Soviet Literature*. Trans. Jesse Savage. Stanford: Stanford University Press, 1997.

———. *The Making of the State Writer*. Stanford: Stanford University Press, 2001.

———. *Aesthetics of Alienation: Reassessment of Early Soviet Cultural Theories*. Evanston: Northwestern University Press, 2005.

Duckworth, J. Herbert. *Autosuggestion and Its Personal Application*. New York: James A. McCann, 1925.

Etkind, Alexander M. "How Psychoanalysis Was Received in Russia, 1906–1936." *Journal of Analytical Psychology* 39 (1994): 191–200.

Fournier, Marijda, Denise de Ridder, and Jozien Bensing. "Optimism and Adaptation to Multiple Sclerosis: What Does Optimism Mean?" *Journal of Behavioral Medicine* 22.4 (1999): 303–26.

Galbraith, John Kenneth. *The Affluent Society*. Boston: Houghton Mifflin, 1958.

Garforth, Lisa. "No Intentions? Utopian Theory After the Future." *Journal for Cultural Research* 13.1 (Jan. 2009): 5–27.

George, Carol V. R. *God's Salesman: Normal Vincent Peale & the Power of Positive Thinking*. New York: Oxford University Press, 1993.

Goffman, Erving. *Gender Advertisements*. New York: Harper and Row, 1976.

Gorky, Maxim. *Untimely Thoughts: Essays on Revolution, Culture, and the Bolsheviks, 1917–1918*. Trans. Herman Ermolaev. New York: Paul S. Eriksson, 1968.

Harris, Gardiner. "Index of Happiness? Bhutan's New Leader Prefers More Concrete Goals." *The New York Times*, Oct. 4, 2013. http://www.nytimes.com/2013/10/05/world/asia/index-of-happiness-bhutans-new-leader-prefers-more-concrete-goals.html?_r=0 (accessed Feb. 6, 2014).

Haven, Joseph. *Mental Philosophy: Including the Intellect, Sensibilities, and Will*. Boston: Gould and Lincoln, 1862.

Helliwell, John, Richard Layard, and Jeffrey Sachs, eds. *World Happiness Report 2013*. New York: UN Sustainable Development Solutions Network, 2013. http://unsdsn.org/files/2013/09/WorldHappinessReport2013_online.pdf (accessed Feb. 6, 2014).

Ho, Samuel, et al. "The Roles of Hope and Optimism on Posttraumatic Growth in Oral Cavity Cancer Patients." *Oral Oncology* 47.2 (2011): 121–24.

Hu Dongyuan 胡东渊. "Qingnian yinggai you shenmayang de xingfuguan?—Xiang Lei Feng tongzhi xuexi ying jiejue de yi ge zhongyao wenti 青年应该有什么样的幸福观?—向雷锋同志学习应解决的一个重要问题 [What Perspective Should Youth Have on Happiness?—An Important Problem That Study of Lei Feng Should Solve]." *Zhongguo qingnian* 中国青年 (China Youth Magazine), 1963, no. 7:15–17, no. 9:20–22.

Hull, Clark L. "Hypnotism in Scientific Perspective." *Scientific Monthly* 2 (1929): 154–62.

Johns, Alfred E. *Scientific Autosuggestion for Personality Adjustment and Development*. New York: Modern Coué Institute, 1952.

Kaye, Herbert. "Why Freud Hated America." *The Wilson Quarterly* 17.2 (Spring 1993): 118–25.

Khullar, D., et al. "Optimism and the Socioeconomic Status Gradient in Adolescent Adiposity." *Journal of Adolescent Health* 49.5 (2011): 553–55.

Kinkley, Jeffrey. "Echoes of Maxim Gorky in the Works of Ding Ling and Shen Congwen." In *Interliterary and Intraliterary Aspects of the May Fourth Movement 1919 in China*, ed. Marian Galik, 179–88. Bratislava: Veda, 1990.

Kirk, Ella Boyce. *My Pilgrimage to Coué*. New York: American Library Service, 1922.

Kotchemidova, Christina. "From Good Cheer to 'Drive-By Smiling': A Social History of Cheerfulness." *Journal of Social History* 39.1 (2005): 5–37.

Kronstrom, Kim, et al. "Optimism and Pessimism as Predictors of Work Disability with a Diagnosis of Depression: A Prospective Cohort Study of Onset and Recovery." *Journal of Affective Disorders* 130.1/2 (2011): 294–99.

Kubzansky, Laura D., et al. "Is the Glass Half Empty or Half Full? A Prospective Study of Optimism and Coronary Heart Disease in the Normative Aging Study." *Psychosomatic Medicine* 63 (2001): 910–16.

Lang, W. "Infectiology and Optimism in Medicine." *Munchener Medizinische Wochenschrift* 127.9 (1985): 191–92.

Larson, Wendy. *From Ah Q to Lei Feng: Freud and Revolutionary Spirit in 20th Century China*. Stanford: Stanford University Press, 2009.

Liu Chengjie 刘成杰, Wang Tianhou 王天后, and Zhang Mingjuan 张明娟. "Xianjin shengchanzhe de xinli tedian: Lun gongchan zhuyi laodong taidu 先进生产者的心理特点:论共产主义劳动态度 [The Psychological Characteristics of Progressive Producers: On the Work Attitude of Communism]." *Beijing daxue xuebao* 北京大学学报 (哲學社會科學版) (Journal of Peking University [Philosophy and Social Sciences]), 1958, no. 4:39–51.

Liu Deyi 刘德一. "Yiku sitian, wengu zhixin: Du *Chuangguan de renmen* 忆苦思甜,温故知新: 读《闯关的人们》 [Remembering Bitterness and Savoring Sweetness, Pondering the Old to Understand the New: On Reading *Those Who Stormed the Gate*]." *Shanhua* 山花 [Mountain Flowers], 1963, no. 10:46–47.

Liu Qingfu 刘庆福. "Gao Erji wenlun zai Zhongguo 高尔基文论在中国 [Gorky's Literary Theories in China]." *Sulian wenxue* 苏联文学 (Soviet Literature), 1988, no. 4:88–96, 73.

Macnaghten, Hugh. *Émile Coué: The Man and His Work*. New York: Dodd, Mead, 1922.

Mangasarian, M.M. *Psycho-analysis and Autosuggestion: Sigmund Freud and Emile Coue*. Chicago: Independent Religious Society, n.d.

Manning, Kimberley Ens, and Felix Wemheuer, eds. *Eating Bitterness: New Perspectives on China's Great Leap Forward and Famine*. Vancouver: University of British Columbia Press, 2011.

Marchand, Roland. *Advertising the American Dream*. Berkeley and Los Angeles: University of California Press, 1985.

Mathewson, Rufus W., Jr. *The Positive Hero in Russian Literature*. Stanford: Stanford University Press, 1975.

McGrath, Jason. "Cultural Revolution Model Opera Films and the Realist Tradition in Chinese Cinema." *The Opera Quarterly* 26.2–3 (2010): 343–76.

Meisner, Maurice. *Marxism, Maoism, and Utopianism: Eight Essays*. Madison: Wisconsin University Press, 1982.

Miller, Martin A. *Freud and the Bolsheviks: Psychoanalysis in Imperial Russia and the Soviet Union*. New Haven: Yale University Press, 1998.

Morton, Debbie, et al. "Reproducibility of Placebo Analgesia: Effect of Dispositional Optimism." *Pain* 146.1/2 (2009): 194–98.

Munro, Robin. *Dangerous Minds: Political Psychiatry in China Today and Its Origins in the Mao Era*. New York: Human Rights Watch; Hilversum, Netherlands: Geneva Initiative on Psychiatry, 2002.

Nikulin, L. "Karnaval molodosti." *Pravda*, July 13, 1936.

Orwig, Sarah Forbes. "Business Ethics and the Protestant Spirit: How Norman Vincent Peale Shaped the Religious Values of American Business Leaders." *Journal of Business Ethics* 38.1/2 (June 2002): 81–89.

Petrovsky, Arthur. *Psychology in the Soviet Union: A Historical Outline*. Trans. Lilia Nakhapetyan. Moscow: Progress, 1990.

Qiu Yunhua 邱运华. "Xiandai Zhongguo wenlun jianshe guocheng zhong de Gao Erji dianxinglun—sanshi niandai Zhou Yang, Hu Feng yu dianxingshuo lunbian 现代中国文论建设过程中的高尔基典型论—三十年代周扬、胡风与典型说论辩 [Gorky's Theory of Typicality in the Development of Modern Chinese Literary Theory: The 1930s Debate on the Theory of Typicality by Zhou Yang and Hu Feng]." *Xiangtan daxue xuebao* 湘潭大学学报(哲学社会科学版) (Journal of Xiangtan University [Philosophy and Social Sciences]), 1997, no. 6:72–77.

Randazzo, Sal. *Mythmaking on Madison Avenue*. Chicago: Probus, 1993.

Rice, James L. *Freud's Russia: National Identity in the Evolution of Psychoanalysis*. New Brunswick: Transaction, 1993.

Scheier, Michael F., and Charles S. Carver. "Optimism, Coping, and Health: Assessment and Implications of Generalized Outcome." *Health Psychology* 4.3 (1985): 219–47.

Schmidt, John R. "Emile Coué: Chicago's Miracle Man." *Chicago History Today*, 2012. http://www.wbez.org/blog/john-r-schmidt/2012-02-06/emile-coue-chicagos-miracle-man-95980 (accessed May 17, 2012, no longer available).

Schudson, Michael. "Advertising as Capitalist Realism." In *Advertising, the Uneasy Persuasion: Its Dubious Impact on American Society*, 209–33. New York: Basic Books, 1984.

Scott, Frank Lincoln. *Autosuggestions and Salesmanship, or Imagination in Business.* New York: American Library Service, 1923.

Shaw, Claire. "A Fairground for 'Building the New Man': Gorky Park As a Site of Soviet Acculturation." *Urban History* 38.2 (2011): 324–44.

Sidel, Ruth. "The Role of Revolutionary Optimism in the Treatment of Mental Illness in the People's Republic of China." *American Journal of Orthopsychiatry* 43.5 (Oct. 1973), 732–36.

Siridonova, Lidiia. "Gorky and Stalin (According to New Materials from A.M. Gorky's Archive)." *The Russian Review* V.54 (July 1995): 413–23.

Smith, Aminda M. "Thought Reform and the Unreformable: Reeducation Centers and the Rhetoric of Opposition in the Early People's Republic of China." *The Journal of Asian Studies* 72.4 (Nov. 2013): 937–58.

Stearns, Peter N. *American Cool: Constructing a Twentieth-Century Emotional Style*. New York: New York University Press, 1994.

Steginga, Suzanne K., and Stefano Occhipinti. "Dispositional Optimism as a Predictor of Men's Decision-Related Distress after Localized Prostate Cancer." *Health Psychology* 25.2 (Mar. 2006): 135–43.

Stibich, Mark. "Top 10 Reasons to Smile." Feb. 4, 2010. http://longevity.about.com/od/lifelongbeauty/tp/smiling.htm (accessed Jan. 9, 2014).

Szasz, Thomas S. "The Myth of Mental Illness: Foundations of a Theory of Personal Conduct." *American Psychologist* 15 (1960): 113–18.

———. *The Myth of Psychotherapy: Mental Healing as Religion, Rhetoric, and Repression*. Cambridge: Oxford University Press, 1978.

Tang, Xiaobing. *Chinese Modern: The Heroic and the Quotidian*. Durham: Duke University Press, 2000.

Tansley, Arthur G. *The New Psychology and Its Relation to Life*. London: G. Allen & Unwin, 1920.

Taylor, Charles. *Sources of the Self: The Making of the Modern Identity*. Cambridge: Harvard University Press, 1989.

Torrey, E. Fuller. *Freudian Fraud: The Malignant Effect of Freud's Theory on American Thought and Culture*. New York: Harper Collins, 1992.

Williams, Raymond. "Advertising: The Magic System." In *Problems in Materialism and Culture*, 170–95. London: Verso, 1980.

Wozniak, Robert H. "Mind and Body: Réne Descartes to William James." *Serendip*, 1995. http://serendip.brynmawr.edu/Mind/ (accessed Jan. 5, 2014).

Yang, Lan. "'Socialist Realism' versus 'Revolutionary Realism plus Revolutionary Romanticism'." In *In the Party Spirit: Socialist Realism and Literary Practice in the Soviet Union, East Germany and China*, ed. Hilary Chung with Michael Falchikov, Bonnie S. McDougall, and Karin McPherson, 88–105. Amsterdam: Rodopi, 1996.

Yip, Kam-Shing. "An Historical Review of the Mental Health Services in the People's Republic of China." *International Journal of Social Psychiatry* 51.106 (2005): 106–18.

Yu, Miin-ling. "From Two Camps to Three Worlds: The Party Worldview in PRC Textbooks (1949–1966)." *The China Quarterly* 215 (Sept. 2013): 682–702.

Yu Zhaoping 俞兆平. *Langman zhuyi zai Zhongguo de si zhong fanshi—Lu Xun, Shen Congwen, Guo Moruo, Lin Yutang* 浪漫主义在中国的四种范式——鲁迅、沈从文、郭沫若、林语堂 [Four Types of Romanticism in China: Lu Xun, Shen Congwen, Guo Moruo, and Lin Yutang]. Guilin: Guangxi shifan daxue chubanshe, 2011.

Zhang Tiexian 张铁弦. "Gao Erji yu wenxue sixiang douzheng 高尔基与文学思想斗争 [Gorky and the Debate on Literary Thought]." *Renmin wenxue* 人民文学 (The People's Literature), 1958, no. 3:10–11.

CHAPTER 3

Metaphors unto Themselves: Mental Illness Poetics and Narratives in Contemporary Chinese Poetry[1]

Birgit Bunzel Linder

> To write prescriptions is easy, but to come to an understanding with people is hard.
>
> FRANZ KAFKA

> Once a poem emerges, the fire is tamed.
> 诗出来了,火就没了。
>
> GUO LUSHENG 郭路生

> An unscathed appearance hides a shattered heart.
> 内心一篇狼籍,却貌似完好无损。
>
> WEN JIE 温洁

Based on the theory that literature can "read the wound,"[2] the medical humanities consider art, poetry, fiction, and other creative writing to be important for understanding and treating patients.[3] In addition to highlighting how illness is experienced, literature and the arts express and address the questions of meaning and suffering. Madness and mental illness in literature not only form a nexus between medicine/psychiatry and literature but are also social

1 A shorter and differently focused version of this article was published in *Literature and Medicine* 33.2 (Fall 2015): 368–92.

2 Geoffrey H. Hartman, "On Traumatic Knowledge and Literary Studies," *New Literary History* 26.3 (1995): 537.

3 The recent discussion of the *critical* medical humanities suggests that in addition to the medical and health related fields, it should also incorporate such non-allied fields and approaches as critical and cultural theories, community-based arts and health, and countercultural practices of activists movement. For a summary of the discussion surrounding the field of medical humanities, the various viewpoints, and a more specific discussion about "critical medical humanities," see Sarah Atkinson et al., "'The Medical' and 'Health' in a Critical Medical Humanities," *Journal of Medical Humanities* 36.1 (2015): 71–81; for a point-by-point summary of the characteristics of critical medical humanities, see William Viney, Felicity Callard, and Angela Woods, "Critical Medical Humanities: Embracing Entanglements, Taking Risks," *Medical Humanities* 41.1 (2015): 2–7.

 | DOI 10.1163/9789004319219_005

indicators that pose challenges to readers. Illness, suffering, pain, and trauma often lead to borderline experiences and form a context within which human beings become conscious of their own limitations and vulnerabilities. The literature of madness articulates such *Grenzerfahrungen*, and, at the same time, can express subjective pain and collective trauma, relay the experience of illness, and offer individual and social insight.[4]

The popularity of illness narratives suggests a strong "representation compulsion" as well as society's desire to read about mental illness experiences in some cultures.[5] When browsing bookshops in China, too, one can find popular psychology sections with self-help manuals and books that explain mood disorders, and among them primarily depression. Many books are translated from English, and the self-help books written by Chinese authors often aim to help people understand their own illnesses or disorders, symptoms, diagnoses, and treatments. The autobiographical bestsellers *Touched with Fire* by Kay Redfield and *Every Day Gets a Little Closer: A Twice-Told Therapy* by Irvin D. Yalom are also readily available in Chinese. However, besides those, illness narratives dealing with mental illnesses are nearly non-existent in China. Sickness has often been aestheticized or spiritualized in literature, but with the onslaught of AIDS narratives, and later mental illness autopathographies, the metaphor has hardened into often bleak portrayals of pathology. Great value is placed on the therapeutic or cathartic function of writing, and on symptoms, medical knowledge, treatment, and coping. Unlike these "authentic" autodiegetic narratives, poetry, like fiction, by virtue of its essentially symbolic nature, performs and signifies differently.[6] Therefore, what is of particular interest for literary

4 "Madness" refers to the kind of eccentric or "mad" behavior on the part of the character or fictional narrator that is not pathological in a clinical sense, but deemed unacceptable or extreme in a certain social or cultural context in literature. Representations of mental illness, by contrast, refer to specific mental disorders of characters that are either diagnosed or readily identifiable as a cognitive or affective disorder.

5 Hartman, "On Traumatic Knowledge and Literary Studies," 551–52. "Illness narratives" are those narrative accounts that take the trajectory of an illness as the plot of the (life) story. To denote specifically autobiographical, autodiegetic narratives, the term has recently been recoined as "autopathographies" by Stephen Moran. For further information, see Arthur Kleinman, *The Illness Narratives: Suffering, Healing, and the Human Condition* (New York: Harper Collins, 1988) and Stephen T. Moran, "Autopathography and Depression: Describing the 'Despair Beyond Despair'," *Journal of Medical Humanities* 27 (2006): 79–91.

6 The term illness "narrative" is often misleading. It is usually an autobiographical account that attempts to be "authentic" rather than fictional. It has to be distinguished not just from poetry, but also from fictional(ized) accounts of illnesses that have defined many pathologies while at the same time preserving their literary nature and function. I am thinking of such

scholars is the related debate by proponents of the critical medical humanities that recommends a more discerning view of what constitutes narrative in various genres and forms, and to study in what ways such genres and forms "speak." This is, of course, at the heart of literary studies, but for the medical humanities, as Angela Woods contends, "a sophisticated account of genre is largely absent from literary and semiotic approaches to medicine-related and illness narrative."[7] In addition, she points out:

> Scholars and practitioners working with narrative in the field of medicine frequently overlook the cultural and historical dimensions of narrative form. Too often particular kinds of narrative are presented as transcultural, transhistorical truths of the human experience, a view that operates at the expense of a more historically and anthropologically grounded approach to understanding the cultural specificity of idioms of distress.[8]

Within such a context, the poets Guo Lusheng, diagnosed with schizophrenia since 1972, and Wen Jie, chronically depressed since childhood, are two convincing examples of a cross-cultural approach to the medical humanities and "illness poetics" in China. I argue for a specific "illness poetics" that is reflected in the illness-related content as much as in the formal aspects inherited from its own Chinese lyrical tradition. Moreover, I argue that in these two cases—and very likely many other cases as well—the delight of writing poetry about one's illness lies less in the attempt at expressing a subjective experience than in finding the devices and forms that integrate individual experience into a collective one, be that one of sorrow and suffering, or of a specific lyrical tradition and its modes of versification.

Considering the lack of information and education about mental illnesses available in China and the stigma still associated particularly with affective disorders,[9] the reception of poetry about mental illness is unsurprisingly

---

defining novels as Joseph Heller's *Catch-22* for PTSD, Ian McEwan's *Enduring Love* for PTDS, Doris Lessing's *Briefing for a Descent into Hell* for psychosis and depression, Sylvia Plath's *The Bell Jar* for depression, Edgar Allan Poe's and Franz Kafka's studies of paranoia, etc.

7 Angela Woods, "The Limits of Narrative: Provocations for the Medical Humanities," *Medical Humanities* 37 (Dec. 2011): 76.

8 Ibid. For the issue of medical humanities as being mostly expressive of Western cultural values, see Hooker and Noonan, "Medical Humanities as Expressive of Western Culture," *Medical Humanities* 37.2 (Dec. 2011): 79–84.

9 For an overview over the link between "face," illness, and Confucianism, see Lawrence Hsin Yang and Arthur Kleinman's illuminating article "'Face' and the Embodiment of Stigma in China: The Cases of Schizophrenia and AIDS," *Social Science and Medicine* 30 (2008): 1–11.

subdued. The poet Zhang Zao 张枣 (1962–2010) praised Wen Jie's poetry, asserting that "her poems display the best of what poetic style of this age has to offer. It is beautifully lyrical and exhibits mastery of cadence and sound."[10] Other readers, however, only see in it the dark side of the aesthetic spectrum and would perhaps prefer to read about beauty or other topics traditionally associated with poetry. Guo, in contrast, although he has always kept his experience of illness private, has become a symbol of cultural schizophrenia and collective *Vergangenheitsbewältigung*, which is unique within Chinese literary history. There are other Chinese poets who occasionally write about madness or mental illness from various perspectives, but Guo Lusheng and Wen Jie have written poetry that courageously represents their own suffering and have become metaphors unto themselves: metaphors of discord within themselves, of a sharpened identity struggle, and of the vulnerability of health, body, and mind. This article examines the relationship between mental illness, identity, and the writing of poetry, as well as the potential value of this poetry for the medical humanities.

Guo Lusheng and Schizophrenia

Guo Lusheng, also known as Shizhi (Shi Zhi) 食指 or Index Finger, was born in 1948 in Shandong 山东 province. His father was a Red Army officer and his mother, a teacher. As an adolescent, Guo had a nervous disposition, but was very studious and engaged in sports and academics. It is said that when he failed his high school exams, some of his hair turned white instantly.[11] In 1965, at age 17, he wrote his first serious poetry and also experienced increased episodes of anxiety. During China's most trying years of the Cultural Revolution (1966–76), Guo was widely admired for his daring and persistent poetry. Following his premature retirement from the army in 1971, he experienced a prolonged period of silence and suicidal depression. Worried, his father admitted him to a hospital, where Guo was subsequently diagnosed with schizophrenia.[12] Guo's hospital stays were intermittent, with the longest stretch of twelve years ending in 2002, when he remarried and returned to his home in Beijing.

10 Zhang Zao, "Wen Jie yu mei ge ren de Bailun 温洁与每个人的拜伦 [Wen Jie and Everyone's Byron]," *Zuojia* 作家 (Writer Magazine), 2001, no. 1:90. Unless indicated otherwise, all translations from the Chinese are my own.

11 Guo Lusheng, *Shizhi de shi* 食指的诗 [The Poetry of Shizhi] (Beijing: Renmin wenxue chubanshe, 2000), 197.

12 Ibid., 205.

Neither his biography nor his own accounts disclose many details about his illness. In 2011, Guo offered a rare explanation:

> After I was demobilized from the army because I could not understand things happening around me—I might even go so far as to say that I no longer knew what was happening at all, and others could no longer understand my words or actions—I was sent to a mental hospital on November 25, 1973. It was a painful time in my life, yet it was only the beginning. I wrote a few poems during this period, two actually: "Pain" and "The Spirit, Part 2" (written in October 1974).[13]

In "The Spirit, Part 2," he aptly expresses his grief in images: "If the deep night is my full black hair/Then the moonlight is my weary face" (假如深夜是我的满头黑发/那么月色便是我一脸倦容).[14] The poem further describes his solitude and pain, but makes no mention of his illness. Schizophrenia was relatively undefined in China when Guo was diagnosed, and it remained so until the first edition of the *Chinese Classification of Mental Disorders* (CCMD; *Zhongguo jingshen jibing fenlei fang'an yu zhenduan biaozhun* 中国精神疾病分类方案与诊断标准) was published in 1979. Although friends and scholars have created an impressive metatext of Guo, they have either refrained from discussing his illness or lacked related information and education.[15] A few biographical details besides his hospitalization have provided insight into his illness. His biography describes two curious instances of "travelling psychoses"[16] during his earlier years, both of which required hospitalization. After being robbed of his wallet and the address of his destination, he was "lost" for twenty days until he

13 Guo Lusheng (Shi Zhi), "To My American Readers," in his *Winter Sun: Poems*, trans. Jonathan Stalling (Norman: University of Oklahoma Press, 2011), 174.

14 Guo, *Winter Sun*, 56.

15 The proliferation of often hyperbolic articles that were published in the early 2000s, when Guo won the literary award, is an indication of the desire to revive his status, be it out of personal support for him or because many people, including many young readers, still uphold him as an example of steadfastness and as someone who was able to overcome his inner and outer demons. Many shorter articles discuss individual poems and never mention his illness. Some overpraise his achievement, putting him on par with Hölderlin, Du Fu 杜甫, and others.

16 It is interesting to note that "travelling psychosis" appears as a culture-specific category of psychosis in the CCMD-3, but not in any Western classifications. For an overview over some of the differences between Western and Chinese classifications see S. Lee, "From Diversity to Unity: The Classification of Mental Disorders in 21st-Century China," *Psychiatric Clinics of North America* 24.3 (Sept. 2001): 421–31.

"regained a clear mind." Both times, he was admitted to a hospital afterwards.[17] Although the account details some aspects of this experience, it does not explain how he survived alone for twenty days. This depiction underscores the general portrayal of him as someone who inadvertently encounters hardship, but remains resilient and true to himself. Neither Guo's own narrative accounts nor his poetry mention these episodes.

Pioneer Poet

Guo's fame rests as much on his poetic *oeuvre* as on his unchanging role as a (mentally ill) poet in a changing society. Most critics do not consider his poetry to be great, but admit that his tenacity and personal resilience are remarkable. Perhaps with the exceptions of his most famous poems "Believe In the Future" ("Xiangxin weilai" 相信未来), "This Is Beijing at 4:08" ("Zhe shi sidian lingbafen de Beijing" 这是四点零八分的北京), or "Mad Dog" ("Feng gou" 疯狗), he does not appear prominently in literary histories or anthologies.[18] Very rarely is there a discussion or analysis of his poetic form. Van Crevel describes Guo's role during and after the Cultural Revolution as "torch-bearer of non-orthodox poetry" and states that Guo, together with his fellow poet Huang Xiang 黄香, has "returned to poetry the ability—and, in a traditional Chinese poetics, the right—to defy political authority rather than function as an artistically shaped extension of its ideology, and to speak with the voice of something like an individual self."[19] In the time-honored voice of a madman, Guo says: "The fate of a poet is determined by the times.... I wrote a few poems and they were well received by the young people of the time."[20] He considers his upholding of freedom during notoriously cruel times to be paramount and believes himself to have been the only writer of "real things" back then.[21] Besides being the *vox*

17 Guo, *Shizhi de shi*, 206.

18 [English translation of "Believe In the Future" and "This Is Beijing at 4:08" by Jonathan Stalling, with the Chinese original, are available in *Push Open the Window: Contemporary Poetry from China*, ed. Qingping Wang (Port Townsend, WA: Copper Canyon Press, 2011), 2–7. Ed.]

19 Maghiel van Crevel, *Language Shattered: Contemporary Chinese Poetry and Duoduo* (Leiden: Research School CNWS, 1996), 29; van Crevel, *Chinese Poetry in Times of Mind, Mayhem and Money* (Leiden: Brill, 2008): 15.

20 Xu Yi 徐熠, "Menglong shi daibiao Shizhi guilai 朦胧诗代表食指归来 [The Representative of Misty Poetry Shizhi Has Returned]," *Qingchun* 青春 [Youth], 2010, no. 1:87.

21 Lei Ming 雷鸣, "Shizhi shige de yiyi 食指诗歌的意义 [On the Significance of Shizhi's Poetry]," *Kaili xueyuan xuebao* 凯利学院学报 [Journal of Kaili College] 28.4 (2010): 66a.

populi, writing also gave him an inner equilibrium, and he credits poetry with saving him during his twelve years in the insane asylum.[22]

Guo divides his poetry into three phases: the early period, when he was often depressed, but paid great attention to poetic style; the second phase, when he "went mad" and wrote to "tame the fire" of anger; and the third phase, when he wrote poetry in the hospital and felt more peaceful and philosophical.[23] He experienced several years of no writing, which he referred to as "years of hell," and which Warren T. Reich has defined as "mute suffering," the first of three phases of suffering when coping with illness.[24] After being diagnosed with schizophrenia, Guo wrote sparingly for a few years. On the one hand, he claims that his insistence on his own ideas frequently prompted his return to the hospital and complains of the unfair treatment he received there.[25] On the other hand, he acknowledges feeling safer in the hospital. In spite of the fact that he is praised for his kindness and consideration, he often talks about his anger and frustration, both before and after his diagnosis. In "Fury" ("Fennu" 愤怒, 1980), he writes that his anger is no longer loud and thunderous but "has been turned into a terrifying silence."[26] He repeatedly complains of the need to control himself for political or medical reasons, or both; although beyond the hospital conditions and likely medication, he does not discuss why he could not write.

His breaks from creativity for over fifty years notwithstanding, he has not varied considerably from his initial source of inspiration, the poetic form of his early mentor He Qifang 何其芳 (1912–77). He Qifang and others postulated a style that departed from traditional Chinese regulated verse, but still adhered to a strict form of rhyme, rhythm, and tone schemes.[27] "Eight Years in

22 Guo, "To My American Readers," 20a.

23 Cui Weiping 崔卫平, "Shishen juangu shouku de ren 诗神眷顾受苦的人 [The Muse Favors Those Who Suffer]," in Liao Yiwu 廖亦武, *Chenlun de shengdian* 沉沦的圣殿 [Sinking Gurdwara] (Urumqi: Xinjiang qingshaonian chubanshe, 1999): 92–93.

24 W.T. Reich, "Speaking of Suffering: A Moral Account of Compassion," *Soundings* 72 (1989): 83–108.

25 Guo, "To My American Readers," 20b.

26 Guo, *Shizhi de shi*, 98.

27 He Qifang and other modern Chinese poets suggested that a poem could have an irregular number of characters, but meter and rhyme should be regular—with typical minor exceptions. In traditional Chinese poetry, metrical rhythm is created by dipodic prosody prevalent in the *Shijing* 诗经 [The Book of Songs] or by a caesura based prosody prevalent in the "Li sao 离骚 [On Encountering Sorrow]" in the "modern regulated poem" propagated by He Qifang and others, and adopted by Guo, lines should have the same number of feet, though each foot (*dun* 顿) need not have the same number of characters. All lines

a Psychiatric Ward" ("Zai jingshenbing fuliyuan de ba nian" 在精神病福利院的八年, 1998) is one of many poems constructed in "modern regulated form" (*xiandai gelüshi* 现代格律诗): four to five stanzas, four lines per stanza, four to five *dun* (feet), parallel grammatical structures, rhyme, and the customary deviation (usually in the number of syllables, *dun*, or rhyme scheme). Although the lines are composed with uneven length, each line is made up of four or five *dun*. The first two lines juxtapose images of summer and winter, hot sweat drops and cold water. Each line ends on a dipodic foot. The rhyme scheme of the first two stanzas is abcb, bdcd, etc.

> I scrub the stairways in summer as sweat falls like rain
> and wash rice bowls in winter with biting cold water.
> Only in the long nights when I try to endure endless fatigue
> does the meager warmth of spring fill my pen.
>
> Sloth, selfishness, crudeness, and unsanitary habits...
> All the weaknesses of the Chinese people concentrated right here.
> Together, they become a brutal hammer on an anvil,
> smashing my mind into a shower of sparks.
>
> 盛夏 如雨的汗 滴下 擦拭 楼道
> 隆冬 冷水中 洗净 饭碗 [rhyme]
> 只有 在支撑着 困倦苦思的 长夜
> 一丝 温暖的 春意 才遣上 笔端 [rhyme]
>
> 懒惰、 自私、 野蛮 和不卫生的 习惯……
> 在这里 集中了 中国人 所有的 弱点 [rhyme]
> 这一切 如残忍无情的 铁砧、 工锤
> 击打得 我 精神的 火花 四溅 [rhyme]

It is obvious that the poet has constructed the poetic form with great care, both in its regularity and irregularity.

---

should end on a two-syllabic foot. Both the number of feet and the rhyme scheme are regulated, although there is not a prescribed rhyme scheme. There is a preference for short lines, for two-line rhyme, for a length of four to five stanzas, and the poem should contain repetition and parallelism. For further explanation about the Chinese metrical system, see Jin Daoxing 金道行, "Lun xiandai gelü shi 论现代格律诗 [On Modern Regulated Poetry]," *Jingchu ligong xueyuan xuebao* 荆楚理工学院学报 (Journal of Jingchu University of Technology) 25.10 (Oct. 2010): 30–36.

Guo is not consciously trying to express his madness, although his style reflects aspects of his mental illness, not in the form of "Janusian" or "homospatial" thinking or "intrapsychic ataxia" (splitting of thought and emotion),[28] but in his formal technical skills. This also does not mean that the use of formal poetry proves that he is mentally ill. Because thoughts and feelings must be manipulated into a structure, form often plays a key role in the ordering effect of poetry and can itself be a mode of reflexivity. However, Guo's poetry does not try to capture the illness that is afflicting him, nor does he want to reflect any symptoms or phenomenological experiences. He does not display the exceptional insight or "forms of translogical thinking" that David Chan describes as typical of schizophrenic thinking,[29] or the exaggerated reflexivity and the diminishment of normal ipseity Louis A. Sass considers characteristic of schizophrenia.[30] Zhang Qinghua 张清华, who is somewhat hyperbolic in his assessment of the poet and is perhaps not aware of the fact that order can reflect inflexibility of thought, doubts Guo's clinical pathology and praises his "perfectly formed and ordered poetry."[31] Michelle Yeh seems to be closer to the truth when she asserts that Guo's poetic form expresses his madness: "Ironically, the central idea of madness is expressed through clear control in form: the regular quatrain, the end rhymes, and the structure of logical progression from cause to result, from argument to counter-argument."[32] Again, one cannot argue that poetic form proves madness in any way; the argument is rather that there seems to be a stubborn holding onto the same form for over fifty years.

---

28 Karl Jaspers, quoted in Louis A. Sass, *Madness and Modernism: Insanity in the Light of Modern Art, Literature, and Thought* (Cambridge: Harvard University Press, 1998), 26.

29 Specifically, translogical thinking refers to a type of conceptualizing in which the thinking process transcends the common modes of ordinary logical thinking. It involves janusian and homospatial processes. Janusian thinking is a conscious process of combining paradoxical or antagonistic objects into a single entity, and homospatial process involves superimposing or bringing together multiple, discrete objects, and is the essence of good metaphor. See David W. Chan, "The Mad Genius Controversy: Does the East Differ from the West?" *Education Journal* 29.1 (Summer 2001): 1–15. For the original article Chan refers to, see Albert Rothenberg, *Creativity and Madness: New Findings and Old Stereotypes* (Baltimore: Johns Hopkins University Press, 1990).

30 Louis A. Sass, "Self and World in Schizophrenia," *Philosophy, Psychiatry, and Psychology* 8.4 (2001): 252.

31 Zhang Qinghua, "The Return of the Pioneer: On Shi Zhi and His Poetry," *Chinese Literature Today* 2 (2011): 10–11.

32 Michelle Yeh, "The Poet as Mad Genius: Between Stereotype and Archetype," *Journal of Modern Literature in Chinese* 6.1 (2005): 134.

According to Sass, the interdependence of language and psychological processes reveals itself "in styles of speaking and interpreting language, and ways in which language ties in with its practical and interpersonal contexts."[33] Another study yields the conclusion that there is no specific personality type associated with outstanding creativity. In fact, Albert Rothenberg finds that writing styles are often rigid and meticulous.[34] Guo Lusheng's poetry also displays such formalized forms of reflexivity and limited variations with regard to rhythm, syntactic complexities, or semantic layering, and critics generally agree that Guo has changed neither his style nor his (admittedly admirable) outlook on life considerably. But even though Guo's poems are often predictable and stereotypical, their design deems purposeful. He has educated himself about poetic theories and traditions and is passionate about reciting poetry aloud. Through meter, tone schemes, and rhyme, he consciously endeavors to reflect the undulations of life and the oscillation between joy and grief.[35] Rhyme creates the illusion of meaningful relations of similarities and contrasts between words and sounds, and repetition becomes a way of expressing meaning.[36] The careful construction of poetry gives Guo a sense of accomplishment and aesthetic delight. His controlled style helps him navigate his internal disillusionment and possible chaos while reflecting Reich's second phase of suffering, "expressive suffering."

Sacrificial Lamb

Leaving aside the episodes of travelling psychoses and his sometimes quixotic behavior, one can make a careful statement that Guo's schizophrenia (and his poetry) is symptom-poor. What then can we glean from his writing? Since his hospitalization, diagnosis, and labeling remain facts, as does the witness to his sometimes contradictory behavior, one can still consider his poetry a reflection of the struggle with his illness. His struggle is not existential and his poetic strife not transcendental. Rather, Guo's main struggles are with his identity as a poet and with his hospitalization. He has grumbled that

33 Sass, *Madness and Modernism: Insanity in the Light of Modern Art*, 176.

34 Albert Rothenberg, *Creativity and Madness: New Findings and Old Stereotypes* (Baltimore: Johns Hopkins University Press, 1990), 8; quoted in Richard M. Berlin, ed., *Poets on Prozac: Mental Illness, Treatment, and the Creative Process* (Baltimore: Johns Hopkins University Press, 2008), 6.

35 Cui, "Shishen juangu shouku de ren," 93.

36 Glenn W. Most, "The Languages of Poetry," *New Literary History* 24.3 (Summer 1993): 557.

readers too often focus on his early poetry, while he prefers his later poetry. In "The Poet's Laurel" ("Shiren de guanjun" 诗人的冠军, 1986), for instance, he complains that his fame rests on his role as a poet during the Cultural Revolution:

> People will ask me, what are you anyway?
> I can be anything except a poet.
> I can only be a smalltime sacrificial lamb
> that lived through those unrighteous times.[37]

> 人们会问你到底是什么
> 是什么都行但不是诗人
> 只是那些不公正的年代里
> 一个无足轻重的牺牲品[38]

While, as noted above, most scholars agree that Guo owes his fame to his individualized lyrical voice in the midst of widespread ideological cant, he considers himself a victim of this reception and of the times. Even after decades of writing poetry, he remains linked to his status as an underground poet during the Cultural Revolution, a "smalltime sacrificial lamb," both persecuted and praised for his poetry. It has been difficult for him to establish himself as a poet in his own right, unrelated to the political context of his early poetry. Guo has become a vicarious, therapeutically honest collective voice, expressing the painful scars of history, the terror of displacement, and the "puzzled anomie" felt by many, especially after Mao's death in 1976.[39] Nevertheless, what have crystallized about Guo are the images he created over time, "of humanity, mental conflict, kindheartedness, firm convictions, sensitive emotions, unshakeable willpower, and a somewhat tragic personality."[40]

If, as in the poem above, he sees himself as victimized by the times, he also considers himself a lunatic and madman who is free to think whatever he

---

37 Guo, *Shizhi de shi*, 129.

38 This poem, for example, has lines with irregular number of characters, but regular meter. The foot (*dun* 顿 or *yinzu* 音组) is arranged by units of meaning (*yi ge* 一个 'one', *bu shi* 不是 'is not', etc.) and this poem yields a meter of four feet per line.

39 Melinda Liu and Katharina Hesse, "Puzzled Anomie," *Newsweek International*, Feb. 14, 2001.

40 Zhang Qinghua, "The Return of the Pioneer," *Chinese Literature Today* 2 (2011): 6–12; repr. in *Winter Sun*, p. xvi.

wants.[41] This likelihood of a mutual interaction between culture and mental illness has long been recognized. However, even in the West, "schizophrenia has long been regarded as the core conundrum of psychiatry,"[42] and some view schizophrenia as a "simulacrum of the modern world in the most private recesses of the soul."[43] Curiously, a poet who has suffered from schizophrenia for over four decades is revered predominantly for his steadfastness and mental resilience. To many of Guo's readers, his schizophrenia symbolizes their collective generational suffering, brought to fruition by an uncommonly susceptible and discerning poet.[44] Particularly in a context still characterized by censorship, the resonance between Guo and his readers also reflects his readership's need for a vicarious (and safe) voice of *Vergangenheitsbewältigung*, the psychological coming to terms with the past.

Hospitalization

Guo describes his years in the hospital as a bitter experience. As Edward Whitmont and Yoram Kaufmann have suggested, "an artist does not create because he is neurotic, but may because he is creative and has to contend with powerful forces within himself."[45] While Guo believes that his hospital stays were necessary to help him cope with his illness, he also complains that the hospital was an uncivilized place without the quietude needed to write; in addition to his powerful internalized emotions, he also had to deal with difficult circumstances in the hospital. He describes the other patients as coarse and messy, as individuals living according to a warped logic, and as "a bunch of loonies, watched over by doctors and nurses."[46] He aptly communicates this

---

41 Yang Zi 杨子, "Shizhi: Jiang tongku biancheng shipian 食指,将痛苦变成诗篇 [Shizhi: Turning Pain into Poetry]," *Nanfang zhoumo* 南方周末 (Southern Weekly), May 25, 2001.

42 Janis Hunter Jenkins and Robert John Barrett, eds., *Schizophrenia, Culture, and Subjectivity: The Edge of Experience* (West Nyack, N.Y.: Cambridge University Press, 2003): 29.

43 Sass, *Madness and Modernism*, 373.

44 Liu Zhirong 刘志荣, "Shizhi yu yidairen de jingshenfenlie 食指与一代人的精神分裂 [Shizhi and a Generation of Schizophrenia]," *Bohai daxue xuebao* 渤海大学学报 (Journal of Bohai University), 2007, no. 4:51.

45 Quoted in Nicholas Mazza, *Poetry Therapy: Theory and Practice* (New York: Brunner-Routledge, 2003), 9.

46 Cui, "Shishen juangu shouku de ren," 90; Lijia Zhang, "Mad Dog: The Legend of Chinese Poet Guo Lusheng," *Manoa* 14.1 (2002): 109.

frustration in the poem "In the Mental Hospital" ("Zai jingshen bingyuan" 在精神病院, 1991):

> To write poetry I am willing to rack my brain.
> But in this sickroom filled with noise, how can I weigh a thought?
> Ribald jokes drop like beads,
> my raised brush unable to finish even one line.
>
> At times I cannot help wanting to vent my anger,
> but the outcome I cannot bear foresee....
> Heavens! What is it that year after year
> makes me idle away my life in a mental ward?
> ....
> When the perils retreat from the mind,
> the heart only harbours emptiness and desolation....
> Afraid to let others notice the tears lingering in my eyes,
> I wander with my head bent, as though at ease.
>
> 为写诗我情愿搜尽枯肠
> 可喧闹的病房怎苦思冥想
> 开粗俗的玩笑，妙语如珠
> 提起笔竟写不出一句诗行
>
> 有时止不住想发泄愤怒
> 可那后果却不堪设想......
> 天呵，为何一次又一次地
> 让我在疯人院消磨时光!
> ....
> 当惊涛骇浪从心头退去
> 心底只剩下空旷与凄凉......
> 怕别人看见噙泪的双眼
> 我低头踱步，无事一样[47]

As in many other poems even before his time in the hospital, his main grievance stems from having to hide his true emotions. What would happen if he vented his anger? He is in a place where he should be able to voice overwhelming emotions. The poem speaks forcefully about the way in which his illness and its treatment have taken control of him. It also discusses the detrimental effect the hospital situation has on him, the same effect, in fact, that

47 Guo, *Shizhi de shi*, 135.

the political circumstances had on him when he first became ill: lack of personal freedom, constant supervision, and a forced lack of agency.

Many of his later poems are influenced by his suffering during and after the Cultural Revolution. After finally gaining recognition for his poetry in 2001, Guo seemingly struggled less with his identity as a poet and switched to addressing his life's pain, which he perhaps then identified as his real pain. In the end of the 2004 poem "Over Fifty" ("Wushi duo sui le" 五十多岁了) he writes:

> I lost myself long ago, but no one knows.
>
> After that, submissive in the psychiatric hospital.
> If there is no fighting in the ward, there is arguing.
> To light a cigarette, brew a cup of tea, even for the news
> one has to kowtow humbly to the nurse.
>
> And produce fake laughter in front of people.
> There is no sense at all of human dignity and pride.[48]
>
> 早就失去了自我可谁都不知道
>
> 之后精神病院里唯唯诺诺
> 病房里不是打架就是争吵
> 为点烟、沏茶甚至为看新闻
> 不得不低三下四地向护士讨好
>
> 一直无奈地在人前装着笑
> 没一点做人的尊严与自豪

Guo views the onset of his illness as a "loss of self" and his treatment a process of "submission." However, his complacent attitude allowed him privileges in the hospital, such as visits, cigarettes, chores, etc. His degree of functionality and mental acuity seem puzzling and have led some to wonder whether he is really mentally ill or feigning part of it. This question requires one to read "between the poems"; Guo has had repeated unproductive periods, and the poems he did write might not embrace the entirety of his experience. In his case, as in that of many others, his silences are as much a marker of his situation as his poems are.

48 Guo, *Winter Sun*, 156.

A few of his poems describe his fear of living in vain, of being unable to leave a legacy, yet he defines himself as a poet who hopes to "offer light to those hungry and cold":

"Eight Years in a Psychiatric Ward"

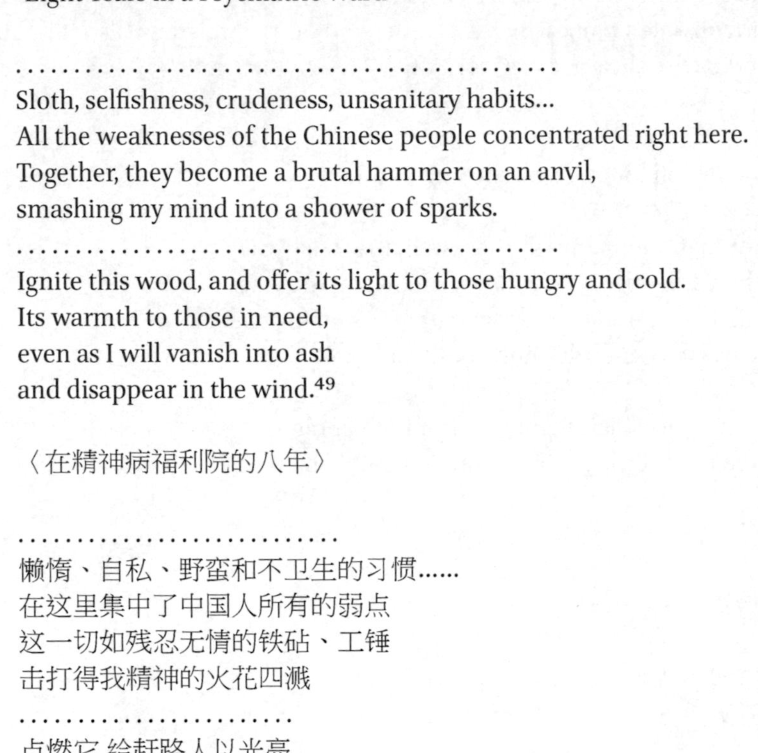

....
Sloth, selfishness, crudeness, unsanitary habits...
All the weaknesses of the Chinese people concentrated right here.
Together, they become a brutal hammer on an anvil,
smashing my mind into a shower of sparks.
....
Ignite this wood, and offer its light to those hungry and cold.
Its warmth to those in need,
even as I will vanish into ash
and disappear in the wind.[49]

〈在精神病福利院的八年〉

....
懒惰、自私、野蛮和不卫生的习惯......
在这里集中了中国人所有的弱点
这一切如残忍无情的铁砧、工锤
击打得我精神的火花四溅
....
点燃它,给赶路人以光亮
让饥寒受冻者来取暖
而我将化为灰烬
被一阵狂风吹散

Placing himself within the context of Romanticism, Guo often reiterates that pain is the wellspring of poetry. Poetry, by its very nature of offering an aesthetic experience, can, through artful construction, elevate sorrow and make sense of suffering. Perhaps it is exactly this poetic ennoblement of his ability to suffer that has subordinated his experience of illness to his image as a "sacrificial" poet. Guo often oscillates between the despair of realizing that this might be all life has to offer and the hope that there is more. Both are linked to his identity as a poet and as someone with a chronic illness. This nexus between

49 Stalling, *Winter Sun*, 129.

hope and despair, and identity and illness, teaches the important lesson that "there are undesired and undeserved pains that must be lived through, that beneath the façade of bland optimism regarding the natural order of things, there is a deeper apprehension of a dark, hurtful stream of negative events and troubles."[50] Optimism and apprehension both want to come into existence in Guo's poetry. There is always a degree of frustration related on the one hand to the lack of an audience and, on the other, to the nature of words that, as Alfred Lord Tenneyson put it, half reveal and "half conceal the Soul within" ("In Memoriam A.H.H.").

Wen Jie

Wen Jie was born in Yan'an in 1963. She studied Chinese literature and has worked as an editor for many years. She began writing poetry in the early 1980s but never belonged to one particular poetry school. In the introduction to her 2003 collection *An Account Given by One Party Only* (*Pianmian zhi ci* 片面之词), her poetry is introduced as an "individualized discourse" (*geti yanshuo* 个体言说) unencumbered by ideological language (or its deconstruction) or didactic purpose—still rare in the contemporary Chinese poetic context.[51] While Guo Lusheng's individual voice represents a *vox populi* that speaks against the hazards and meaninglessness of the times, Wen Jie's individualized discourse focuses on the way in which she uses language to express herself with original metaphors and artful subjectivity. Her poetry is not marked by the same stubborn formalism as Guo's, but by the use of other poetic devices such as personalization, metaphors, objectification, repetition, parallelism, enjambment, etc. Her poetry cycle "My Psychiatrist" ("Wo de jingshenbing yisheng" 我的精神病医生, 2001), for example, has an interesting structure: it is eight poems long, each poem followed by a chorus. However, the chorus is not a repetitive stanza. The "main" poems are all addressed to her doctor, while the choruses express her feelings, fears, and doubts, asking questions of herself and remembering painful moments. She juxtaposes the very clear medical diagnosis and treatment described in the four main poems with the chaos and fragmentation felt inside. This cycle impresses upon the reader the distance between medical reality and the experience of the patient.

---

50 Arthur Kleinman, *The Illness Narratives: Suffering, Healing, and the Human Condition* (New York: Harper Collins, 1988): 54–55.

51 See Ni Weiguo's 倪为国 introduction to Wen Jie, *Pianmian zhi ci* 片面之词 [An Account Given by One Party Only] (Shanghai: Shanghai sanlian shudian, 2003), n.p.

Depression

Wen Jie's biography is simple, and rather than focusing on specific events, she prefers to present a general feeling about life—the kind of dejection Guo expresses in his poetry, but does not discuss directly in conversations or interviews. In her own words, Wen Jie explains:

> My mother is a teacher, and my father works in a mine. During the 1960s and 1970s many couples lived and worked apart in China. In addition, my father's work required him to travel all over the place to find ore. Sometimes we would not see him more than once in a year or two, and so I basically grew up without a father at home.
>
> My parents never got along, and because of that, they were both unhappy and in turn treated us children cruelly and coldly. My childhood experiences have had a great impact on me, particularly the feeling that my own parents did not love me. Of course, this carried over into my adult life and relationships. I had very little interest in or understanding of the world around me, and my views of things always seemed to diverge from that of other people.[52]

Nearly all of Wen Jie's poems express this isolation and coldness. In "Saturday Night Glove" ("Libailiu yewan de shoutao" 礼拜六夜晚的手套, 1986), she describes a lost glove "you" gave her and the need to live since then with one cold hand all the time, even in the heat of summer. She concludes the poem:

> Possibly, it won't snow all winter long.
> Possibly, I will still stretch my hand out to you.
> But there still is one glove missing.
> All the Saturdays of my life will forever
> be a frozen hand that lost its glove
>
> 也许整个冬天都不会下雪
> 也许我的手还会伸向你
> 但是有一只手套再也找不到
> 我一生中的礼拜六
> 永远是一只丢失手套的寒冷的手[53]

---

52 Wen, e-mail message to author, Sept. 16, 2010.

53 Wen, *Pianmian zhi ci*, 28.

The glove is a metaphor for protection and belonging, and the frozen hand a metaphor of herself. She uses repetition and grammatical parallelism (anaphora) to juxtapose her hope that not all is lost and the reality of what has already been lost.

She explains that her depression started in childhood and has interfered with her life since. In particular, she bemoans her inability to experience happiness the way other people do and her failure to find contentment even in a warm family life. She reflects this ever-present pain in a 1994 poem, "Gaze" ("Ningwang" 凝望):

> Pain has me suspended like a glowing red fruit
> that hangs too high for reach. What you have cultivated in me
> is so rich. Smelling the breath you have left behind
> like an injured wolf. I live on to gaze at you, and because of it
> I have already lived many years,
> lived in the midst of my own madness.
>
> 痛苦把我悬挂起来,像一枚红透的果实
> 在树的顶端高不可及,你已将我培育得
> 如此丰腴,嗅着你遗留的气息像一只
> 受伤的狼,我之所以活下来是为了
> 能够凝望你,凭借它我已活过多年
> 活在自身的疯狂之中[54]

She addresses her depression and equates its richness to that of madness. Whether perceived as glowing or smelling, her depression is perceptible with all her senses, has filled and unwittingly inhabits her life. In "Hidden Depression" ("Yinnixing yiyuzheng" 隐匿性抑郁症, 1991), Wen Jie describes the feeling of illness that is always secretly lingering and her unwillingness to be treated. The poem expresses her unhappiness with her illness and foreshadows many other poems in which Wen effectively argues that her illness is not an evil that needs to be exorcized, but a part of her that needs to be accepted. This "argument" is particularly important to her, considering that her depression is chronic and will remain part of her throughout her life. In the Chinese context, Wen is a highly courageous poet. As an affective disorder, depression remains highly stigmatized and is rarely discussed; for her to lay bare her innermost feelings is both instructive and unusual.

54 Ibid., 61.

Identity

Many of her poems speak of the stigma associated with depression, even in front of doctors. Her early poems, like the one above, mostly discussed denial. In the later poem below from the cycle "My Psychiatrist," her illness becomes her identity.

"Mental Health Center"

I know in this world, some people
are doctors, others are patients;
some are the enemies of others.
They are like good and evil, mutually

serving as each other's *raison d'être*, just like
two sides of a coin, of the same material,
yet showing different faces; do you
have iron bones of everlasting rebar?
....
What kind of strength is needed to harbor havoc in my heart
and yet appear unsullied? I see most people's
faces, they are at perfect ease like yours.
They are this world's most proper part,

the most common, but also the most powerful.
My face, however, is the reverse of your face.
It caves in on its own flesh and blood, and in its
rottenness and decay emits a reeking stench,

a stench rejected by this world.[55]

〈心理卫生中心〉

我知道这个世界上，一些人
是医生，另一些人是病人
一些人是另一些人的敌人
他们就像好和坏，彼此

55 Wen, "My Psychiatrist," trans. Birgit Linder, *Renditions* 62 (2004): 94.

互为存在的依据，就像是
一枚银币的两面，质地相同
却以不同的面目示人，是否你
有永远不坏的钢筋铁骨
....
[需要]何等的力气，才能心中一遍狼籍
却貌似完好无损，我看到大多数人
他们的脸，像你的脸一样游刃有余
他们是这个世界正确的部分

最普遍，也最有力量
而我的脸，却是你的脸的反面
它凹陷在自己的血肉里，在其中
腐烂，变质，发出令人掩鼻的气味

也就是被这个世界弃绝的气味

Here, the regularity of form—uncharacteristic of her poetry—reflects the order imposed by the world. The last line stands alone as much as the poet-patient stands alone. Wen's poetry exhibits considerably more defiance than Guo's, yet both "harbor havoc" in their hearts and do not question the validity of such feelings, nor does either poet engage in deeper "soul searching" to discover reasons for their illnesses. Guo's struggle mostly concerns trying to contain his anger, and he makes his own vulnerability known. Wen struggles instead for an existential identity amidst her illness and positions the patient uniquely against the world. When addressing the doctor in "Psychoanalytical Therapy" ("Jingshen fenxi liaofa" 精神分析疗法, 2001), she goes so far as to suggest that the world needs both the sick and the healthy:

[I am] a specimen urgently needing cure, but who is the one
who can cure me, who can from this world
take away pain and only leave behind happiness, who can
take away me, and leave behind
all of you?[56]

[我]是一个岌待救治的标本，但谁是可以
救治我的人，谁可以从这个世界上
拿走痛苦，只留下欢乐

56 Wen, "Psychoanalytical Therapy," trans. Linder, ibid., 98.

拿走我，只留下
你们

This poem adopts an almost scrupulous yin/yang philosophy: without the sick, the healthy cannot exist. The poem is a plea to reconsider her illness as part of her life history (and future) and a plea not to vilify that in her that she cannot change. She realizes her "otherness," but claims that she can be "other" to the healthy only if both are accepted as worthy. Moreover, in this poet's identity struggle, this is the first representation of mental affliction that assigns value to the condition. She longs to transcend her illness and achieve a strengthened identity that is colored, but unconquered, by depression.

Medication

Her poems about medication also reflect her defiance of this negative identification. Her self-narrative explains:

> I have to take medication. I have taken a lot of this type of medication. For a certain time and to a certain degree, they can lessen or even treat various symptoms. I also have friends who have become healthy on medication. But I personally feel that the stronger the spirit of a person, the less effect medication has. And that is me. The function of this medication is to lessen the impact of the symptoms; it's a numbing kind of drug. But as soon as there is an opportunity, it declares war again. Therefore, although I have seemed normal on the surface for years, my heart has been empty most of the time. As I said in my poem, "An unscathed appearance hides a shattered heart."[57]

Wen Jie's struggle with the power of medication is obvious. Her resistance seems to result from the interference of another individual, who lacks a complete understanding but assumes to know her needs and "prescribes" her a feeling. In "Diagnosis" ("Zai zhenduan shi" 在诊断室, 2001) Wen describes, with force, the beginning phase in which medication produces side effects without demonstrated benefits. The poem also expresses her anxiety about being viewed as a patient instead of a person. In "Prescription Pad" ("Chufang jian" 处方笺, 2001), she expresses her dismay at her own powerlessness and the side-effects of taking such medication:

57 Wen, e-mail message to author, Sept. 16, 2010.

Medicine that piles up in my body
accumulates, until it develops unexpectedly
a will of its own, replacing me,
running amok in the world, this body of medicine
becomes my body.

Oh, doctor, you who sets pen to paper like a knife,
crazed champion of pills, star subjugator of disease,
I sincerely hope you run into trouble,
I wish you bad luck.[58]

药物堆积在身体里
日积月累，出人意料地长出它
自己的意志，代替我
在世上横行，药的身体
成了我的身体 ，
嗳，医生，你这下笔如刀的人
药物的狂热拥护者，疾病的克星
真心地希望你遭受厄运
祝你倒霉

Although the doctor is the "healer" and medication is supposed to help, the above poem—addressed to her psychiatrist—is accusatory. Medically speaking, it is clear that she does not feel that the medication enhances her wellness. This speaks to the difficult and painful issue of medication often being prescribed generically and without individualized care, at least in the 1990s. But more importantly, she writes of an alienated body, a body symbolic of social alienation. Pills are felt to silence the voice of the body, separating her from her social self. Instead of constituting an effective treatment, they contribute to the alienation of self and body, and she resents that the doctor loses sight of her as a social being.

Roslyn Wallacli Bologh explains that many patients feel this way, and "among other things, this means that the class of physicians does not address itself to the social conditions that contribute to the illness or to those that might contribute to curing that social body."[59] In other words, this kind of treatment

58 Wen, "My Psychiatrist," 90.

59 Roslyn Wallacli Bologh, "Grounding the Alienation of Self and Body: A Critical, Phenomenological Analysis of the Patient in Western Medicine," *Sociology of Health & Illness* 3.2 (July 1981): 190.

prescribes a disease to a body that she feels inhabit her self, while the doctor treats it like an object. It is most acutely felt in patients with mental illnesses, perhaps because of the way medication can interfere with both the mind and the body and render an otherwise physically healthy person incapacitated in unexpected ways. On the one hand, it reminds of the close connection between body and mind; on the other hand, this very connection is ignored when patients are treated like objects. This objectification is clearly felt as a subordination of the patient to the doctor in the second stanza, and therefore constitutes a loss of autonomy and dignity. Bologh further explicates the physician-patient relationship:

> While the patient is reduced to the level of a thing, a body, the physician is raised to the level of super-human. The physicians' sense of entitlement, which contrasts with the patients' vulnerability, derives from the treatment they are accorded and come to accept as natural and to be expected. The treatment they receive is one of respect that takes the form of deference in the literal sense of the deferment of other needs to the needs and commands of the physicians in their role as curer of illness.[60]

These poems evoke a deep feeling of loneliness and helplessness. Those who are able and willing to help her are looked upon as enemies. However, without their help, she cannot survive.

Will to Meaning

Although the poems on medication are the most obstinate ones, the issue of medication is not what has saddened her most.

> What saddens me most is that I have the feeling that I can never be emotionally satisfied. Already as a child I never experienced nurturing love, and after I grew up, I looked for that missing love in my husband. I have been married twice.... When I think about it now, it seems clear that leaving my first husband is also a reflection of my depression. It is as though I felt that I didn't need this kind of happiness, and that there must be something better out there. I didn't know what, but I left to search for it.... After so many years, I discovered that I still haven't found the happiness I have been looking for.[61]

60 Ibid., 197.

61 Wen, e-mail message to author, Sept. 16, 2010.

A chorus in "My Psychiatrist" expresses this tiresome pain:

> "Chorus: Yellow Letters from an Alien City"
>
> The one-dimensional scene of my life, the unchanging living room,
> directs me toward the old chronic disease. I bow faint-heartedly,
> to avoid being seen by the past. My steps keep to one side.
> Besides, I'm accustomed to walking by night.[62]
>
> 〈副歌:异城的黄色信答〉
>
> 我平面的生活场景，不变的客厅
> 通向陈年的宿疾，我低首衽衽
> 不愿被往事看见。脚步靠边
> 并且习惯夜行

This poem describes her grief over her deteriorated health and her mourning for the bodily foundation of daily behavior and self-confidence. Geoffrey Hartman suggests that such poetry

> grapples, again and again, with issues of *reality*, *bodily integrity*, and *identity*. It is a doubt (sometimes a brooding ecstasy) which afflicts reference (is this the real or at least a sign of the real?), subjectivity (saying "I" and the possibility of meaning it), and memory or story (being in control of the "plot" of one's life rather than part of some other, unknown but fatal, narrative).[63]

Being part of the plot of her life is a repeated theme in Wen Jie's poetry that is also echoed by the medical humanities' attempt to account for the connection amongst physical, psychological, social, and spiritual manifestations. The doctor, no longer merely a practitioner, is expected to have a more personalized relationship with the patient and to display "compassionate solidarity suffering."[64] The poet's ability, for example, to articulate his or her suffering is important for remaining rooted in the self. Otherwise, the absence of this ability might give rise to the feeling that "something has eaten itself

62 Wen, "My Psychiatrist," 96.

63 Hartman, "On Traumatic Knowledge and Literary Studies," 547–48.

64 For a defining article of the concept, see Jack Coulehan, "Compassionate Solidarity Suffering, Poetry, and Medicine," *Perspectives in Biology and Medicine* 52. 4 (Autumn 2009): 585–603.

into life."[65] In this context, Arthur Kleinman describes the need to develop perspective:

> When we are shocked out of our common-sensical perspective on the world, we are then in a transitional situation in which we must adopt some other perspective on our experience. We may take up a moral perspective to explain and control disturbing ethical aspects of our troubles, or a religious perspective to make sense of and seek to transcend misfortune, or, increasingly, a medical one to cope with our distress.[66]

Wen Jie respects the cathartic aspect of poetry. Like Guo Lusheng, she credits her pain in life and her sensitivity as her muses. However, unlike Guo, whose greatest frustrations were the stifling hospital situation and his reception as a poet, Wen seems to want to "transcend misfortune," such that poetry is more than a "temporal fix"; she seeks spirituality as a longer lasting, deeper-reaching cure.

> I would say that depression has actually made me a poet. Had I ever been able to experience common happiness like other people, I would not have become a poet. For a very long time, writing poetry was cathartic for me, like a self-help therapy. With every poem I released some of the complicated feelings that accumulated in my heart. But, looking at it in retrospect, this kind of release only temporarily postponed my pain; it never eliminated it. My [Buddhist] faith seems to have a better and more lasting effect.... At least I feel that I have a direction in life.[67]

The issues of spirituality and healing have become important aspects of health humanities research. One of the goals of this new patient/person and doctor/healer relationship is to help the afflicted to transcend his or her suffering. Thomas R. Egnew explains: "Suffering is transcended when invested with meaning congruent with a new sense of personal wholeness. Wholeness of personhood is facilitated through personal relationships that are marked by continuity."[68] Wen Jie longs for such transcendence, and her newly found Buddhist faith clearly distract her in a healthy way and gives her a sense of

---

65 David Le Breton, *Schmerz* [Pain], trans. Maria Muhle, Timo Obergöker, and Sabine Schulz (Berlin: diaphanes, 2003): 268.

66 Kleinman, *The Illness Narratives*, 27.

67 Wen, e-mail message to author, Sept. 16, 2010.

68 Thomas R. Egnew, "The Meaning of Healing: Transcending Suffering," *Annals of Family Medicine* 3.3 (2005): 258.

meaningful "strife." But they have also sensitized her in ways that have not been healthy and have caused severe psychotic episodes that she had not experienced before. The idea of poetry as a "temporal fix" rather than as a part of a lasting therapy highlights its efficacy as a tool, not a cure. By the same token, spirituality as a human expression of the desire to find meaning cannot always be considered or experienced as a cure, although it might be a valuable motivational force akin to what Viktor Frankl defined as "will to meaning."[69] As Wen Jie's case shows, whether poetry, spirituality, and the transcendence of one's suffering are "successful" and result in a *lasting* "wholeness of personhood" and "personal relationships that are marked by continuity" can only be said for sure in retrospect. It is a vulnerable place to be, which is perhaps why Wen yearns to be accepted "as is" rather than to have to rely on a changeable context.

Conclusion

Glenn Most explains that "the language of poetry responds to two kinds of fundamental needs, one psychological in nature and the other social."[70] He adds a philosophical twist and asserts that the mastery of language is a satisfactory reflection of the mastery of one's destiny:

> Those who most succeed in optimizing their lives and achieving their desires are usually not the ones who direct their efforts to excluding chances but who have the wit and flexibility to adept chance and their needs to one another, not excluding shocks but instead exploiting them. Control of the materiality of language on the one hand can provide the (illusory) satisfaction of suggesting the possibility of our mastering chance and dominating its empire over our bodies; generation and transformation of repetitions on the other hand can yield the (delusive) consolation of hinting that we might after all be capable of rationalizing time, of breaking its ineluctable cycles (our days which are numbered) and creating *ours* (a circle which cannot be broken, an infinite repetitive series: immortality).[71]

69 The idea is related to Frankl's concept of logotherapy, a form of existential analysis and psychotherapeutic method that was first introduced in his *Man's Search for Meaning: An Introduction to Logotherapy* (London: Random House, 2004). Frankl suggests that suffering is easier to bear when one can find philosophical or personal meaning in it.

70 Most, "The Languages of Poetry," 558.

71 Ibid., 558–59.

Writing is inarguably a therapeutic form of self-expression for those inclined toward narrative expression or poetry. Albert Rothenberg's study found that although all creative people are not the same, they share one characteristic: motivation that results from a "direct, intense, and intentional effort on the creator's part."[72] Hence, the ability to write poetry can often be considered a marker of wellness rather than an immediate expression of a poet's deepest pain. Both poets, Guo Lusheng and Wen Jie, grapple with long periods of creative muteness and with identity issues directly related to health and well-being. However, when they possess enough motivational force to write, both experience "an aesthetic delight in imposing narrative structure on chaos."[73] For readers, such poetic representation may be the closest understanding and interpretation of what still seems so inexplicable.

The works of these two poets, disparate in style and language, reflect the aims of the medical humanities: "Exploring the contexts of medicine; gaining insight into the experiences of health, illness, and health care; and examining the relationship between embodiment, thought, and spirit."[74] Guo's tendency to compress all emotions into the same poetic form reflects an admirable constraint that in turn might also reflect the way in which he deals with his illness and his life. Wen Jie also constructs her anger and helplessness in expressive language and gives shape to her experience using a variety of poetic devices, including anaphora, personalization, indirect dialogue, poetic cycles, and choruses. In spite of both poets' rapt attention to form, the "lyric glow of illness" Michel Foucault ascribed to the literature of (romanticized) madness is absent. Rather, the poetry of both poets is marked by a bold will to vulnerability. It offers glimpses into the potential experience of a mental illness and enables us to share the concern for healing and acceptance. Pain and illness are often subjective and cultural, and both poets provide valuable insights into historical and medical contexts. If pain and suffering are not only subjective but also cultural, Western concepts, theories, and therapies are not absolute. The still neglected area of cross-cultural Health Humanities could possibly open this field to new thoughts and therapies, considering more carefully, for example, the advantages of a healthy acceptance of the "givenness of life."[75]

---

72 Quoted in Berlin, *Poets on Prozac*, 4.

73 Crawford and Baker, "Literature and Madness," 238.

74 Caleb Gardner et al., "People Say There Are No Accidents: Poetry and Commentary," *Journal of Medical Humanities* 31 (2010): 258.

75 Yi-fu Tuan 段义孚, *Segmented Worlds and Self: Group Life and Individual Consciousness* (Minneapolis: University of Minnesota Press, 1982), 139. Tuan has argued that Western culture's encouragement of intense self-awareness could result in an exaggerated belief

In the poetry of Guo Lusheng and Wen Jie, one essential point to consider is the chronic nature of illness and, therefore, its link to life-long suffering and meaning construction. The examination of mental illness from a literary viewpoint sheds light on the trajectory of mental illness that, as a chronic illness, becomes one's life course and is inseparable from the meaning of life and suffering. Perhaps because both poets' life perspectives and feelings were influenced by the suffering of a sustained condition without the hope of healing, the clearest universal message these poets offer readers is that "the question is not to cure or be cured, but how to live."[76]

Guo Lusheng and Wen Jie are first and foremost poets who strive to express themselves artfully. Poetic formalism is often linked to social practices, and in the case of these two poets it metaphorically mirrors the disorders of society. Guo's poems are not merely about his illness (in fact, only a dozen or so directly address his mental illness), they are primarily about living an authentic life in an often diseased and inauthentic society. Whether he complains about the uncivilized behavior of his fellow inmates, his role as a poet hailed as well as stigmatized because of his disorder, or the rampant materialism in today's world, the poet speaks from the moral standpoint of an honest and refined self in search of authenticity and simplicity. Likewise, Wen Jie's poetry is an expression of her illness experiences as much as it is a metaphor of social alienation and stigmatized "otherness." Her lack of control and agency in the face of all-powerful doctors and pills reflects the helplessness generally felt in the face of overwhelming (even if sometimes necessary) power relationships. Both poets make insightful contributions to the medical humanities and to poetry in general. Any reader who faces difficulties in life can find inspiration in the stubborn tenacity of Guo Lusheng and the expressive capability of Wen Jie.

References

Atkinson, Sarah, Bethan Evans, Angela Woods, and Robin Kearns. "'The Medical' and 'Health' in a Critical Medical Humanities." *Journal of Medical Humanities* 36.1 (2015): 71–81.

---

in the power and value of the individual. It can provide a sense of independence and personal responsibility, but can also cause isolation and loneliness, or "a loss of natural vitality and of innocent pleasure in the givenness of the world."

76 Vickers, *The Other Side of You*, 18.

Berlin, Richard M., ed. *Poets on Prozac: Mental Illness, Treatment, and the Creative Process*. Baltimore: Johns Hopkins University Press, 2008.

Bologh, Roslyn Wallacli. "Grounding the Alienation of Self and Body: A Critical, Phenomenological Analysis of the Patient in Western Medicine." *Sociology of Health & Illness* 3.2 (July 1981): 188–206.

Chan, David W. "The Mad Genius Controversy: Does the East Differ from the West?" *Education Journal* 29.1 (Summer 2001): 1–15.

Coulehan, Jack. "Compassionate Solidarity Suffering, Poetry, and Medicine." *Perspectives in Biology and Medicine* 52.4 (Autumn 2009): 585–603.

Crawford, Paul, and Charley Baker. "Literature and Madness: Fiction for Students and Professionals." *Journal of Medical Humanities* 30 (2009): 237–51.

Cui Weiping 崔卫平. "Shishen juangu shouku de ren 诗神眷顾受苦的人 [The Muse Favors Those Who Suffer]." In Liao, *Chenlun de shengdian*, 85–96.

Egnew, Thomas R. "The Meaning of Healing: Transcending Suffering." *Annals of Family Medicine* 3.3 (2005): 258–60.

Frankl, Viktor. *Man's Search for Meaning: An Introduction to Logotherapy.* London: Random House, 2004.

Gardner, Caleb, et al. "People Say There Are No Accidents: Poetry and Commentary." *Journal of Medical Humanities* 31 (2010): 257–63.

Guo, Lusheng (Shi Zhi). *Shizhi de shi* 食指的诗 [The Poetry of Shizhi]. Beijing: Renmin wenxue chubanshe, 2000.

———. *Winter Sun: Poems*. Trans. Jonathan Stalling, with an introduction by Zhang Qinghua. Norman: University of Oklahoma Press, 2011.

Hartman, Geoffrey H. "On Traumatic Knowledge and Literary Studies." *New Literary History* 26.3 (1995): 537–63.

Hooker, Claire, and Estelle Noonan. "Medical Humanities as Expressive of Western Culture." *Medical Humanities* 37.2 (Dec. 2011): 79–84.

Jenkins, Janis Hunter, and Robert John Barrett, eds. *Schizophrenia, Culture, and Subjectivity: The Edge of Experience*. West Nyack, N.Y.: Cambridge University Press, 2003.

Jin Daoxing 金道行. "Lun xiandai gelü shi 论现代格律诗 [On Modern Regulated Poetry]." *Jingchu ligong xueyuan xuebao* 荆楚理工学院学报 (Journal of Jingchu University of Technology) 25.10 (Oct. 2010): 30–36.

Kleinman, Arthur. *The Illness Narratives: Suffering, Healing, and the Human Condition.* New York: Harper Collins, 1988.

Le Breton, David. *Schmerz* [Pain]. Trans. Maria Muhle, Timo Obergöker, and Sabine Schulz. Berlin: diaphanes, 2003.

Lee, S. "From Diversity to Unity. The Classification of Mental Disorders in 21st-Century China." *Psychiatric Clinic North America* 24.3 (Sept. 2001): 421–31.

Lei Ming 雷鸣. "Shizhi shige de yiyi 食指诗歌的意义 [On the Significance of Shizhi's Poetry]." *Kaili xueyuan xuebao* 凯利学院学报 [Journal of Kaili College] 28.4 (2010): 65–67.

Liao Yiwu 廖亦武. *Chenlun de shengdian* 沉沦的圣殿 [Sinking Gurdwara]. Urumqi: Xinjiang qingshaonian chubanshe, 1999.

Liu, Melinda, and Katharina Hesse. "Puzzled Anomie." *Newsweek International*, Feb. 14, 2001.

Liu Zhirong 刘志荣. "Shizhi yu yidairen de jingshenfenlie 食指与一代人的精神分裂 [Shizhi and a Generation of Schizophrenia]." *Bohai daxue xuebao* 渤海大学学报 (Journal of Bohai University), 2007, no. 4:45–51.

Mazza, Nicholas. *Poetry Therapy: Theory and Practice*. New York: Brunner-Routledge, 2003.

Moran, Stephen T. "Autopathography and Depression: Describing the 'Despair Beyond Despair'." *Journal of Medical Humanities* 27 (2006): 79–91.

Most, Glenn W. "The Languages of Poetry." *New Literary History* 24.3 (Summer 1993): 545–62.

Reich, W[arren]. T. "Speaking of Suffering: A Moral Account of Compassion." *Soundings* 72 (1989): 83–108.

Rothenberg, Albert. *Creativity and Madness: New Findings and Old Stereotypes*. Baltimore: Johns Hopkins University Press, 1990.

Sass, Louis A. *Madness and Modernism: Insanity in the Light of Modern Art, Literature, and Thought*. Cambridge: Harvard University Press, 1998.

———. "Self and World in Schizophrenia." *Philosophy, Psychiatry, and Psychology* 8.4 (2001): 251–70.

Tuan, Yi-fu 段义孚. *Segmented Worlds and Self: Group Life and Individual Consciousness*. Minneapolis: University of Minnesota Press, 1982.

Van Crevel, Maghiel. *Language Shattered: Contemporary Chinese Poetry and Duoduo*. Leiden: Research School CNWS, 1996.

———. *Chinese Poetry in Times of Mind, Mayhem and Money*. Leiden: Brill, 2008.

Vickers, Sally. *The Other Side of You*. London: Harper Perennial, 2007.

Viney, William, Felicity Callard, and Angela Woods. "Critical Medical Humanities: Embracing Entanglements, Taking Risks," *Medical Humanities* 41.1 (2015): 2–7.

Wang, Qingping, ed. *Push Open the Window: Contemporary Poetry from China*. Port Townsend, WA: Copper Canyon Press, 2011.

Wen Jie. *Pianmian zhi ci* 片面之词 [An Account Given by One Party Only]. Shanghai: Shanghai sanlian shudian, 2003.

———. "Wo de jingshen yisheng 我的精神医生 [My Psychiatrist]." *Huacheng* 花城 [Flower City], 2001, no. 2:128–31. Trans. Birgit Linder. *Renditions* 62 (2004): 86–102.

Woods, Angela. "The Limits of Narrative: Provocations for the Medical Humanities." *Medical Humanities* 37 (Dec. 2011): 73–78.

Xu Yi 徐熠. "Menglong shi daibiao Shizhi guilai 朦胧诗代表食指归来 [The Representative of Misty Poetry Shizhi Has Returned]." *Qingchun* 青春 [Youth], 2010, no. 1:87–89.

Yang, Lawrence Hsin, and Arthur Kleinman. "'Face' and the Embodiment of Stigma in China: The Cases of Schizophrenia and AIDS." *Social Science and Medicine* 30 (2008): 1–11.

Yang Zi 杨子. "Shizhi: Jiang tongku biancheng shipian 食指,将痛苦变成诗篇 [Shizhi: Turning Pain into Poetry]." *Nanfang zhoumo* 南方周末 (Southern Weekly), May 25, 2001.

Yeh, Michelle. "The Poet as Mad Genius: Between Stereotype and Archetype." *Journal of Modern Literature in Chinese* 6.2 (2005/06): 119–44.

Zhang, Lijia. "Mad Dog: The Legend of Chinese Poet Guo Lusheng." *Manoa* 14.1 (2002): 105–13.

Zhang, Qinghua. "The Return of the Pioneer: On Shi Zhi and His Poetry." *Chinese Literature Today* 2 (2011): 6–12.

Zhang Zao 张枣. "Wen Jie yu mei ge ren de Bailun 温洁与每个人的拜伦 [Wen Jie and Everyone's Byron]." *Zuojia* 作家 (Writer Magazine), 2001, no. 1:90.

PART 2

Drugs and Cancers: From Nation to Fiction

CHAPTER 4

Unmaking of Nationalism: Drug Addiction and Its Literary Imagination in Bi Shumin's Novel

Haomin Gong 龚浩敏

The "genesis" of modern Chinese literature is closely connected with disease. Lu Xun's 鲁迅 symbolic shift from medical studies to literature has, over the years, become a myth in the narrative of the rebuilding of a national literature. His relentless critique of the corrupt Confucian tradition and the defective Chinese national character, best exemplified in his short stories such as "A Madman's Diary" ("Kuangren riji" 狂人日记), "The True Story of Ah Q" ("Ah Q zhengzhuan" 阿Q正传) and, more manifestly, "Medicine," constitutes a starting point for much modern Chinese literature and serves to shape its most striking characteristic, which is, in C.T. Hsia's influential phrase, "an obsession with China." What characterizes modern Chinese literature, in Hsia's view, is "its burden of moral contemplation: its obsessive concern with China as a nation afflicted with *a spiritual disease* and therefore unable to strengthen itself or change its set ways of inhumanity."[1]

This concern with *spiritual* disease, so prominent in Lu Xun's works, as well as those of his followers, is inevitably in wedlock with *national* concerns, given modern Chinese literature's "obsessive concern with China as a nation." Recent studies have shown that writing of diseases in modern China is deeply shaped by sociocultural conditions and, as a result, diseases are often used as a metaphor and become highly ideological.[2] However, drug addiction, a disease that is so central to Chinese national crisis, has unfortunately yet been adequately explored. As I will show below, this disease, if it is so called, has been written and rewritten especially firmly within the paradigm of nationalism. It is only normal, given its critical role in modern Chinese history, that this disease be viewed as such. However, this nationalistic imagination of drug addiction (and, arguably by extension, many other diseases) is facing certain remodulations in contemporary time, due mainly to the new sociocultural conditions under which the disease is written about and read. To be more specific,

1 C.T. Hsia, *A History of Modern Chinese Fiction*, 3rd ed. (Bloomington: Indiana University Press, 1999), 533–34; my emphasis.

2 See, for instance, Carlos Rojas, ed., *Modern Chinese Literature and* Culture 23.1 (Spring 2011), a special issue on discourses of disease.

 | DOI 10.1163/9789004319219_006

the postsocialist condition has rendered the nationalistic understanding of drug addiction less than adequate, and required that it be "consumed" in a more diverse and less political fashion.

Bi Shumin's novel, *The Red Prescription* (*Hong chufang* 红处方, 1997), provides an intriguing case about how drug addiction is reimagined and refashioned in contemporary Chinese literature. Situating this novel in her writing career and reading it in the context of postsocialism, I examine how the dimension of nation-state, which used to be predominant in narratives of disease, makes place for the discourse of multiplicity and de-politicization, and in what way gender, particularly fashioned in the crisscross of nationalism and scientism, stages prominently in this transition to the postsocialist condition.

Bi Shumin is a prolific woman writer active since the 1980s, and she is best known for her medical fiction, most notable among them five novels: *The Red Prescription*, *A Blood Treatment Project* (*Xue linglong* 血玲珑, 2001), *Save the Breast* (*Zhengjiu rufang* 拯救乳房, 2003), *The Female Psychologist* (*Nü xinlishi* 女心理师, 2007), and *Corolla Virus* (*Huaguan bingdu* 花冠病毒, 2012), each dealing with a type of controversial disease in contemporary China—drug addiction, leukemia, breast cancer, psychological problems, and a SARS-like epidemic caused by an imaginary virus.[3] It is intriguing that, like Lu Xun, Bi also turned from her career as a physician to writing. Before becoming a professional writer, she had served as a military doctor in western border areas for over a decade. Her experience of medicine has a strong impact on her writing, not only in the sense that her professional knowledge provides her with subject matter, but that it also influences her writing style and informs her perspective on the problematic of disease in particular and human lives in general. Her medical experience is not merely "one of a wide repertoire of subjects" enabling the author to probe her "own selfhood and imagination" but rather, a "*force majeure*." This concept, an integral part of the "externalist" view put forward by George Sebastian Rousseau, is grounded in his observation that "all types of writers enthusiastically read nonliterary works and consequently 'import' subject matter, and… [this] importation permits those materials to be transformed into the stuff of great imaginative literature."[4] I argue that disease, for Bi, is not *used* as a means, a backdrop, or a metaphor, but its very *physical* existence constitutes the subject of her writing.

3 [For a detailed discussion of *Save the Breast*, see the next chapter by Howard Y. F. Choy. Ed.]

4 George Sebastian Rousseau, "Literature and Medicine: The State of the Field," *Isis*, no. 72 (1981): 408–9.

Moreover, the postsocialist condition in China, under which Bi writes and against the backdrop of which she sets most of her stories, shapes her writing at various levels. Bi's approach to disease, particularly drug addiction, is remarkably different from those of her predecessors, be they of the May Fourth, revolutionary, or socialist period. Her writings are almost apparently free of the nationalistic and moralistic burdens assumed by her predecessors. With her, diseases seem to register as *de-politicized* characteristics—characteristics, that is, to be viewed not in terms of national honor, but of an urge to separate from it. Along with this change of emphasis appears a re-fashioned gender consciousness, because as disease is reimagined and redefined in today's world, a certain gendered nationalism comes under sharp scrutiny in her work. However, this apparent feature of de-politicization, paradoxically, precisely reveals the ideological complexities specific to the postsocialist condition. The increasingly commercialized and ideologically diversified society serves as the very politics that mark the characteristics of the reimagination of drug addiction.

Beyond the National: Contouring Drug Addiction

Studies of literature and disease over the past decades have become a burgeoning field in the Western academic world. With the publication of the journal *Literature and Medicine* in the U.S. in the 1980s, this promising area began to attract increasing attention, and has by now grown into a fertile field. Mapping this field, Charles E. Rosenberg sees it as an interactive system between the distinctions—"ontological versus physiological, disease versus illness, biological event versus socially negotiated construction."[5] More specifically,

> disease is at once a biological event, a generation-specific repertoire of verbal constructs reflecting medicine's intellectual and institutional history, an occasion of and potential legitimation for public policy, an aspect of social role and individual—intrapsychic—identity, a sanction for cultural values, and a structuring element in doctor and patient interactions. In some ways disease does not exist until we have agreed that it does, by perceiving, naming, and responding to it.[6]

5 Charles E. Rosenberg, "Framing Disease: Illness, Society, and History," Introduction to *Framing Disease: Studies in Cultural History*, ed. Charles E. Rosenberg and Janet Lynne Golden (New Brunswick, N.J.: Rutgers University Press, 1992), xxiii.

6 Ibid., xiv.

Insightful as this observation is, however, one important dimension (or "frame," to use Rosenberg's term) in the Western articulations of disease remains underaddressed—that is, nationalism.[7] While nationalism does not play as a prominent role in the Western discourses of disease as in China, it predominates and shapes Chinese people's lives and imagination. For example, the "Sick Man of East Asia" (*Dong Ya bingfu* 东亚病夫), among other terms, may be the most vociferous expression of Chinese nationalism with respect to disease. The Chinese, as a nation, were regarded as being weak and sick physically, and by extension, spiritually. Remarkably foreign in its origin, the term had been detailed in both real and imagined ways, so as to spur a nationalistic sentiment. Understandably, its *foreign* character was markedly stressed, and as a result, the Sick Man of East Asia has become a national unconscious, the specter of which has to be exorcised repeatedly on various occasions thereafter.[8]

The modernization of medicine in China, as an integral part of the efforts to shed this humiliating title, is also tightly locked with the Chinese nation-state. Ruth Rogaski has shown in her seminal book, *Hygienic Modernity: Meanings of Health and Disease in Treaty-Port China*, how the term *weisheng* 卫生 "hygiene/sanitary/health" in modern China was discursively formulated in the course of national liberation and strengthening. The nation-state played a determinant role in the formulation of the term because the idea of *weisheng* originated in Chinese people's internalization of their national deficiency; almost all of the campaigns to achieve *weisheng* were orchestrated at a national level by the state, and the aim of being *weisheng* was, besides individual welfare, ultimately a modern nation, be it a capitalist or socialist. As Rogaski insightfully remarks, "in an uncanny way, the single modern Chinese term *weisheng* encompasses what Foucault called 'biopower', a series of techniques through which the

7 In his "Framing Disease: Illness, Society, and History," Introduction to *Framing Disease: Studies in Cultural History*, ed. Charles E. Rosenberg and Janet Golden (New Brunswick, N.J.: Rutgers University Press, 1992), xiii–xxvi, Rosenberg first used the term "frame" to map out the intersection of disease and culture, though from the history rather than literature discipline. The last section of his edited volume, "Disease as Social Diagnosis," deals with the ways in which disease is used as a gauge for assessing social, or *national*, illness. See also George Sebastian Rousseau, Introduction to *Framing and Imagining Disease in Cultural History*, ed. George Sebastian Rousseau et al. (Houndmills: Palgrave Macmillan, 2003), 1–48. I would like to thank the anonymous reader who brought this point to my attentions.

8 See Yang Jui-Sung 杨瑞松, "Xiangxiang minzu chiru: Jindai Zhongguo sixiang wenhua shi shang de 'Dong Ya bingfu' 想象民族耻辱：近代中国思想文化史上的'东亚病夫' [Imagining National Humiliation: 'Sick Man of East Asia' in the Modern Chinese Intellectual and Cultural History]," *Guoli Zhengzhi Daxue lishi xuebao* 国立政治大学历史学报 [The Journal of History], no. 23 (2005): 1–44.

state undertakes the administration of life, and 'governmentality', the idea that individuals internalize disciplinary regimes and thus harmonize their own behaviors with the goals of the state"; thus, "*weisheng* as hygienic modernity becomes a definitive example of a 'derivative discourse' of nationalism."[9]

However, when "modernity" becomes a term in which national honor is much less at stake as China grows into a major player in the world since the 1990s, the imagination and narration of disease take on new features with respect to nation-state. The "Reform and Opening-up" (*gaige kaifang* 改革开放) initiated in the late 1970s does not simply bring about China's economic take-off but further causes deeper sociocultural transformations. Socialist ideology becomes increasingly ineffective while the spread of commercialization gains momentum; and neo-liberalism, patronized by the state, pushes economic development on a high-speed track, which ironically weakens the grip of the state, whereas neo-conservatism seeks to validate the rule of the regime. This constitutes a scene of ideological ambiguity and complexity that is characteristic of postsocialism.

As national crisis is no longer a major concern of this period, nationalism, if not waning in intensity and urgency, is staged in many other forms than national liberation and strengthening.[10] On the other hand, de-politicization, as a result of the market economy and the influence of Western liberalism, is burgeoning rapidly. The discourse of disease, accordingly, reflects this change. In what follows, I examine how *The Red Prescription*, a transitional work as I would call it, fleshes out the ideological complexity and ambivalence of postsocialist China in its quite heteroglossic narrative of disease.

Bi Shumin's works draw heavily on her personal experience as a soldier and doctor. Her early writings, such as the novella "Eulogy of the Kunlun Mountains" ("Kunlun shang" 昆仑殇, 1987), are based on military lives in Ah Li area in Tibet, where she used to work. Foregrounding the deadly hardships that soldiers endure and the sacrifice that they have made for the country, these works convey a sentiment of sublimation that smacks of revolutionary and

9 Ruth Rogaski, *Hygienic Modernity: Meanings of Health and Disease in Treaty-Port China* (Berkeley and Los Angeles: University of California Press, 2004), 300, 9.

10 See, for example, Peter Hays Gries, *China's New Nationalism: Pride, Politics, and Diplomacy* (Berkeley: University of California Press, 2004); Yingjie Guo, ed., *Cultural Nationalism in Contemporary China: The Search for National Identity under Reform* (London: Routledge, 2004); Christopher R. Hughes, *Chinese Nationalism in the Global Era* (London: Routledge, 2006); Jonathan Unger, ed., *Chinese Nationalism* (Armonk, N.Y.: M.E. Sharpe, 1996); and Yongnian Zheng, *Discovering Chinese Nationalism in China: Modernization, Identity, and International Relations* (Cambridge: Cambridge University Press, 1999).

socialist realism. But her focus shifts to medical subjects with the publication of "An Appointment with Death" ("Yuyue siwang" 预约死亡) in 1994, a novella regarded as a representative work of the "new experience fiction" (*xin tiyan xiaoshuo* 新体验小说).[11] Her following novels continue this "new experience" of writing, which probes social, cultural, and, more importantly, psychological problems centering on medical issues. This shift of subject matter, as well as thematic focuses, coincides with her increasing interest in psychology and her subsequent pursuit of a Ph.D. degree in this field.

The Red Prescription certainly reflects this transition. The topic, drug addiction, is such a significant and intriguing issue in China that, besides medical and therapeutic concerns, it involves a wide range of other concerns of a historical, sociological, moral, ideological, and political nature. In the discussions of drug addiction, nationalism has always been a theme that could not be circumscribed or, even further, an almost exclusive theme.[12]

Arguably, Chinese nationalism has its origin in drugs. In the orthodox historiography of China, the First Opium War between the United Kingdom and the Qing Dynasty in 1839–42 marked the beginning of modern Chinese history. This event has often been construed in tight relation with the rise of Chinese nationalism, because the forced introduction of modernity by Western powers generated the modern idea of nation among the Chinese, and

---

11 Jason McGrath believes that labels like this are problematic: "The very proliferation of new 'schools' of literature—each championed by one or another literary journal—was as much a reflection of the journals' efforts to attract attention and appear on the cutting edge as it was a result of real, significant changes or distinctions within literature itself. In other words, such labels were appearing no longer as positions taken on an ideological or aesthetic battleground, but rather as name brands to help journals and critics compete on the cultural market." Jason McGrath, *Postsocialist Modernity: Chinese Cinema, Literature, and Criticism in the Market Age* (Stanford, Calif.: Stanford University Press, 2008), 61.

12 Huang Hongzhao 黄宏昭 calls this exclusive focus on the dark and sick side of opium in relation to grand discourses of national humiliation and Chinese modernity in the narratives of opium in China "repressive production" and "productive repression." Huang further reads this discursive exclusion (and inclusion) in parallel with similar maneuvers in the fabrication of Chinese modernity ("inclusive exclusion" and "exclusion inclusion"). By so reading, the author intends to lay bare the constructedness of this discursive process and thus opens it up to more narrative possibilities. Huang, "Yapian de xiandaixing yayi: Baohan/paichu yu yayi de shijie 鸦片的现代性压抑: 包含/排除与压抑的试解 [The Repressiveness of Modernity of Opium: Inclusion/Exclusion and an Analysis of Repressiveness]," *Wenhua yanjiu yuebao* 文化研究月报 (Cultural Studies Monthly), no. 50 (Sept. 2005), http://www.cc.ncu.edu.tw/~csa/journal/50/journal_park381.htm (accessed June 13, 2012).

this nation was inevitably linked with the senses of weakness and deficiency vis-à-vis their Western invaders. The national humiliation culminated in the spread of the humiliating term of the "Sick Man of East Asia" at the turn of the twentieth century, and this sense of sickness was further metaphorized into the spiritual bankruptcy of the nation. Thus, anti-drug crusades in China were not simply efforts usually taken on the national scale to save individuals but also highly symbolic of the grand cause of national liberation and strengthening.

In the nationalistic narratives of drugs, foreignness was often discursively stressed. From discovering drugs' foreign origins to the National Anti-Opium Association's acts that often resorted to Chineseness in the Republican era, further to the Communists' strategy of propaganda that always put drugs in conjunction with Western imperialism and liberalism, anti-drug crusades were never short of foreign targets, which is reminiscent of what Susan Sontag calls "imagining foreignness" in narrating illness in general.[13] On the other hand, foreign imagination of China with respect to drugs also helps cast China into an Orientalist stereotype as the backward and the unenlightened.[14] Foreign devils, in either way, are essential to Chinese nationalism with regard to drugs. As Yongming Zhou remarks,

> Anti-drug crusades are closely intertwined with nationalism in modern China. Nationalism provides motivation, legitimacy, and the requisite emotional charge for the Chinese to take an anti-drug stance. Nationalism plays a major role in the making of a mainstream, anti-drug discourse in modern China, in the interpretations of the history of the Opium Wars, in the mobilization of the social elite and general public in the cause of

---

13 See Su Zhiliang 苏智良, *Zhongguo dupin shi* 中国毒品史 [A History of Drugs in China] (Shanghai: Shanghai renmin chubanshe, 1997); Wang Jinxiang 王金香, *Zhongguo jindu shi* 中国禁毒史 [A History of Drug Prohibition in China] (Shanghai: Shanghai renmin chubanshe, 2005); Yongming Zhou, *Anti-Drug Crusades in Twentieth-Century China: Nationalism, History, and State Building* (Lanham, Md.: Rowman & Littlefield, 1999); and Yongming Zhou, *China's Anti-Drug Campaign in the Reform Era* (Singapore: World Scientific, Singapore University Press, 2000). Susan Sontag, *Illness as Metaphor and AIDS and Its Metaphors* (New York: Picador, 2001), 136.

14 See Zhou Ning 周宁, "Yapian diguo: Langmanzhuyi shidai de yi zhong Dongfang xiangxiang 鸦片帝国：浪漫主义时代的一种东方想象 [The Opium Empire: An Oriental Imagination of Romanticism]," *Waiguo wenxue yanjiu* 外国文学研究 [Foreign Literature Studies], 2003, no. 5:88–95; and Zhou Ning, *Yapian diguo* 鸦片帝国 [The Opium Empire] (Beijing: Xueyuan chubanshe, 2004).

> drug suppression, and even in the linking of drugs to the survival of the Chinese nation in the face of foreign aggression and threat.[15]

Yet, this nationalistic narration of drugs and drug-addiction encountered serious challenges in the postsocialist period. In particular, the Communist regime tended to depoliticize its drug-related maneuvers gradually after 1989, although the national discourse had already become decreasingly effective since 1952.[16] In the depoliticized narrative, drugs' serious harm to individuals and the society (rather than to the nation-state) comes to the fore, while nationalistic sentiments manifestly retreat. In fact, commercialization and globalization have rendered nationalist discourse on drugs rather contradictory—the foreignness that this discourse is largely based on is incompatible with the dominant tone of opening-up, and is thus shied away from.

Moreover, the state, as a result of liberalization, is gradually losing its iron-handed control of the society and capacity for continuous mass mobilization. Thus, the mass mobilizations of anti-drug campaigns formerly seen in Chiang Kai-shek's New Life Movement (1934), for example, are becoming increasingly irrelevant, except in some scattered cases such as the outbreak of epidemics of SARS (2003) and H1N1 (2009). For contemporary Chinese people, the military metaphors implied in such disease management, similar to the case that Sontag talks about in the West, arouse a resistance to the repressive power of the state and are thus gradually losing ground.[17]

Still further, the ideological complexity in postsocialist China makes understanding of drug abuse and drug addiction ambivalent. While nationalistic preaching is decidedly waning, moralistic teachings persist in line with socialist ideology. Meanwhile, loosening of state control on both physical and spiritual levels, as well as social liberalization, renders possible a re-imagining of drug (ab)use. For instance, for some people, use of drugs is more a lifestyle and a personal choice, signifying coolness and uniqueness, rather than moral bankruptcy. As Yongming Zhou explains the situation of heroin in contemporary China:

---

15 Zhou, *Anti-Drug Crusades in Twentieth-Century China*, 170.

16 Ibid., 128. 1952 was the year, as remarked in Zhou's book, when the CCP's mobilization of the masses based merely on nationalism began to be less effective. This argument might be debatable.

17 Sontag, *Illness as Metaphor and AIDS and Its Metaphors*, 96–99. Rousseau also remarks: "Until recently the history of medicine has largely focused on disease as seen from the top down (this was certainly true until the last generation), generally without listening to private voices." This is also partly true of the Chinese situation. Rousseau, Introduction, 14.

> On the one hand, heroin has been depicted as a drug with mysterious effects, able to make the user have unspeakable euphoric feelings, fulfill all wishes, and elevate out of the real world. On the other, it has also been described as untouchable and destructive, producing universal and irresistible dependency among all its users. Numerous stories have been written describing how heroin made good people turn evil, made a good woman a prostitute, and drove a healthy person to death. Yet despite the stories describing the terrible fate of addicts, sometimes readers could easily come away with the impression that addicts were adventurous and curious people whose explorations just went sour.[18]

Bi Shumin's *The Red Prescription*, against this background, exhibits a cultural uniqueness reflective of postsocialist ideological ambivalence and complexity. The novel tells a story of Shen Ruoyu 沈若鱼, a retired nurse practitioner, passing off as a drug addict to examine the lives of patients in a rehabilitation hospital headed by her friend Jian Fangning 简方宁. During her stay in the hospital, Shen gets to know about a variety of people and their stories with drugs. The most important person is Zhuang Yu 庄羽, a young talented woman, who gets addicted in youth as she is disillusioned by fake respect from her seniors and peers. After she has been released from the hospital free of drug, she soon retakes drugs as she found Jian, not unlike other people, reluctant to show her respect. Thus, out of a love-hate complex, she contrives a vindictive plan against Jian and, as a result, Jian is inadvertently addicted to a terminal drug. Another inmate, Beiliang 北凉, is also addicted because of an overindulgence in everything, including sex, since his childhood. Satiated, he uses drugs to fill up the emptiness left by unrestrained supply, only to find a deeper emptiness. Qiren 琪仁, similarly, takes drugs because of an oversupply of maternal love, which causes his distorted sexuality.

Apart from these addicts, some other patients and caretakers also have interesting stories. Third Uncle 三大伯, for instance, passes off as an addict in order to "do business" in the hospital, including selling drugs to other inmates; Madame Meng 孟妈 works in the hospital as a nurse practitioner for the purpose of stealing patients' personal information and medicines for her own rehabilitation business; the nurse Li Qiu 栗秋 hangs on in the hospital so that she can take advantage of this experience to get married to a rich addict; Qin Bing 秦炳, a local resident, holds a mysterious traditional cure that his grandfather has left him, which he intends to sell to the hospital, but a foreign company

18 Zhou, *Anti-Drug Crusades in Twentieth-Century China*, 118.

pays a much larger sum for the cure and shelves it in order to maximize their profits. The novel ends with Jian Fangning's death, as she realizes that to save herself from drug addiction she will have to lose her ability to feel happiness and sadness; so she chooses to end her life in dignity.

Weaving multiple story lines, this novel as a whole can be read as an effort to come to term with the definition of drug addiction. Drug addiction, strictly speaking, is not simply a disease as such but also a highly culturally resonant diagnosis. In the novel, the characters' lack of understanding of, or refusal to understand, this "disease" signals not only an inveterate and corporate discrimination against drug addiction but also an ambiguity and difficulty in articulating this discourse. The semi-episodic structure of the novel allows a variety of voices to tell their own stories, and these vignettes form a heteroglossic narrative.

The moralistic judgment of drug addiction as dehumanizing, quite understandably, constitutes a starting-point, or a background, for the novel's exploration of the disease's meanings. From time to time throughout the novel, a variety of people on different occasions express such a view, showing a prevalent understanding of, if not a discrimination against, drug addiction: Dr. Teng 滕 thinks that drug addicts have "lost the basic sentiments of human beings" and are an "entirely different species" (82); Fan Qingke 范青稞, i.e., Shen Ruoyu, shares this belief—the world consists of two kinds of people: drug addicts and non-drug addicts (307); Zhou Wu 周五 says blatantly that they are creatures of the "most poisonous features," of the "lowest of all of the sick people," and the sooner they die, the better-off this world will become (170, 172); and Fan/Shen reiterates this opinion: their best contribution to the society is to die (316); she desperately calls the rehabilitation hospital an inferno-like "dirty and helpless" corner where human sins are condensed (315).[19] Drugs, in this view, are naturally associated with crimes and prostitution. Most intriguing and thrilling in this novel, however, is the story-within-story about a Russian called Mikhalin, who works as a so-called "man-beast" (*renshou* 人兽), a man serving as a prey in hunting games because he needs the high pay for his drug use. The allegorical overtone here is quite obvious: the drug turns a human being into a beast. This judgmental stance is reminiscent of the overwhelmingly critical tone conventionally manifest in Chinese literature from the late Qing to the contemporary period in regard to drugs.[20]

---

19 Page numbers in parentheses are from Bi Shumin 毕淑敏, *Hong chufang* 红处方 [The Red Prescription] (Guilin: Lijiang chubanshe, 2008).

20 Huang Hongzhao discusses this "repressive" unanimity in narratives of opium, especially in the late Qing. This "repression" does not change much in later historical periods. Yet the author also notes some exceptions, including Zhang Changjia's 张昌甲 (b. 1827) booklet, *Opium Talks* (*Yan hua* 烟话, 1878). See Huang, "Yapian de xiandaixing yayi." For

Yet, excoriating as this point of view sounds, such a critique remains ambiguous, if not altogether ironic, in the novel. Those emotional expressions appear rather weak when juxtaposed with more "rational" and "objective" ideas, although almost all the opinions in this novel are the characters' subjective voices. More notably, however, nationalist judgment, which usually dominates this moralistic view in China, is considerably subdued or treated as irrelevant. For instance, the Opium Wars are referred to, but only in an offhand fashion, not arousing any significant nationalistic feeling. History, in Dr. Cai's 蔡 words, is only "a roll of bad-quality toilet paper" (211). Intriguingly, references to Lin Zexu 林则徐 (1785–1850), a significant symbol of the Chinese anti-drug cause, are cast into certain tension with his traditional image as a national hero.[21] This novel focuses much more on Lin's unremitting but failed experiments with rehabilitative medicine than on his glorified deeds, such as burning opium in Canton. Indeed, though Lin is still portrayed as a tragic figure, his failure is depicted more in the medical sense at a personal, as well as national, level than metaphorized as a national humiliation. In addition, the *historical* story of Lin's medical experiments that Dr. Cai tells is juxtaposed with a *fictional* grotesque story that Cai also recounts of growing poppies in the Philippines out of human bodies and a legend about Qin Bing's traditional Chinese medicine. The juxtaposition of these stylistically different stories simply makes this narration ideologically ambiguous.

Perhaps the only place where nationalism is definitely fleshed out in the novel is along the thread of traditional Chinese medicine. The cure "No. 0" tried on Zhuang Yu and Zhi Yuan 支远, Zhuang's husband, is such a medicine, whose formula has been passed down from Qin Bing's grandfather, and it is said to be the only effective medicine in the area of drug rehabilitation in the world so far. This description conforms to the popular nationalistic imagination that a cure of an incurable disease by Western medicine can often find an

---

discussions of how Zhang's work describes the experience of smoking opium otherwise and the cultural significance of such description, see Keith McMahon, *The Fall of the God of Money: Opium Smoking in Nineteenth-Century China* (Lanham, Md.: Rowman & Littlefield, 2002), 105–37.

21 Lin Zexu and his anti-opium feats are repeatedly celebrated in modern Chinese literature and art, and are constructed into one of the most important symbols of Chinese anti-drug crusades, as well as anti-imperialism campaigns. Works that are especially devoted to Lin include the films *Lin Zexu* (dir. Zheng Junli 郑君里 and Cen Fan 岑范, 1959) and *Yapian zhanzheng* 鸦片战争 (*The Opium War*, dir. Xie Jin 谢晋, 1997), the TV series *Lin Zexu* (dir. Song Zhao 宋昭, 1997) and *Yapian zhanzheng yanyi* 鸦片战争演义 (*The Opium War*, dir. Huang Jun 黄军 and Meng Hongfeng 孟洪峰, 1997), and Cai Dunqi's 蔡敦祺 historical novel *Lin Zexu* (Xiamen: Lujiang chubanshe, 2002).

alternative solution in traditional Chinese medicine. In fact, this rather clichéd assertion of nationalism disappears in Bi's later works. (In her second novel, *A Blood Treatment Project*, for instance, she describes the so-called elixir folk prescriptions as utterly mysterious, self-contradictory, and unreliable.) Foreign capital's coveting of this resource and cheating Qin Bing out of it in the name of a "supra-national" science, touches another popular issue of science versus nationalism. Rhett Butler, who gives himself a Chinese name Bi Ruide 毕瑞德, is depicted unfavorably as a typical foreign comprador: he offers a very high bid to buy Qin Bing's formula, only to seal it off, so that foreign capitalists can continue to reap tremendous profits from their own products. Surely, this familiar episode arouses a strong nationalistic feeling; yet, it concludes in an optimistic belief in internationalism of science. This episode, in my view, also highlights an important understanding of drug addiction—the parallel of drugs with human greed: in order to gain an undue and excessive sense of "happiness," drug addicts resort to drugs, while to fulfill their insatiable demand for unlimited profits, capitalists are willing to risk anything and sell their souls.[22]

Bi Shumin's critique of this greed, however, is delivered more at the level of the personal and the societal than the national. What the drug destroys, as shown in the "beast-man" story of Mikhalin, are mainly individuals and a society that consists of these individuals, much less the national honor. Shen Ruoyu sees in those drug addicts "inborn weaknesses" (307) and "innate defects" (315) of human beings. These weaknesses and defects are mainly the inability of human beings to reject dark lures and evil satisfactions and, therefore, lose their humanity. Humanity here, obviously, is used in a universal sense that is devoid of national characters among other things. Moreover, this collective entity in postsocialist China consists of individuals atomized by the market economy. As Zhuang Yu declares, taking drugs is her own choice and nobody but she herself is responsible for her own life (251). This individualistic view is supported by Rhett Butler who, turning to a "Nobel Prize Laureate and economic authority on the free market," believes that drug taking "is not a crime, but a

22 This reminds me of Alai's 阿来 novel, *Red Poppies* (*Chen'ai luoding* 尘埃落定, 1988), which depicts the destruction of the chieftain (*tusi* 土司) system in Tibet in the early twentieth century. One important factor contributing to this destruction, as its English title indicates, is the growing of poppies in Tibet under the warlords' influence during the Republican period (1912–49). As Gang Yue 乐刚 has it, poppies function as a trope for the unlimited, dark "desire," and this novel demonstrates capitalists' "addiction" to the desire to destroy the primitive indigenous Tibetan culture. Gang Yue, "As the Dust Settles in Shangri-La: Alai's Tibet in the Era of Sino-Globalization," *Journal of Contemporary China*, no. 56 (2008): 543–63.

character, a personality"; it is just a "personal hobby" (326). Drug addiction, for him, becomes a social issue only starting from this stand.

If drug taking is a personal choice, the drug, once one is addicted to, becomes the agent that destroys a person's ability to choose and deprives him/her of humanity. Jian Fangning's final fight against her own addiction, viewed in this sense, is a heroic assertion of the human will against this utterly dehumanizing power. In Jian's case, the only treatment available for her addiction to the so-called "Seven," the strongest of all kinds of heroin, is to remove her locus coeruleus, a nucleus in the brain stem involved with physiological responses to stress and panic. That is to say, in order to save her life from this deep drug addiction, she has to sacrifice the basic human feelings of happiness and pain a normal person possesses. She becomes a walking puppet then, as she sees it, and the meaning and value of life are therefore lost to her. "I am an independent individual," Jian writes in her last letter, "and I do not live for anybody else, I only live for myself" (379–80). This loud cry for self, which is rarely seen in Jian, is not simply an assertion of individualism but, instead, an acknowledgement of her previous selfless life, in which she has somehow refused those feelings of happiness and pain. By *choosing* to die with honor, Jian defeats "Seven" on the grounds of human dignity.

Obviously, Jian's choice cannot serve as a common cure for drug addiction. Moreover, the individualistic view of drug addiction is equally problematic because it ignores social factors involved in this issue. An alternative view, then, is to consider the sociality of the disease. It is surely simplistic to think of crime and prostitution, as moralists do, when the social issues raised by the drug are being addressed. Things are more complicated than this. In Beiliang's case, it is his parents' overindulgence, which demystifies everything for him, including sex, that causes him to take drugs as a gesture of defiance, as well as a means by which to seek novelty. For Qiren, he is addicted to drugs as a result of the psychological pain he suffers from the oedipal complex. Above all, Zhuang Yu initially takes drugs, as she confesses, as a self-destructive retaliation because she "has lost all hope" for this society, whose hypocrisy kills the innocence in her heart first and exposes in front of her all kinds of its dirtiness and ugliness later (89–93). "A drug addict is not a person who has necessarily lost her wisdom and morality, as people think them to be," Zhuang tells Jian (311). Perhaps it is not only that the drug makes its addicts lose morality, but the society should also take the responsibility.

A cure for this social problem is, as the novelist proposes, a community. Once, Professor Jing Tianxing 景天星, a pioneer expert of drug rehabilitation in China, shows Jian Fangning the latest information about drug rehabilitation treatment in developed countries. For Jing, TC (Therapeutic Communities) and NA (Narcotics Anonymous) represent the future trend in this field. The aim of these communities and programs is to cure drug addiction by cutting its psychological dependence on old environments and encouraging individuals to enter into the care of new communities. To be admitted to a therapeutic community, according to Jing's description, drug addicts have to have their deranged and inescapable old selves seriously exposed, so that they can build up an entirely new life blueprint with the help of others. One important step in this cure, moreover, is sharing with other members their happy memories and experiences (281–82). These practices, in their efforts to restructure human relations, recognize communal responsibilities and power in the treatment of drug addiction.

This communal power is also much based on individual members. To join a therapeutic community, a drug addict must have an extremely strong will to be away from drugs. The reason that a strong will is a prerequisite is: as another important line of understanding goes in this novel, drug addiction is essentially more a psychological problem than a physiological one (128).[23] As Jian Fangning explains to Shen Ruoyu, the most important thing in drug rehabilitation research is to find a way to cure addicts' "psychological addiction" (*xinyin* 心瘾), a psychological dependence caused by the sense of happiness—"undeserved happiness" (*wuli de xingfu* 无理的幸福) in Jian's words—in drug (ab)use (133). And her experiments with animals seem to have proved this point. Jian's failure to cure Zhuang Yu, in fact, rests precisely in her disregard for Zhuang's psyche. She understands that an effective method of those therapeutic communities is their "care of the [patients'] heart" (278), but she somehow refuses to try to understand their "heart" (311). Zhuang wants to have a "heart-to-heart talk" (*cuxi tanxin* 促膝谈心) with Jian, but Jian deliberately keeps a distance from Zhuang in a "professional" manner or, in Zhuang's view, assuming an air of a "messiah." When Zhuang proposes to make friends with Jian, the latter, remembering therapeutic communities and wanting to give this relationship a try, agrees hesitantly (312–13). But she fails to keep their "friendship," partly due to her husband's interference, partly due to the doubt of and prejudice against her patients from the depths of her heart.

In all, it is intriguing that Bi Shumin brings to Jian's, as well as the readers', awareness of the psychological understanding of drug addiction—and, in fact, this is the understanding that the novel very much highlights—but she also lets Jian fail on exactly the same ground. This self-contradictory design helps to create a melodramatic ending that is essential to the popularity of this novel,

---

23 This novel, however, also offers a physiological view of drug addiction, which is in line with new evidence of effect on the brain and physiology of addiction.

but it also reflects an ideological ambivalence in Bi's writing. Manifest in this final drama is a rare assertion of heroism through martyrism, resonant of socialist realism and romanticism. "Rare" because, as Shen Ruoyu's husband says, in this age, when everyone chooses to lead a life as s/he wishes to, there are no heroes, generally speaking (371). Yet, in spite of this prevalent individualism, Jian's death dramatically arouses a collective sentiment among the characters and converts Shen to her unfinished, "glorious cause" of rehabilitation. The novel ends in a reemphasis of the state's role in concerted maneuvers of drug prohibition, the Chinese government's efforts being especially foregrounded. Accompanying this reassertion of the dimension of the nation-state, further, a moralistic view is also reaffirmed: there is no reconciliation or compromise between drugs and drug addiction on the one side, and the power that eliminates them on the other (384).

Critic Huang Hongzhao suggests that once opium was defined as a prohibited narcotic in the medical sense and thus exclusively managed in the professional field of medicine, the human body affected by opium then was no longer regarded as a national/ethnic body, but instead as a medical body.[24] What Huang emphasizes here is that no matter whether defined in the medical or the national sense, imaginations and articulations of opium have constantly been discursively oppressed. Yet, the transition indicated by Huang never occurred in China. As Ge Hongbing 葛红兵 and Song Geng 宋耕 point out, in Lu Xun's world, national and medical/sick bodies are "interchangeable" (*huwen* 互文), and this view has influenced modern Chinese intellectuals.[25] Drug addiction, as a special disease, has never been entirely separated from the nation-state in modern China. Rehabilitation centers in China today, according to Zhou Yongming, are still run singly by the authorities of public security, although civil administration and public health departments used to participate in it.[26] This state management, or state control, is hailed at the end of this novel, despite that the psychological narrative, in my view, constitutes the most important and interesting dimension of it. This psychological narrative, crisscrossing with many other ones, will have to wait until it is adequately fleshed out in Bi's later novels, *Save the Breast* and *The Female Psychologist*. Yet, as Sabina Knight insightfully points out in her seminal study of *Save the Breast*, psychotherapy, which is the central concern in the novel, instead of confirming an individualistic therapy culture, in fact celebrates a communicative method

24 Huang, "Yapian de xiandaixing yayi."

25 Ge Hongbing and Song Geng, *Shenti zhengzhi* 身体政治 [Body Politics] (Shanghai: Sanlian shudian, 2005), 72–73.

26 Zhou, *Anti-Drug Crusades in Twentieth-Century China*, 141.

based on collective relationships. Yet still, the novel embodies a constant tension between individualistic ideologies and collective ones.[27] It is also true that *The Red Prescription* exemplifies a similar cognitive ambiguity in its narratives of drugs, which marks the ideological complexity of contemporary China.

Yet, the significant ebb of the formerly predominant narrative of drug addiction along the line of the national is clear, and with this ebb, other narratives find their ways to define this disease and problem. The individual, social, psychological, even the spiritual (Narcotics Anonymous), along with the national, speak together and form a polyglossic narrative in recounting this disease. For instance, the socialist ideology, although still officially orthodox, is becoming increasingly residual. But on the other hand, its ideological power remains an indispensable social factor. On several occasions in Jian Fangning's translation of English material, she unconsciously uses expressions of the socialist period and is immediately corrected by her academic supervisor Jing Tianxing. This is not surprising because Jian spent her prime time in that period in an army of the western border, and her mindset is shaped by the socialist ideology. However, this socialist background does not make her idiosyncratic but, instead, it empowers her in her heroic fight and death. In Zhuang Yu's case, contrarily, her background as an heir of red aristocrats (*hongse guizu* 红色贵族) distorts her psyche, and becomes the target of her self-destructive retaliation.

Perhaps Third Uncle's story best speaks of the social transformation from socialism to commercialism. He passes off as a drug addict and stays in the hospital in order to make money by working as a contact person for other inmates. His only goal is to make more money, so that his children will not suffer from poverty and social discrimination that he has had to endure. He understands the immorality of this business, but he gets into it anyway because, as he says, it brings him the "power" and "money" that this age most values (266). As a member of the *laosanjie* 老三届 and an "educated youth," he sacrificed his youth in the countryside, but the high socialist morality he had gained therein was smashed to pieces when this society was overtaken by commercialism and the morals of the market economy.[28]

This postsocialist condition is the socio-historical background against which the stories in the novel unfold. Most notable among the disparate narratives of drug addiction, the national shame that used to be tied to drugs is mostly

27 Sabina Knight, "Cancer's Revelations: Malignancies and Therapies in a Recent Chinese Novel," *Literature and Medicine* 28. 2 (Fall 2009): 351–70.

28 *Laosanjie* refers to junior and senior high school graduates of 1966–68, who, due to the start of the Cultural Revolution in 1966, did not finish their education at school and were sent down to the countryside as "educated youth" to be "re-educated" and "remodeled."

replaced by their dehumanizing effects; both of the nationalist and individualist understandings are questioned because the former is becoming increasingly ineffective and the latter problematic; what is foregrounded, instead, is a narrative of a social and communal nature, which is based on ever-deepening understanding of psychology under the specific contemporary Chinese social conditions.

Gender, Science/Scientism, and Nation-State

Sontag, in another context, writes about the othering in discourses of disease: "Interpreting any catastrophic epidemic as a sign of moral laxity or political decline was as common until the later part of the last century [i.e., the 19th century] as associating dreaded diseases with foreignness. (Or with despised and feared minorities.)"[29] Indeed, foreignness, as well as ethnic minorities, is often taken as an important other in the nationalist discourse of drug addiction in China.[30] The female, as a perennial minority, is also given a similar role along this line of narration. In addition to some clichéd narratives, which hold that prostitution in drug addiction is always closely and almost exclusively associated with female addicts, gender can also be seen to play a more complex part in the narration of this disease. In his seminal studies of opium smoking in nineteenth-century China, Keith McMahon investigates, among other things, "gender hierarchies, family relationships, and sexual economies" involved in this social phenomenon, not only in the domestic social order but also registered in the gendered relationship between China and the West.[31] Gender, as McMahon shows, is a significant factor both in the articulation of drug addiction as a disease and of nationalism in China.

Indeed, nationalism in China is often gendered.[32] In modern Chinese literature, various, even contending, discourses of nationalism tend to take advantage of stereotypical images of Chinese women.[33] However, as the sense of the

---

29 Sontag, *Illness as Metaphor and AIDS and Its Metaphors*, 142.

30 See Zhou, *Anti-Drug Crusades in Twentieth-Century China*, esp. Chapters 1, 2, 5, and 8.

31 McMahon, *The Fall of the God of Money: Opium Smoking in Nineteenth-Century China*, 9.

32 Perhaps the most well-known example of gendered nationalism is Yu Dafu's 郁达夫 "Sinking" ("Chenlun" 沉沦).

33 See Meng Yue 孟悦 and Dai Jinhua 戴锦华, *Fuchu lishi dibiao: Xiandai funü wenxue yanjiu* 浮出历史地表: 现代妇女文学研究 [Emerging from the Horizon of History: Modern Chinese Women's Literature] (Beijing: Zhongguo renmin daxue chubanshe, 2004); and Amy D. Dooling, *Women's Literary Feminism in Twentieth-Century China* (New York: Palgrave Macmillan, 2005).

national is decidedly waning yet not disappearing in postsocialist China, and a variety of other forces are coming to the fore of the society, gender is coming to be fashioned in different and disparate ways.

Arguably, Bi's works on disease can also be characterized as feminist writing. Gender constitutes an indispensable dimension in articulating drug addiction in particular, and other diseases in general. *The Red Prescription* exhibits a conspicuous gender consciousness: Jian Fangning once specifically notes how the gender ambiguity of the pronoun *ta* 他/她 "he/she", in spoken Chinese helps her cover her identity. This incident also shows how sensitive Jing Tianxing is to the gender of drug addicts (364). In *Save the Breast*, which has been promoted as the "first psychotherapeutic novel in China," breast cancer, as the focal issue of the novel, is particularly gender specific. Yet, the double identities of Cheng Mumei 成慕梅/Cheng Muhai 成慕海, a male patient contracting breast cancer passing off as a female, besides dramatizing the story, renders the issue of gender identity with respect to this disease highly ambiguous and intriguing. In *The Female Psychologist*, as the title indicates, Bi's gender awareness is as manifest as her specific devotion to the psychological approach of medical writing. For the female protagonist, He Dun 贺顿, a plain-looking, poorly educated girl coming from the countryside, who has been violated by her stepfather at a young age, her professional achievements as a psychotherapist parallel her growth into an independent, strong, and unique woman.

Apparently, Bi is writing against what Lu Tonglin 吕彤邻 calls the "misogynist" trend (mainly in men's writing) in contemporary Chinese literature.[34] Women, in her novels, are not victims of the scapegoat policy of Communist China but, instead, are depicted as being (or becoming) strong and independent individuals.[35] Specifically in *The Red Prescription*, women are not represented as a political or ideological other in regard to drugs.[36] Men and women are equally susceptible to drug addiction, cause similar social problems, and need the same amount of treatment and care. Even the main "antagonist," Zhuang Yu, is not depicted as a purely evil woman. Her drug taking is more a defiant attitude towards the corrupt society; she sets Jian up because of

34 Tonglin Lu, *Misogyny, Cultural Nihilism and Oppositional Politics: Contemporary Chinese Experimental Fiction* (Stanford, Calif.: Stanford University Press, 1995), 2.

35 Yang Xin, in "Configuring Female Sickness and Recovery: Chen Ran and Anni Baobei," *Modern Chinese Literature and Culture* 23.1 (Spring 2011): 170, talks about how "sickness is a narrative strategy and imaginative tool for women writers to explore identity in times of rapid social change."

36 The most telling and thrilling example that ties women with drugs in Chinese literature is perhaps Zhang Ailing's 张爱玲 "Golden Cangue" ("Jin suo ji" 金锁记).

her destructive possessiveness—she wants friendship from Jian, but when it is not granted, she destroys herself in order to setback Jian's professional accomplishment, and also destroys the subject that she cannot possess out of a distorted affection. Being a female, Zhuang shows a particularly dominant and cynical relationship with the male, as she claims that drugs provide more pleasure than men do in sex (100). The novel seems to suggest that distorted love and independence, for women, are as poisonous as drugs, which provide a spurious pleasure.[37]

Gender problems, in Bi's work, are more intriguingly fleshed out in a woman's professional credibility as a physician, especially in terms of modern medicine as a scientific discipline, than in the ideologized association of the female with diseases, no matter how demonized or romanticized it is.[38] Science, or scientism, is arguably a crux in the interrelationship among disease, nation-state, and gender in *The Red Prescription*. In this part, I proceed to investigate how gender is refashioned in the narration of drug addiction and inevitably intertwined with "science"/"scientism" and nationalism in this novel. Involved in this investigation are the entanglement of gender, the national, and the scientific, and the challenge to and reinstatement of the dichotomies embedded in their relationships.

I argue that Bi's portrayals of independent women in their scientific pursuits, who are at the same time able to bring "non-scientific" emotions to their professions, question the wedlock of the male and science as well as that of the

37 The Chinese term for narcotics, *dupin* 毒品, indicates a "poisonous" (*du* 毒) feature of them.

38 Some diseases are romanticized in China and are usually associated with the female. For instance, leukemia has become one of the most romanticized diseases in recent years, due primarily to the high popularity of Korean TV dramas in East Asia. Zhang Wei 张维 argues that the romanticization of leukemia is closely connected with the aestheticization of this disease and the "virgin complex" deeply rooted in the Confucian culture. Zhang also parallels this romanticization with the case of tuberculosis in the nineteenth and twentieth centuries (mostly in the West), which Sontag has discussed vigorously. In fact, in modern Chinese literature there are a few works in which tuberculosis is romanticized, such as Ding Ling's "Miss Sophie's Diary" ("Shafei nüshi de riji" 莎菲女士的日记). Bi Shumin's second novel, *A Blood Treatment Project*, centers on leukemia. Although the female sexuality is key in this novel, the disease is not particularly gendered. See Zhang, "Ai yu si de tonghua: Jiedu Han ju zhong de baixuebing xianxiang 爱与死的童话: 解读韩剧中的白血病现象 [The Fairy Tale of Love and Death: An Analysis of the Leukemia Phenomenon in Korean TV Drama]," DialogNet, 2006, http://www.dialognet.net:70/Item/6089.aspx (accessed May 5, 2014); and Sontag, *Illness as Metaphor and AIDS and Its Metaphors*, 3–87, *passim*.

West and science, which inevitably marginalize the Chinese female. By extension, Chinese nation and its traditional medicine are also feminized in this discourse of scientism, and because of this, a reassertion of the role that the nation/state plays in a concerted fight against drug addiction in the end ironically turns back to the nationalism that the author has been making effort to dislodge.

Quite assertively, Bi shows an unquestionable belief in women's ability in science, a field that has been dominated by men until recently. However, the price that women have to pay for their professional accomplishment in this field is equally obvious. Jing Tianxing, Jian Fangning (*The Red Prescription*), Cheng Yuanqing 程远青 (*Save the Breast*), and He Dun (*The Female Psychologist*), though successful professionally in different ways, do not have a happy family. Jing has devoted her whole life to the cold scholarship; for her, a love relationship is simply a waste of time, and her identity as an old maid somehow helps her with professional development (4–5). Jian marries her husband simply for the sake of becoming a doctor; her profession further alienates her from sexual life as she sees the latter in purely medical terms (156) and as a result, her husband develops an extramarital affair with their maid. Embedded in their failure in sex, which is in contrast to their professional success, there lies a mechanism of compensation: the lack in the former inevitably makes up for fulfillment in the latter. In other words, it is the female's very lack of certain characteristics, such as emotionality, that makes her suitable for science.

There is a consistent effort throughout the novel to understand drug addiction scientifically (read rationally, or even in entirely physical terms), which the female is also capable of, or sometimes even obsessed with. One such theory goes that drugs, particularly morphine, generate a sense of pleasure and excitement in their users because of the resemblance of their molecular structure with that of enkephalin, a peptide in human brain that is said to be the material causing the sense of happiness (133–35). Jian insists on this physical interpretation of drug addiction and tries to reduce human feelings to different "existential forms of substances" (132). For her, complex social and psychological problems can find scientific explanations in the laboratory, and the animals that she experiments with offers "pure and clear"—that is, simplified—answers to human problems (121). She claims that the human body is a "highly ordered, delicate machine" (136), resonant of Dr. Teng's treatment of drug addicts as if they were "products" on a production line (18), and Dr. Cai's remark that patients are simply "capsules" with diseases inside, not human beings (213).

Dehumanizing indeed, implied here is also a notion of "certainty," a perception, as Rousseau remarks, "by patients that physicians consider themselves practitioners of a science rather than an art that has fueled patients' attacks on doctors."[39] This notion, in addition, constitutes a determining factor in modern science's assault on traditional Chinese medicine. One problem about the medicine that Qin Bing provides is that it is almost impossible to determine its ingredients by modern technologies, although the novel seems to imply that Jing's research group is close to success in the end. This episode reflects a tension, if not incompatibility, between traditional Chinese medicine in general and modern medical science; and this tension is also indicative of the debates in China on such large issues as the East vs. the West and tradition vs. modernity.[40]

While the limits of scientism have been quite extensively discussed,[41] and Bi's ironic tone also belies the truth-value of these scientistic ideas, the very emphasis on the importance of these ideas bespeaks the author's serious concern about distortion and destruction of science, not a rare case in modern Chinese history. For example, Jing's initial distrust of Jian's ability is because of the latter's academic background as a worker-peasant-soldier student (*gongnongbing xueyuan* 工农兵学员); in Jian's view, this is not a "tragedy of a generation, but a trick of history"—a history of man-made tragedies (6). Also in the novel, the Communists' rehabilitation method of "naturally" cutting off the drug supply in the 1950s is referred to several times. Although a method that has possibly achieved the best effect in human history, at least on a social level for a nascent state, this "temporary moment of pride" in human civilization is more a political victory than a medical success (152–53). Scientific rationality, over the modern history of China, has thus been disturbed and disrupted by state power. Dr. Cai believes that a good doctor will make a good state leader (213). Against this background, his words make much sense: although, unlike what Dr. Teng claims, science is not always "neutral" or value-free (148),

39 Rousseau, "Literature and Medicine: The State of the Field," 417. Rousseau's observation of the rather confrontational relationship between physicians and patients is mainly based on his investigation of the condition in the West (Ibid., 421). In China, people's views of physicians vary and change. Doctors, especially in the socialist period, used to be regarded as one of the most respected careers, and were given the name "angels in white clothes" (*baiyi tianshi* 白衣天使). Tensions began to build up between physicians and patients as corruption appeared and became prevalent in the 1990s, when commercialization swept China.

40 See Rogaski, *Hygienic Modernity*, esp. Conclusion.

41 Nathan Sivin points out that scientism is antithetical to "medical pluralism." Wang Hui 汪晖 details the limits of scientism in the Chinese context. See Sivin, "The History of Chinese Medicine: Now and Anon," *positions: east asia cultures critique* 6.3 (1998): 746; and Wang, *Xiandai Zhongguo sixiang de xingqi* 现代中国思想的兴起 [The Rise of Modern Chinese Thought], 2nd ed. (Beijing: Sanlian shudian, 2008), 1424–38.

a divorce of nation-state, politics, and other ideological factors from it, in the Chinese context, will only make science healthier. To extend this conclusion further, in regard to the relationship between gender and science, the point of departure of my discussion, dislodging the wedlock, though a negative one, of women and science, therefore, will benefit both in China.

Or, perhaps women have more to offer to science—that is, a humanistic outlook, which is seemingly incompatible with hardcore rationality of science. Affection, in Bi's view, is not to be excluded from science, but on the contrary, is an indispensable part of it. Early in the novel, Jian protects a pregnant woman from the interrogation by the head doctor/political leader during the operation of a forced abortion. She says calmly in response to Shen Ruoyu's praise, "I am happy only if my patients are happy" (49). Her self-denying pursuit of medicine, quite paradoxically, is based on her ideal of the human value in this scientific study. One important factor in Jing's decision to take Jian as her assistant is the latter's experience in dealing directly with patients, a skill, as Jing acknowledges, that she herself lacks: Jing can "repair" them, but cannot makes friends with them, nor talk with them, heart-to-heart (10). Towards the end of the novel, Jian is reminded of a well-known saying among doctors: "It is more important to know what kind of person a patient is than what disease s/he has contracted" (332). An affective bond in science is reaffirmed here, whereas the affectionless understanding of science appears more questionable. In fact, Jing looks at her own loveless life not without regret; and Shen's decision in the end to take Jian's place after her death, in the sense of a balance between rationality and affection, is a moderate correction to the latter's scientific but regrettable life.

To be sure, by bringing an affectionate side, which is conventionally associated with femininity, into the rational science, Bi intends to debunk the dichotomies of female/male, humanity/science and, by extension, tradition/modern and Eastern/Western. Still, some contradictions in this regard emerge. For instance, Jian's use of a psychological method on drug addicts is an attempt to establish a humanistic bond between doctors and patients, but at the same time she shows a certain degree of resistance to this method, especially in Zhuang Yu's case. What is called for, at her heroic death, is the state's re-assumption of the leading role in campaigns and movements against drug addiction. This call is resonant of Beiliang's and Qiren's cases, in which the inadequacy, or lack, of a father's role and an excess of mother's presence (as well as too great a supply of women) symbolically and virtually cause them to become "sick" in both personality and psyche, and as a result, make them subject to drug addiction. It is thus understandable that a "strict hierarchy" and "obedience to the authority" in therapeutic communities are essential for the process of rehabilitation (283).

Jian's contradictory attitude towards psychotherapy, a medical method that becomes the focus of Bi's later works, moreover, not only reflects ambiguity and hesitance on the author's part towards this method at this stage of her evolution as a writer, but also reveals some deeper ambivalence in the Chinese discourses of science with regard to nation and gender.[42] Jian's understanding of psychotherapy is arguably shaped by the discourse of science; in other words, she takes psychology more as a scientific discipline that takes human psyche as an object of study than as a channel for heart-to-heart communication. As Wang Hui 汪晖 argues, through categorization of disciplines and institutionalization of education, social sciences and humanities, disciplines related to the spiritual sphere to varying degrees, are incorporated into the discourse of science in China.[43] Jian, though a caring doctor, is overburdened by her determined pursuit of professionalism. This assertion of scientism, moreover, coincides with the rise of nationalism/statism at the time when she "victorious" commits suicide. Embedded in this rise of nationalism/statism is a national anxiety about emasculation still existing today. Although implicit in this novel, nationalism is still connected with gender—Bi's efforts to debunk this connection, not only often run into self-contradictions but also paradoxically reveal the very discursive power of this connection.

Conclusion: De-metaphorizing Drug Addiction

Rosenberg writes about the importance of naming/negotiating a disease as follows: "disease classifications serve to rationalize, mediate, and legitimate

42 Science, as one of the two Western ideals ("science" and "democracy") adopted by the May Fourth intellectuals, plays a significant role in the formation of modern Chinese thought. Wang Hui, in his four-volume work, *The Rise of Modern Chinese Thought*, discusses in detail how the "community of scientific discourses" (*kexue huayu gongtongti* 科学话语共同体) shaped Chinese modernity: science "closely connects a universalist worldview with a nationalist/globalist social system, and finally, through a rationalized taxonomy of knowledge and social division, encompasses in its wide genealogy various forms and statuses of human lives"; specifically in China, through the debates on the modern vs. the traditional, the West vs. the East, and knowledge vs. ethics/culture, "universal principles" (*gongli* 公理) of science took the place of "principle of the heaven" (*tianli* 天理) of traditional China and thus established its predominant status in modern Chinese thought and formulated Chinese modernity. Notably in the formation of this discourse, women played virtually no role except that, in a nationalistic view, the female symbolized Chinese deficiencies vis-à-vis the West with respect to scientific development. See Wang, *Xiandai Zhongguo sixiang de xingqi*, 1395.

43 Ibid.

relationships between individuals and institutions in a bureaucratic society," in which a disease "becomes an actor in that social setting, legitimating and guiding social decision-making."[44] Drug addiction, however, is a disease that has many different definitions in China—for along the whole stretch of modern Chinese history it has been elaborately intertwined with a variety of issues including economics, politics, international relations, ideologies, gender, nationalism, medical studies, and so on. Yet efforts have been constantly made, almost in every period, to define this disease in the service of certain specific ideological purposes. Inevitably, drug addiction, similar to cancer and AIDS in Sontag's studies, becomes metaphorized, although in a more uniform fashion mainly as a poisonous and evil product.

Sontag cautions the reader against viewing illness "otherwise," that is, metaphorizing it, and attaching inappropriate meanings to it. She wrote two essays on cancer and AIDS in order to "de-mythicize" them, to de-metaphorize them, and to deprive them of accrued extrinsic meaning.[45] To a certain degree, Bi Shumin's work achieves the same effect. *The Red Prescription* provides a range of disparate, even contending, views of drug addiction—including professional ones ("drug abuse" [*yaowu lanyong* 药物滥用], 311), scientific ones (substitutive mechanism of a peptide), "liberal" ones (a "character," a "personal hobby"; a "mistake," not a "disease" or "sin," 184), psychological ones ("psychological addiction," "distorted personality"), sociological ones (a "problem of public health" vs. crime, 325), moralistic ones (moral lapse), and nationalistic ones (national honor)—so that the disease does not remain mysterious in this effort of dissemination of meanings. Further, the semi-episodic structure of the novel, plus supplementary sections of "Material" (*ziliao* 资料), helps a variety of views to be more evenly presented and juxtaposed. The mainly detached speech of the third person narrator, in addition, creates a friendly environment for the reader to reflect on these views.

However, as a popular novel, *The Red Prescription* also embodies certain features that undermine the de-metaphorizing effect. Its sentimental ending, for instance, renders the final assertion of the much played-down statism almost a natural outcome. The emotional catharsis achieved in this episode significantly dilutes its potential for constructive reflection. Moreover, its highly dramatized plots, though essential for attracting readers, play on

44 Rosenberg, "Framing Disease: Illness, Society, and History," xxi.

45 Sontag, *Illness as Metaphor and AIDS and Its Metaphors*, 4, 7, 102.

their voyeuristic instinct.[46] For example, the Holmesian opening dialogues appear a little out of place even though the main plot does have something of a detective-story feeling; and Zhuang Yu's intricately designed scheme, in this regard, does tend to re-mystify drug addiction, contradicting the novel's overall de-mystifying effect.

In fact, Bi is quite conscious of the status of her works, as well as her own writing per se. In a self-referential episode, Shen seeks to take advantage of her knowledge and experience in the medical field and write literature on this subject. She models her writing after the works of "median levels" (39), that is, not high-brow literature, but something for popular consumption. Jian agrees to let Shen stay in her rehab center, passing her off as a drug addict, to observe the life there, because she intends to make drug addiction less mysterious to Shen's general readers. However, while deciding to demystify constructed halos usually found in literary works, Shen reveals her voyeuristic intent in writing—peeping at Jian's world through a "hole" (58)—and invites her readers to identify with her prying eyes. This contradiction precisely reflects that of Bi's own writing.

There are many such contradictions in and about this novel, as well as in and about the articulation of disease in the postsocialist condition in general. Postsocialism, after all, is a period marked by ideological intermingling and ambivalence. However, these contradictions do not prevent us from enjoying this novel. On the contrary, if disease, as Rosenberg has it, is "both the occasion and the agenda for an ongoing discourse concerning the interrelationship of state policy, medical responsibility, and individual culpability," contradictions in articulating disease serve as a productive site where the politics of disease are more intriguingly unfolded.[47] In the case of drug addiction exemplified in this novel, as I have discussed, discourses of nation, gender, science, and humanity come to contend and form a scene of interesting dynamics. This constitutes an epitome of postsocialist writings in China.

---

46 In fact, drugs have become a hot subject of the popular literature, film, and TV drama of mainland China since the late 1990s. For instance, in addition to the 1997 TV drama that is based on this novel (dir. Dong Zhiqiang 董志强), the TV dramas *Never Close My Eyes* (*Yong bu mingmu* 永不瞑目, 1999) and *Jade Bodhisattva* (*Yu Guanyin* 玉观音, 2009), the latter of which also has an earlier filmic version directed by Ann Hui (2003), all adapted from Hai Yan's 海岩 novels of the same titles, were among the most popular works addressing drug smuggling, abuse, and addiction. These works supply ample opportunities for popular curiosity and voyeurism on the subject.

47 Rosenberg, "Framing Disease: Illness, Society, and History," xxii.

References

Bi Shumin 毕淑敏. *Hong chufang* 红处方 [The Red Prescription]. Guilin: Lijiang chubanshe, 2008.

———. *Xue linglong* 血玲珑 [A Blood Treatment Project]. Guilin: Lijiang chubanshe, 2008.

———. *Zhengjiu rufang* 拯救乳房 [Save the Breast]. Guilin: Lijiang chubanshe, 2008.

———. *Nü xinlishi* 女心理师 [The Female Psychologist]. Guilin: Lijiang chubanshe, 2008.

———. *Huaguan bingdu* 花冠病毒 [Corolla Virus]. Changsha: Hunan wenyi chubanshe, 2012.

Dooling, Amy D. *Women's Literary Feminism in Twentieth-Century China*. New York: Palgrave Macmillan, 2005.

Ge Hongbing 葛红兵 and Song Geng 宋耕. *Shenti zhengzhi* 身体政治 [Body Politics]. Shanghai: Sanlian shudian, 2005.

Gries, Peter Hays. *China's New Nationalism: Pride, Politics, and Diplomacy*. Berkeley: University of California Press, 2004.

Guo, Yingjie, ed. *Cultural Nationalism in Contemporary China: The Search for National Identity under Reform*. London: Routledge, 2004.

Hsia, Chih-tsing. *A History of Modern Chinese Fiction*. 3rd ed. Bloomington: Indiana University Press, 1999.

Huang Hongzhao 黄宏昭. "Yapian de xiandaixing yayi: Baohan/paichu yu yayi de shijie 鸦片的现代性压抑：包含/排除与压抑的试解 [The Repressiveness of Modernity of Opium: Inclusion/Exclusion and an Analysis of Repressiveness]." *Wenhua yanjiu yuebao* 文化研究月报 (Cultural Studies Monthly), no. 50 (Sept. 2005). http://www.cc.ncu.edu.tw/~csa/journal/50/journal_park381.htm (accessed June 13, 2012).

Hughes, Christopher R. *Chinese Nationalism in the Global Era*. London: Routledge, 2006.

Knight, Sabina. "Cancer's Revelations: Malignancies and Therapies in a Recent Chinese Novel." *Literature and Medicine* 28.2 (Fall 2009): 351–70.

Lu, Tonglin. *Misogyny, Cultural Nihilism and Oppositional Politics: Contemporary Chinese Experimental Fiction*. Stanford, Calif.: Stanford University Press, 1995.

McGrath, Jason. *Postsocialist Modernity: Chinese Cinema, Literature, and Criticism in the Market Age*. Stanford: Stanford University Press, 2008.

McMahon, Keith. *The Fall of the God of Money: Opium Smoking in Nineteenth-Century China*. Lanham, Md.: Rowman & Littlefield, 2002.

Meng Yue 孟悦 and Dai Jinhua 戴锦华. *Fuchu lishi dibiao: Xiandai funü wenxue yanjiu* 浮出历史地表：现代妇女文学研究 [Emerging from the Horizon of History: Modern Chinese Women's Literature]. Beijing: Zhongguo renmin daxue chubanshe, 2004.

Rogaski, Ruth. *Hygienic Modernity: Meanings of Health and Disease in Treaty-Port China*. Berkeley and Los Angeles: University of California Press, 2004.

Rojas, Carlos, ed. *Modern Chinese Literature and Culture* 23.1 (Spring 2011). Special issue on discourses of disease.

Rosenberg, Charles E. "Framing Disease: Illness, Society, and History." Introduction to *Framing Disease: Studies in Cultural History*, ed. Charles E. Rosenberg and Janet Lynne Golden, xiii–xxvi. New Brunswick, N.J.: Rutgers University Press, 1992.

Rousseau, George Sebastian. "Literature and Medicine: The State of the Field." *Isis*, no. 72 (1981): 406–24.

———. Introduction to *Framing and Imagining Disease in Cultural History*. Ed. George Sebastian Rousseau et al Houndmills: Palgrave Macmillan, 2003. 1–48.

Sivin, Nathan. "The History of Chinese Medicine: Now and Anon." *positions: east asia cultures critique* 6.3 (1998): 731–62.

Sontag, Susan. *Illness as Metaphor and AIDS and Its Metaphors*. New York: Picador, 2001.

Su Zhiliang 苏智良. *Zhongguo dupin shi* 中国毒品史 [A History of Drugs in China]. Shanghai: Shanghai renmin chubanshe, 1997.

Unger, Jonathan, ed. *Chinese Nationalism*. Armonk, N.Y.: M.E. Sharpe, 1996.

Wang Hui 汪晖. *Xiandai Zhongguo sixiang de xingqi* 现代中国思想的兴起 [The Rise of Modern Chinese Thought]. 2nd ed. Beijing: Sanlian shudian, 2008.

Wang Jinxiang 王金香. *Zhongguo jindu shi* 中国禁毒史 [A History of Drug Prohibition in China]. Shanghai: Shanghai renmin chubanshe, 2005.

Yang Jui-Sung 杨瑞松. "Xiangxiang minzu chiru: Jindai Zhongguo sixiang wenhua shi shang de 'Dong Ya bingfu' 想象民族耻辱：近代中国思想文化史上的 '东亚病夫' [Imagining National Humiliation: 'Sick Man of East Asia' in the Modern Chinese Intellectual and Cultural History]." *Guoli Zhengzhi Daxue lishi xuebao*国立政治大学历史学报 [The Journal of History], no. 23 (2005): 1–44.

Yang, Xin. "Configuring Female Sickness and Recovery: Chen Ran and Anni Baobei." *Modern Chinese Literature and Culture* 23.1 (Spring 2011): 169–96.

Yue, Gang. "As the Dust Settles in Shangri-La: Alai's Tibet in the Era of Sino-Globalization." *Journal of Contemporary China*, no. 56 (2008): 543–63.

Zhang Wei 张维. "Ai yu si de tonghua: Jiedu Han ju zhong de baixuebing xianxiang 爱与死的童话：解读韩剧中的白血病现象 [The Fairy Tale of Love and Death: An Analysis of the Leukemia Phenomenon in Korean TV Drama]." DialogNet, 2006. http://www.dialognet.net:70/Item/6089.aspx (accessed Aug. 3, 2015).

Zheng, Yongnian. *Discovering Chinese Nationalism in China: Modernization, Identity, and International Relations*. Cambridge: Cambridge University Press, 1999.

Zhou Ning 周宁. "Yapian diguo: Langmanzhuyi shidai de yi zhong Dongfang xiangxiang 鸦片帝国：浪漫主义时代的一种东方想象 [The Opium Empire: An Oriental Imagination of Romanticism]." *Waiguo wenxue yanjiu* 外国文学研究 [Foreign Literature Studies], 2003, no. 5:88–95.

———. *Yapian diguo* 鸦片帝国 [The Opium Empire]. Beijing: Xueyuan chubanshe, 2004.

Zhou, Yongming. *Anti-Drug Crusades in Twentieth-Century China: Nationalism, History, and State Building*. Lanham, Md.: Rowman & Littlefield, 1999.

———. *China's Anti-Drug Campaign in the Reform Era*. Singapore: World Scientific, Singapore University Press, 2000.

CHAPTER 5

Narrative as Therapy: Stories of Breast Cancer by Bi Shumin and Xi Xi*

Howard Y. F. Choy 蔡元丰

With Lu Xun's 鲁迅 celebrated stories "A Madman's Diary" ("Kuangren riji" 狂人日记, 1918) and "Medicine" ("Yao" 药, 1919), modern Chinese literature started off in a medical approach often interpreted by critics as national allegory.[1] Taiwanese literary scholar Lin Xiu-rong 林秀蓉 has pointed out that during the May Fourth era (1915–27) "especially evident in the process of constructing a modernistic nation, the 'illness' discourse had been transformed into a cultural practice and entrusted a more realistic curative function."[2] In this regard, the therapeutic function of narrativity and storytelling at the personal level has been overshadowed by political concerns.[3] As health becomes more of a social as well as an individual issue in China today, writers have finally reexamined the private experience of psychological and physiological problems in their recent works. The importance of "individual voices" or "private voices" in the construction and discourse of

* Earlier versions of this essay was presented at the joint conference of the Association for Asian Studies & International Convention of Asia Scholars in Mar. 2011, the Institute for Chinese Studies at the Ohio State University in May 2012, and the Chinese Cultural Heritage Center at Hong Kong Baptist University in Dec. 2013. I am grateful for the suggestions and questions by Nicole Elizabeth Barnes, Carlos Rojas, Hu Ying 胡缨, Kirk Denton, and Zhang Enhua 张恩华.

1 Among these critics the best known is Fredric Jameson. In his seminal essay "Third-World Literature in the Era of Multinational Capitalism," *Social Text* 15 (Fall 1986): 69–70, he considers "A Madman's Diary"—read in the psychological language as a protocol of "nervous breakdown"—to be the "supreme example" of national allegory in third-world literature.

2 Lin Xiu-rong, *Zhong shen xianying: Taiwan xiaoshuo jibing xushi yihan zhi tanjiu (1929–2000)* 众身显影:台湾小说疾病叙事意涵之探究 [Developing the Bodies: An Inquiry of the Implications of Illness Narratives in Taiwanese Fiction] (Kaohsiung: Chunhui chubanshe, 2013), 7. I thank Sujane Wu 吴愫珍 for the reference.

3 A good example is the *shanghen wenxue* 伤痕文学, "scar literature" or "wound literature," of the late 1970s and early 1980s that rendered personal pains during the Cultural Revolution as national trauma, with which the individual's catharsis can only be brought about by the political experience of a collective catastrophe.

 | DOI 10.1163/9789004319219_007

disease through imagination has been stressed by cultural historian George Sebastian Rousseau.[4]

This chapter focuses on the breast cancer narratives by two contemporary Chinese women writers, namely, Xi Xi's 西西 *Elegy for a Breast* (*Aidao rufang* 哀悼乳房, 1992) and Bi Shumin's 毕淑敏 *Save the Breast* (*Zhengjiu rufang* 拯救乳房, 2003). At the turn of the millennium when Xi Xi and Bi wrote their novels, it was found that "Hong Kong has the highest breast cancer incidence in Asia" with an overall increase from the early 1980s to the end of last century, and China's most common cancer for women was also breast cancer, according to the GLOBOCAN 2002 database, with 426,057 females diagnosed and living with the disease.[5] The "Westernized way of life" in affluence, diet, and fertility was believed to be responsible for the trend in Hong Kong and attributed to "an emerging epidemic of breast cancer" in China.[6] The births of these two works indicate the awareness of the situation.[7]

Within the three areas of medical narrative identified by European social psychologist Lars-Christer Hydén, Bi's psychotherapeutic work reflects "narrative as a clinical tool" to work on a patient's mental problem, whereas Xi Xi's autobiographical account of her suffering belongs to the kind of "illness narrative" that uses storytelling as a way to regain her body and reconstitute her identity from the dominations of both the dreaded disease and the medical system or, in the words of Hydén, to "restore a sense of personal agency lost through the objectifying procedures of clinical care and treatment."[8] In

4 George Sebastian Rousseau, Introduction to *Framing and Imagining Disease in Cultural History*, ed. George Sebastian Rousseau et al. (New York: Palgrave Macmillan, 2003), 12–14.

5 See G.M. Leung et al., "Trends in Breast Cancer Incidence in Hong Kong between 1973 and 1999: An Age-Period-Cohort Analysis," *British Journal of Cancer* 87.9 (Oct. 2002): 982, 988, http://www.ncbi.nlm.nih.gov/pmc/articles/PMC2364319/ (accessed May 5, 2014); Margaret McDonald, Robin P. Hertz, and Susan W. Pitman Lowenthal, "The Burden of Cancer in Asia," *Pfizer Facts*, Dec. 2008, 81, http://www.pfizer.com/files/products/cancer_in_asia.pdf (accessed May 5, 2014).

6 Leung, "Trends in Breast Cancer Incidence in Hong Kong between 1973 and 1999," 982.

7 The awareness is also evidenced in 2004, one year after the publication of *Save the Breast*, by the Chinese Ministry of Public Health's initiation of a special fund focusing on screening programs on breast cancer, cervix cancer and digestive tract cancers for early detection and treatment. See Ping Zhao et al., "Cancer Trends in China," *Japanese Journal of Clinical Oncology* 40.4 (Jan. 2010): 284, http://jjco.oxfordjournals.org/content/40/4/281.full.pdf+html (accessed May 5, 2014).

8 David Herman, Manfred Jahn, and Marie-Laure Ryan, eds., *Routledge Encyclopedia of Narrative Theory* (London: Routledge, 2005), s.v. "Medicine and Narrative," by Lars-Christer Hydén.

light of the post-Freudian,[9] Foucauldian deconstruction practices of narrative therapy, I argue that the two masto-texts have emerged as investigative reports beyond physical pain to "re-story" fe/male fears of the malignant neoplasm that is not only incurable but also unspeakable, publicly unnarratable because of its perceived relation to sexual characteristics. When speaking of mammary cancer, the health problem immediately becomes a narrative problem.

Buttressed by postmodern literary and poststructuralist therapy theories, this research undertakes a narratological rather than allegorical analysis of the clinical stories or, as resisted by Susan Sontag, metaphoric thinking of illness, to address issues of ethics and subjectivity.[10] Promoted as the first Chinese psychotherapy novel by a psychologist, *Save the Breast* relates an experimentation of talk therapy with a group of patients to deal with the biopolitics of breast cancer as both social stigma and physio-psychic trauma against the tide of medical marketing in today's China. Its precursor from Hong Kong, *Elegy for a Breast*, the first work of Chinese women's cancer literature, draws readers into discovering their physical corpora as well as the textual corpus per se, suggesting an alternative authorship in the first-person narrative of a patient text. Although a critic may follow the allegorical tradition to argue that "breast cancer is also a metaphor for sickness at the heart of a nation racked by rapid social and economic change" and that Bi's novel "allegorize[s] the cultural distress caused by large-scale market transitions" in mainland China,[11] I am more interested in how these two "fictional treatments" seek therapy in narrative and reinvent narrative as therapy.

The third area is "narrative about illness" employed by health professionals to formulate and communicate medical knowledge among themselves.

9 Harvard psychiatrist and medical anthropologist Arthur Kleinman, in his *The Illness Narratives: Suffering, Healing, and the Human Condition* (New York: Harper Collins, 1988), 42–43, while acknowledging "Freud's great contribution…to authorize the interpretation of the biography of the patient and the interpersonal context of disorder as an appropriate component of the practitioner's craft" and "to construct a new language of general health care that addresses the deeply private significance of illness," problematizes psychoanalysts' "reach for 'deeper' meanings [that] can dehumanize the patient every bit as much as the numbing reductionism of an obsessively biomedical investigation."

10 For Susan Sontag's literary effort to strip cancer of its metaphoric mistreatment, see her *Illness as Metaphor and AIDS and Its Metaphors* (New York: Anchor Books, 1990), 3–87.

11 Sabina Knight, "Cancer's Revelations: Malignancies and Therapies in a Recent Chinese Novel," *Literature and Medicine* 28.2 (Fall 2009): 354.

Narrative Therapy: A Counter-Practice of Psychotherapy

Narrative therapy was first theorized by Australian family therapist Michael White and his New Zealand colleague, David Epston, as seen in their 1990 book *Narrative Means to Therapeutic Ends.* Instructed by John McLeod's description of narrative therapy as "postpsychological," educationist A.C. Tina Besley points out that the "narrative turn" in psychotherapy is actually a "countertherapy" or an "anti-psychiatry" grounded less in psychological discourse than in poststructuralist theory, particularly Foucault's philosophy.[12] A form of social psychology, narrative therapy does not target a "correct diagnosis" by identifying pathology, but rather aims to "[open] space for the authoring of alternative stories," "unique accounts" or "unique redescriptions" that would yield "unique possibilities" instead of an absolute solution.[13] In narrative therapy, solutions are derived from personal experiences and imagination rather than expert views and knowledge. Based on American psychologist Jerome Bruner's two modes of cognitive learning, White and Epston prefer the narrative to the logico-scientific mode of thought because "the narrative mode leads, not to certainties, but to varying perspectives" and "the particulars of experience" that serve as links between aspects of life, past and present, in the creation of a "unique context" for new possibilities and alternative meanings, which are excluded by the logico-scientific mode.[14] While the logico-scientific mode uses quantitative descriptions and technical language "to reduce the risks of polysemy," the narrative mode embraces qualitative descriptions and poetic

---

12 McLeod, Foreword to *Narrative Therapy: An Introduction for Counsellors*, by Martin Payne (London: SAGE, 2000), x; A.C. Besley, "Foucault and the Turn to Narrative Therapy," *British Journal of Guidance and Counselling* 30.2 (2002): 126, 140. In the opening paragraph of his and David Epston's *Narrative Means to Therapeutic Ends* (New York: W.W. Norton, 1990), 1, Michael White acknowledges the importance and influence of Foucault's reflections on knowledge and power.

13 White and Epston, *Narrative Means to Therapeutic Ends*, 6, 41. At the end of a discussion dated 1998 in his *Reflections on Narrative Practice: Essays and Interviews* (Adelaide: Dulwich Centre Publications, 2000), 115, White expressed his discontent with the pathologizing practices of psychotherapy:

> … I have always questioned the pathologizing discourses that are so routinely dishonoring of people's lives, and that marginalize and disqualify the knowledges and skills that people bring with them into the therapeutic arena, knowledges and skills that have been generated in the history of their lives and their relationships with others. And I have continued to challenge the taken-for-granted practices of immodesty of the culture of psychotherapy.

14 White and Epston, *Narrative Means to Therapeutic Ends*, 78–81.

or picturesque language to encourage "more than one line of interpretation or reading at any one time."[15] Unique meanings are thereby performed in the therapeutic process of enfolding, unfolding, and interplaying of stories, which "are full of gaps and inconsistencies."[16]

It is important to understand that White's narrative metaphor "should not be confused with that which proposes that stories function as a reflection of life or as a mirror for life"; rather, that "stories are shaping of life, and that they have real, not imagined, effects—and that these stories provide the structure of life."[17] White is less interested in human nature than in narrative practice, for it is in the latter that life can be understood as one possible way among many others instead of one single truth with no exit. On the text analogy, people "live their lives by stories"; they are both writers and readers of day-to-day lives. White's patient-centered "text therapy," as we may call it, empowers patients to take over the authorship of their own lives actively through the narrativization of illness. "Indeed," as Linda Mills points out, "the force of NT [narrative therapy] is in the power it gives to clients to rename and reclassify their suffering."[18]

When White interviews and is being interviewed by his clients (i.e., "*inter*view" in its true, mutual sense), he does not treat them as "patients"; instead, they are "protagonists" in their life stories and "participants" in their life worlds: "This is a world of interpretative acts, a world in which every retelling of a story is a new telling, a world in which persons participate with others in the 're-authoring', and thus in the shaping, of their lives and relationships," and so they have become "the privileged authors" in a position to restructure their identities and reimagine their lives.[19] In storied therapy, story sharing has a dual function:

> Firstly, in the act of witnessing the performance of a new story, the audience contributes to the writing of new meanings; this has real effects on the audience's interaction with the story's subject. Secondly, when the subject of the story "reads" the audience's experience of the new performance, either through speculation about these experiences or by a more

---

15 Ibid., 81–82.

16 Michael White, "Deconstruction and Therapy," in *Therapeutic Conversations*, ed. Stephen Gilligan and Reese Price (New York: W.W. Norton, 1993), 38.

17 Ibid., 36.

18 Herman, Jahn, and Ryan, *Routledge Encyclopedia of Narrative Theory*, s.v. "Narrative Therapy," by Linda Mills.

19 White and Epston, *Narrative Means to Therapeutic Ends*, 82–83.

> direct identification, he or she engages in revisions and extensions of the new story.[20]

As life stories are told and retold, the self-narratives are constantly revised with sub-plots, "alternative plot[s] or counterplot[s]."[21] Notice that the self is constructed not only by the multiple stories of personal lives but also by socio-politico-cultural discourses in the realities. Once a discourse becomes a "dominant plot" of life, problems arise. These problems include the binary oppositions of healthy/unhealthy, normal/abnormal, male/female, so on and so forth. As perceived by Chan Chitat 陈智达, a Hong Kong counseling researcher and a student of Michael White, the therapeutic process of narrative therapy is "to deconstruct and subvert the dominant narratives that trouble the clients."[22] Canadian psychiatrist Karl Tomm speaks of White's clinical method as one of protest: "His approach is to carefully direct the protest against problematic beliefs and practices rather than against the persons who hold those beliefs and enact those practices."[23]

By archaeologizing and objectifying or, in the terminology of narrative therapy, "externalizing" the problem from within the person, the person's identity is non-essentialized, rather deconstructed, and can be reconstructed and redeemed through marginal discourses. In order to distance the person from, so as to reduce, the problem, narrative therapy would encourage her/him to write "a 'success' story rather than the 'sad tale' format of many psychotherapy narratives," as White claims: "I do not believe that it is acceptable for therapeutic conversations to contribute to re-traumatization or renewed distress, or to the reinforcement of people's negative identity conclusions," which are often drawn from single-storied conversations; instead, White advocates "double- or multi-storied conversations" to provide space for previously untold lived experience or suppressed storylines, so as to draw positive outcomes or "alternative identity conclusions."[24]

---

20 Ibid., 17. According to Arthur W. Frank, *The Wounded Storyteller: Body, Illness, and Ethics* (Chicago: University of Chicago Press, 1995), 2, new stories are needed by the body "when its disease disrupts the old stories"; therefore, disease is not only the topic of a story but the condition of storytelling.

21 White, "Deconstruction and Therapy," 43.

22 Chitat Chan, "Narrative Practice with Youth: A Heuristic Case Study on a Youth-Centre Drama Workshop," *Journal of Social Work Practice* 26.2 (June 2012): 197.

23 Karl Tomm, "The Courage to Protest: A Commentary on Michael White's Work," in Gilligan and Price, *Therapeutic Conversations*, 63.

24 White and Epston, *Narrative Means to Therapeutic Ends*, 163; White, *Reflections on Narrative Practice*, 41.

Narrative therapy is therefore, according to Besley's Foucauldian definition, "a lifestyle and political project…that is concerned with different ways of producing the 'self'."[25] Foucault's focus on one's relationship to and constitution of oneself as an ethical existence has supported a poststructuralist identity project in narrative therapy.[26] Since identity is a product of "narrative negotiations,"[27] that is, negotiation and renegotiation within oneself as well as between the self and the other in a narrative frame or plot, therapeutic narratives are necessarily dialogical and conversational. "Re-membering conversations" are often used to relate the past with the present, to re-engage with the personal history of life, so as to become "other than who one was."[28] White does not adopt the practice of reframing history, for he is afraid that such practice can only replace established totalizations with new ones in "the development of single-storied experiences of life and of identity"; instead, he approaches identity in "a multi-layered and multi-voiced sense."[29] He proposes:

> Rather than reproducing a practice that has the effect of substituting one frame for another, and rather than engaging with a practice that is revisioning of the familiar historical records of people's lives, the practices of narrative therapy that contribute to options for a re-engagement with history bring forth multi-storied experiences of life and of identity. These practices not only contribute to an expansion of people's narrative resources, but also make it possible for them to alter their relationship with their own histories.[30]

Multi-voiced identities are developed from the sense of community "that is the outcome of experiencing some of the stories of our lives joined with the stories of the lives of others around shared themes and values."[31] Accordingly, White understands all descriptions as "relational, not representational" for their double-sidedness: the visible, seemingly representational "presence" and

25 Besley, "Foucault and the Turn to Narrative Therapy," 135.

26 White, *Reflections on Narrative Practice*, 164–65.

27 Ibid., 62.

28 Ibid., 75.

29 Ibid., 35, 76.

30 Ibid., 35–36.

31 Ibid., 171. White critiques single-voiced identities as "the vogue of contemporary western culture." His sense of community follows Frank's Preface to his *The Wounded Storyteller*, xi: "The ill person who turns illness into story transforms fate into experience; the disease that sets the body apart from others becomes, in the story, the common bond of suffering that joins bodies in their shared vulnerability."

the “absent but implicit” in the Derridean “traces of a multiplicity of unstated signs” or hidden voices.[32] The deconstructive method of reading in narrative therapy brings forth the unstoried, yet storyable, experiences of living, and in practice it often points to further retellings at the end of a person’s story in a rather formulaic and suggestive conclusion: “But that is another story.”[33] In effect, there are endless stories in narrative therapy.

While participants are asked to narrate their experiences, which are witnessed, interpreted or even interrogated by the narrative therapist and other team members, the narrative therapist’s power is demystified in the “decentered sharing” of a story.[34] The therapist is not so much an arbitrator as a collaborator who “takes initiative to co-create new enlivening stories to replace the old oppressive ones.”[35] In effect, stories are co-authored by the therapist and the client(s) with a consciousness of their power relations during the process of their joint construction of a new narrative. White sees no possession of “an objective and unbiased account of reality” or “truth discourses of the psychotherapies” on the part of the therapist: “Therapists can contribute to the deconstruction of expert knowledge by considering themselves to be ‘co-authors’ of alternative and preferred knowledges and practices, and through a concerted effort to establish a context in which the persons who seek therapy are privileged as the primary authors of these knowledges and practices.”[36]

Narrative as Group Therapy: *Save the Breast*

Bi Shumin began her writing career in 1987 after twenty-two years of practice in internal medicine and psychology, including eleven years of service as a medic in the People’s Liberation Army in Tibet. Veteran writer Wang Meng 王蒙 calls her a “writer-doctor” who “has a way of thinking, a mode of writing and behaving that prescribes the humanistic concern, passion and compassion into calmness, that combines conscience, literature, and science into an organic whole.”[37] Bi’s writings can indeed be regarded as medical prescriptions for

32 White, *Reflections on Narrative Practice*, 36–37.

33 Ibid., 48, 53.

34 Ibid., 75.

35 Tomm, “The Courage to Protest,” 65.

36 White, “Deconstruction and Therapy,” 56–58.

37 Wang Meng, Preface to *Bi Shumin zixuan jingpin ji* (*xiaoshuo juan*) 毕淑敏自选精品集(小说卷) [Self-selected Best Works of Bi Shumin: Fiction] (1995; Beijing: Zhongguo shehui chubanshe, 2002), n.p.

the morbid modern man. Chinese critics have characterized her first novel *The Red Prescription* (*Hong chufang* 红处方, 1997) in terms of its "sorrowful sympathy and rescue" which, unlike the postrevolutionary *shanghen wenxue* or "scar literature," extends humanistic concerns beyond the limits of times to "transcend social history, politics" and policies.[38] It is suggested that the writer's focus on human nature in this tragic story of drug rehabilitation was the turning point of her career prior to her pursuit of Master's in psychology.[39] Yet there is another turn from the nature of human to the narrative of life in her work later.

Because of the novelty of her subject matter and personal experience found in her representative work "An Appointment with Death" ("Yuyue siwang" 预约死亡, 1994), Bi Shumin is labeled a "new experience" (*xin tiyan* 新体验) writer in China.[40] While there are few theorizations about "new experience fiction," the literary phenomenon that emerged from the decline of "neorealist fiction" (*xin xieshi xiaoshuo* 新写实小说) allows the writer to appear in the text not as a first-person narrator or an implied author, who is only an "other-presence" (*ta zai* 他在), but as a "self-presence" (*wo zai* 我在) of the real author who guides the real reader to "directly comprehend the meanings of existence and life" through what Deng Hanmei 邓寒梅 describes Bi's fiction as "a kind of present narrative that focuses on the 'illness spot'."[41] For the existential experience, I would like to point out the *ti* in *tiyan* that is both "bodily" and "personal" in the biopolitical sense.

Bi Shumin's *Save the Breast* is promoted as "the first Chinese psychotherapy fiction by a psychologist" on its red-and-black cover with writer-healer and

---

38 Ren Xianghong 任向红, "Beimin yu jiudu [shu]—Bi Shumin xiaoshuo *Hong chufang* qianxi 悲悯与救渎[赎]——毕淑敏小说《红处方》浅析 [Sorrowful Sympathy and Rescue: Brief Discussion on *The Red Prescription* Written by Bi Shumin]," *Xibei minzu daxue xuebao* (*zhexue shehui kexue ban*) 西北民族大學學報(哲學社會科學版) (Journal of Northwest University for Nationalities [Philosophy and Social Sciences]), 2007, no. 2:104; Liu Lili 刘俐俐, *Tuibai yu zhengjiu—Bi Shumin yu yi lei wenxue zhuti* 颓败与拯救——毕淑敏与一类文学主题 [Decline and Salvage: Bi Shumin and a Literary Theme] (Beijing: Huaxia chubanshe, 2000), 130, 134.

39 Liu, *Tuibai yu zhengjiu*, 134–35.

40 He Zhenbang, "Bi Shumin's Stories: Submersed in Reality," trans. Chen Haiyan, *Chinese Literature* (Spring 1997): 61. In fact, Bi's "An Appointment with Death" is collected in and appears as the book title of the "new experience fiction" series edited by Fu Yonglin 傅用霖 (Beijing: Zuojia chubanshe, 1995).

41 Yu Hong 于泓, "Qianyi 'xin tiyan xiaoshuo' 浅议'新体验小说' [Brief Remarks on 'New Experience Fiction']," *Liaoning shizhuan xuebao* (*shehui kexue ban*) 辽宁师专学报(社会科学版) (Journal of Liaoning Teachers College [Social Sciences]), 2005, no. 3:41; Deng Hanmei, *Zhongguo xiandangdai wenxue zhong de jibing xushi yanjiu*, 304.

cancer survivor Deena Metzger's photo portrait "Tree" by Hella Hammid (*The Warrior*, 1980) at the center.[42] The title, while adopted by the People's Literature Publishing House lest the word "cancer" in the original designation *Cancer Group* (*Aizheng xiaozu* 癌症小组) intimidate potential readers, is charged by literary critics for its sensationalism.[43] Indeed, both "breast" and "cancer" are still taboos in early twenty-first century China.[44] Nevertheless, as the 2003 SARS (severe acute respiratory syndrome) outbreak in Beijing has reportedly "brought about an unprecedented fusion of diverse cultural strata, making concern for physical and mental health and the living environment a new literary trend,"[45] the doctor-turned-writer was inspired by a terminal illness.

Sponsored by a pharmaceutical manufacturer Lü Kezha 吕克闸, female psychologist Dr. Cheng Yuanqing 程远青 puts together a medical "encounter group" of eight breast cancer sufferers from different social classes, plus a male assistant from the biomedical company. Facing mortality, the patients each have their own stories to tell in the 32-chapter novel. Sex worker Lulu's 鹿路 tumor is discovered during a surgery to remove the saline-filled implants inserted for her breast augmentation, which have been strip off by a boorish client. Graduate student Zhou Yunruo 周云若, after offering her virginity to her boyfriend the night before she was admitted to the tumor hospital, plays fast and loose with her wooers' affections but never develops intimate relations with them. Public servant Bu Zhenqi 卜珍琪 fears that the diagnosis, once announced, would jeopardize her chance of promotion. Veteran cadre An Jiang 安疆 has been so loyal to her leader-turned-husband, even after his death, that she cannot make up her mind about the cancer treatment until he instructs her in a dream. School principal Yue Ping 岳评 witnessed the pains of her daughter and does not understand why the patient was so impatient about her motherly concerns. Bank employee Hua Lan 花岚 suspects that her husband has been

42 For an analysis of the appropriation of Deena Metzger's image, see Knight, "Cancer's Revelations," 367–68; for further information about Deena Metzger and the "Tree" poster, see her homepage http://deenametzger.net/the-poster/ (last accessed Dec. 18, 2013).

43 Wu Fei 吴菲, "Bi Shumin: Weishenme tuoxie, weishenme fangqi 毕淑敏:为什么妥协, 为什么放弃 [Bi Shumin: To Compromise or to Give up]," *Beijing qingnian bao* 北京青年报 (Beijing Youth Daily), May 28, 2003.

44 In the case study of personal narratives of breast cancer in his *Recovering Bodies: Illness, Disability, and Life Writing* (Madison: University of Wisconsin Press, 1997), 79n, G. Thomas Couser notes that even in modern English literature authors and publishers are "subconsciously affected by the taboo against naming the disease" in the narratives' titles.

45 Xu Hong, "Epidemic Heralds Humanistic New Wave," *China Today*, Sept. 2003, http://vod.sxrtvu.edu/englishonline/bjzs/chinatoday/chinatoday2003/20039/9p34.asp (accessed Mar. 30, 2016).

having an affair since she was diagnosed with malignancies. Laid-off worker Ying Chuncao 应春草 accepts domestic violence as a norm. Most dramatically, male patient Cheng Muhai 成慕海 (a.k.a. Cheng Mumei 成慕梅), disguising himself as a woman, her brother, and an anonymous informant, is planning a suicidal bombing from the very beginning of the novel.

Dr. Cheng initiates the first group gathering by admitting that she feels herself "inferior" (*zibei* 自卑) to other members in terms of her marriage failure, middle age and, most intriguingly, lack of personal experience with breast cancer. This strategy of self-abasement aims not only to create a sense of equality between the therapist and her clients but also to shift the authority and authorship of cancerous experience onto the patients. Upon signing their contracts, Dr. Cheng insists, "everyone is an actor and a spectator at the same time."[46] Yet Cheng is not portrayed as, to follow the drama metaphor, a godlike director: "Psychologists are not gods; they are only more aware of and [willing to] reconstruct themselves" (365). While Lü Kezha cashes in on her affective weakness to trick her into advertising his new drug, Cheng Muhai deceives her over the phone throughout the narrative. She is attracted, distracted by them and, as a result, her power is subtracted. In fact, she herself is also undergoing psychotherapy with her clients, especially when Cheng Muhai's phone calls serve as what Karl Tomm terms "the meta-conversation about the therapeutic conversation."[47]

Being a common theme of the personal stories revealed in the novel, breast cancer is identified as a "killer of women" due to its "devastating destruction of the secondary sexual characteristic" (9) which, as the young student Zhou Yunruo has confessed when asked to retell her genuine feelings, weighs heavier than life. While the female patients suffer from post-surgical scarring along with discrimination as asexual after the removal of their breasts, the male patient develops split personalities from a popular misunderstanding of mastocarcinoma as a gynecological disease. Both are related to the biopolitics of gender identity. Zhou no longer regards herself as a girl: "I've become a monster neither female nor male" (125). On the contrary, Bu Zhenqi attempts to cover up her "gynecological disease" in the male-dominated realm of officialdom lest it remind people of her very femininity. And the "transsexual" Cheng Muhai's statement reveals illnesses as indicators of gender and class:

> Illnesses do have genders and ranks. If you're a boss, you could get high blood pressure, heart disease, and diabetes, which are patrician maladies,

46 Bi Shumin, *Zhengjiu rufang* [Save the Breast] (Beijing: Renmin wenxue chubanshe, 2003), 59. Further page numbers appear in the text; all translations are mine.

47 Tomm, "The Courage to Protest," 73.

> synonyms of luxuries and comforts, nothing to be ashamed about. But you shouldn't get hepatitis. With hepatitis, people would immediately lower your social status, thinking that you must have got the infectious disease as a frequent patron of street-side food stalls. If you got a VD, that's okay—as long as it's not AIDS, all men could laugh it off. Yet I got a women's disease. If I told people about it, instead of having their sympathy and concern, I'd become a bizarre tale for entertainment at their leisure. [359]

Thus, for the male patient, breast cancer is more a shame than a sickness. With mastectomy, his masculinity is castrated or, in his own words, "removed on the operating table" (362). He is cut into two: an isolated feminine self without womanliness (Cheng Mumei) and an idolized masculine self without manliness (Cheng Muhai).

During the subsequent group and private meetings held at special places such as a cemetery, tumor hospital, and assembly hall, Dr. Cheng consistently encourages her clients to work with her in the quest for a second life. She employs "re-membering" conversations and "re-authoring" dialogues to help them spot omissions in their stories that are essential to their life struggles. The therapeutic narrative conversations are often begun by her asking questions that would create an opening to retrieve forgotten events or suppressed memories and to recruit alternative experiences. For example, after unlocking "the door of memory" (325) at an assembly hall built in the 1960s and redeeming herself from the death of her mother for which she felt responsible, Bu Zhenqi stops hiding her illness and starts a new treatment program. And when Lulu reveals her story of selling her virginity to pay the medical bills for her half-brother, with whom she secretly falls in love, she is encouraged to call him; upon finding that he only cares about her money, not her, she decides to abandon her sacrificial fantasy and begin a new life for herself. In both cases, the female patient-protagonists are released from the prison of the past and regain the authorship of their lives. They have reached the final step of narrative therapy, that is, the very high-level task of "making plans to act upon the newly understood concepts they have formed."[48]

Moreover, through the interactions of group therapy, Yue Ping has learned to be a good listener at her school administration meetings. Zhou Yunruo

48 Chan, "Narrative Practice with Youth," 199–200. In practice, the narrative therapist would categorize the clients' utterances into five levels, from "nam[ing] and characterize[ing] the problem or initiative" (low) to "expand[ing] intentions into plans for action" (very high) according to Michael White's framework.

finally utters the term "breast cancer," a taboo she has put on the biological disease even in front of her doctor and now successfully breaks it with the team's support. Ying Chuncao, with a simple rhetorical switch of her substitutive second-person narrative to first-person, retells her story and recognizes herself as a victim of her husband's abusive behavior. Hua Lan is persuaded to verify her suspicion about a mistress' phone number, which is proven to be a case of mistaken identity: the number is that of a business account. An Jiang is empowered to make her own decision to discontinue her painful treatments for a peaceful end of her long life. The cross-dresser Cheng Muhai's schizophrenia is overcome by being allowed to disrobe to expose his scarred body and acknowledging its/his existence as one and real. His destruction of the explosive device at the end signifies that he has found a way of living with the fatal—not necessarily female—illness. As Sabina Knight has pointed out: "The novel thus shifts from a medical paradigm, focusing on the individual, to a social paradigm emphasizing relational factors."[49]

Dr. Cheng realizes that cancer patients are a disadvantaged minority, particularly helpless in the increasingly tense practitioner-patient relationship. To deconstruct the relation that is described as "an immeasurable black hole, even more unfathomable than the black hole of death" (184), she adopts play therapy by dressing up a white chair with a white gown in a consulting room and inviting the cancer patients to comment on their doctors. To the patients, these white-coated people are "familiar strangers" (180).[50] On the one hand, their contacts are as close as allies; on the other, their conflicts arise from their power and economic relationships. The game turns into a call for complaints about physicians' arrogance, indifference, inhumaneness and, most seriously in mainland China, corruption, reflecting a general mistrust of doctors.

People have now become conscious that they are not only patients but also patrons in a clinical encounter; they are clients or, more precisely, customers in the market economy of what Arthur Kleinman describes as the amoral "commoditization of the healer-sick person relationship as an economic transaction."[51] As patients, they want their doctors to respect them and their

49 Knight, "Cancer's Revelations," 360.

50 This is reminiscent of Rita Charon's portrayal of the alien and yet close doctor-patient relationship from the perspective of an internist in her Afterword to *Psychoanalysis and Narrative Medicine*, ed. Peter L. Rudnytsky and Rita Charon (Albany: State University of New York Press, 2008), 292: "We are at the same time *alone* and *with*, strange and intimate. The presence of the other is both mysterious and known." For a further study of doctor-patient interactions, see Howard Waitzkin, *The Politics of Medical Encounters: How Patients and Doctors Deal with Social Problems* (New Haven: Yale University Press, 1991).

51 Arthur Kleinman, *The Illness Narratives*, 54.

privacy; they do not want to be dehumanized and their breasts displayed as an object of biomedical study or, in Hua Lan's vivid figuration, "a rotten pineapple" that draws the "flies" of medical students (191–192). As patrons, they demand equality and consumers' right to know their health conditions. In a multi-storied structure, the chapter critiques the agent of medical science and challenges its authority or, as the author reflects during an interview, its "rights" (*faquan* 法权) and "discursive power" (*huayuquan* 话语权).[52] Although it ends with Dr. Cheng leading her group to bow their thanks and hopes in front of the white frock, it also allows a member, the male patient Cheng Muhai, to maintain his resistant gesture.

The ultimate confrontation, however, is not with the doctor, but with the entrepreneur Lü Kezha. Facing the biomedical company's coercion and bribery to film a commercial for its new herbal medicine, Dr. Cheng calls for a vote in the support group that has been divided due to different backgrounds of its members. Consequently, at the climax of the novel, they unite together against their sponsor's imposition, announcing the comic triumph of the cancer patients reborn with a group identity. The dramatic turn directs the attack on the technologically facilitated ruse of medical marketization and commercial exploitation. As the 400-page novel concludes in a farewell of the old patient An Jiang at her deathbed, it has become a requiem rehearsal that constructs death as dignity.

The narrative functions as a group therapy for the patients-personae and the psychologist-protagonist within, as well as the physician-poet without. In her inquiry of narratives of illness, American physician and literary scholar Rita Charon observes: "When health care professionals write reflectively about their practice, they learn how interwoven are stories of patients and story of self.... As these authors wrote the biographies of their patients, they came to understand how urgent it is for them as health care professionals to reflect on and tell of their own lives."[53] Bi Shumin reveals to us the postmodern "several selves" as described by Arthur W. Frank in his case study of Sue Nathanson, who narrates her traumas of an abortion and a tubal ligation: "She is a *writer* telling how she as a *therapist* spoke to her client about what she as a *woman*

52 Zhou Xiaoli 周晓丽, "Bi Shumin de zui xin changpian xiaoshuo *Zhengjiu rufang* 毕淑敏的最新长篇小说《拯救乳房》 [Bi Shumin's Latest Novel *Save the Breast*]," interview with Bi Shumin, Renminwang 人民网 (people), Aug. 1, 2003, http://www.people.com.cn/GB/14738/14754/21862/1995449.html (accessed May 27, 2012).

53 Rita Charon, *Narrative Medicine: Honoring the Stories of Illness* (Oxford: Oxford University Press, 2006), 75.

who had suffered learned about the *multiple sides* of herself."[54] Bi's stories of sickness not only deconstruct and reconstruct the patients-characters' biographies to re-narrativize their experiences but also share the clinician-writer's autobiography to re-navigate her life. Such sharing suggests an intersubjectivity in Charon's "narrative vision for health care": "Through narrative effort, we achieve first the subject position and then, with luck, the intersubjective bond between ourselves and others, thereby inaugurating and framing the therapeutic relationship."[55] Four years after the appearance of *Save the Breast*, Bi published another psychotherapy novel, *The Female Psychologist* (*Nü xinlishi* 女心理师, 2007). But that is another story.

Narrative as Self-therapy: *Elegy for a Breast*

If Bi Shumin's therapeutic game is largely set between the therapist-author and her clients-characters, Xi Xi's earlier metafiction playfully engages the patient-writer with her "you"-readers. Whereas *Save the Breast* is rather sentimental and well knit, *Elegy for a Breast* is loosely plotted and considered by critics to be a fiction of fusion that blends narrative with dialogue, essay, poetry, report, and exposition into a kaleidoscope.[56] The I-narrator appears to be a dramatis persona, a translator, a poet, a critic and, most importantly, an analysand and an analyst at once, who examines her own ailing health like a piece of translation or artwork. The process of narration becomes a process of self-therapy and self-discovery at the same time.

In the general editor's note to the collection of Xi Xi's stories in English translation, Eva Hung points out that *Elegy for a Breast* is "the first literary work in which a Chinese woman writer deals with the experience of breast

---

54 Frank, *The Wounded Storyteller*, 70; italics in the original. Nathanson's story is published under the title *Soul Crisis: One Woman's Journey through Abortion to Renewal* (New York: New American Library, 1989).

55 Charon, *Narrative Medicine*, 236.

56 See Ho Fuk Yan 何福仁, "Shuxie de Ajian—du *Aidao rufang* 书写的阿坚——读《哀悼乳房》 [Ah Kien as a Writer: On *Elegy for a Breast*]," *Shun po* 信报 (Hong Kong Economic Journal), Nov. 11, 1992, 6. Stephen C. Soong 宋淇, "Building a House: Introducing Xi Xi" (1985), trans. Kwok-kan Tam 谭国根, in Xi Xi, *A Girl Like Me and Other Stories* (1986; enlarged ed., Hong Kong: Chinese University of Hong Kong, 1996), 134, has observed that sentimentalism is not a characteristic of Xi Xi's works. This is also true of *Elegy for a Breast*, which has inspired Hong Kong film director Law Wing Cheong 罗永昌 in making the romantic comedy *2 Become 1* (*Tiansheng yidui* 天生一对, 2006), in a reading scene of which the book appears briefly. But that is a sentimental story.

cancer."[57] Being both the author and subject of her novel, Xi Xi has published what White and Epston call a "self story" or, in a broader sense of the term, a "counter document"—an alternative to the official diagnosis that ascribes to her the "problematic identity" of a "patient," who is to be marginalized, if not fully ostracized, from the "healthy" population.[58] Unlike the institutionalized therapies that are oral-oriented, narrative therapy also emphasizes written accounts including "letters, statements, certificates and creative writing."[59] As it is informed by Michael Stubbs' socialinguistics, "recourse to the written tradition in therapy promotes the formalization, legitimation, and continuity of local popular knowledges, the independent authority of persons, and the creation of a context for the emergence of new discoveries and possibilities."[60] Xi Xi decided and desires to write down her treatments and reflections, so as to reclaim her "narrative identity" from the subordination of herself to "diagnostic identity," as she alerts her readers, "not from an expert's perspective, but in a patient's identity."[61]

Inspired by the playful form of Argentinean novelist Julio Cortázar's 1966 novel *Hopscotch* (*La Rayuela*), Xi Xi engages her readers by encouraging them to select or skip certain passages.[62] In her preface, which opens with a direct address to the reader by imagining her/him in a bookstore, she suggests that one should feel free to choose among the thirty non-chronically composed

57 In Xi Xi, *A Girl Like Me and Other Stories*, 6.

58 White and Epston, *Narrative Means to Therapeutic Ends*, 163, 190.

59 Martin Payne, *Narrative Therapy: An Introduction for Counsellors* (London: SAGE, 2000), 127.

60 White admits that due to time pressures they still "privilege the oral tradition" in daily practice. White and Epston, *Narrative Means to Therapeutic Ends*, 35, 37.

61 Xi Xi, *Aidao rufang* [Elegy for a Breast] (Taipei: Hongfan shudian, 1992), ii. While some English excerpts of *Elegy for a Breast* by Caroline Mason are found in Xi Xi, *A Girl Like Me and Other Stories*, 113–25, no full rendition of the novel is available; all translations here are mine. Hereafter page references are given in the text. For the concept of "narrative identity" as the "definition of subjectivity" to seek for "a narrative understanding of ourselves," see Paul Ricoeur, "Life: A Story in Search of a Narrator," trans. J.N. Kraay and A.J. Scholten, in M.C. Doeser and J.N. Kraay, eds., *Facts and Values: Philosophical Reflections from Western and Non-Western Perspectives* (Dordrecht: Martinus Nijhoff, 1986), 131–32. Unlike White who works to "re-author" our life, however, Ricoeur realizes the sedimentation of cultural tradition in play and limits the possibility "to become the *narrator of our own story* without completely becoming the author of our life" (originally in italics).

62 In fact, the pen name Xi Xi is related to hopscotch as the writer has explained it: "The Chinese character 西 'xi' looks like a girl in a skirt, her two feet planted in a square. Put two of them side by side, and they are like two frames of a film, a girl in a skirt playing hopscotch in two squares." See Soong, "Building a House," 128–29.

chapters that interest one or concern one's sex, age, profession, or health condition. With hints and cross references passim in the end of chapters, at least seven paths—some long, some short—are found in the order of reading. For example, at the end of "Doctors' Sayings" the author suggests: "What to do if your family or friend finds a lump in her breast? Please tell her to avoid the mistakes I made as described in 'Silly Things', p. 85"; a special note is made for male readers: "If you are not female and want to learn something about breast cancer in men, please turn to page 207 and read 'Beard and Eyebrows'"; a reminder of a previous passage: "How to resist cancer? Prevention is better than cure, yet in case you had it, you have no choice but to fight it. Remember 'Counterattack' on page 167?"; and a less inviting case: "The next chapter is about a fool doing math, pretty boring and repetitive—skip it if you are in a bad mood" (25, 31, 209, 248).

The same strategy is also found in the very beginning of *Narrative Means to Therapeutic Ends*, where Michael White tries to present to his reader Foucault's complex ideas: "I'm not sure how successful I have been—this can only be determined by you, the reader. Some readers might find it preferable to skip this chapter, go immediately to chapters 2, 3 and 4, and then return to the first chapter at a later stage…."[63] The change of reading habit facilitates alternative stories in life, "alternative stories that incorporate vital and previously neglected aspects of lived experience."[64] It is through author-reader interactions that a new story is co-constructed and that the novel, with its informative chapters, reads rather like a women's health guide such as the American bestseller *Our Bodies, Ourselves*, which "drew the reader's attention to the sensation of investigating herself."[65] With this strong sense of instructiveness, Xi Xi's autopathography not only concerns about the self, but also encourages other people in similar situations.[66]

---

63 White and Epston, *Narrative Means to Therapeutic Ends*, 1–2.

64 Ibid., 31.

65 Susan Wells, Our Bodies, Ourselves *and the Work of Writing* (Stanford: Stanford University Press, 2010), 135.

66 Couser, in his *Recovering Bodies*, 44, defines "autopathographies as much in response to discourse about disease as to the diseases themselves" and argues: "the most threatening discourse is not medical discourse; it is the general cultural discourse that ascribes stigma to a bodily dysfunction" because "disease is always culturally constructed." Anne Hunsaker Hawkins, in her *Reconstructing Illness: Studies in Pathography* (West Lafayette, Ind.: Purdue University Press, 1993), 178n, traces the use of the word "pathography" to Freud's *Leonardo da Vinci and a Memory of His Childhood* (1910), trans. Alan Tyson (New York: W.W. Norton, 1964), 81, in which da Vinci's sexual life is related to his artistic activity, whereas Hawkins borrows the word simply "to refer to an autobiographical or biographical narrative about an experience of illness."

Elegy for a Breast is not without a typical cancer sufferer's sensitivity and helplessness. The author once (mis)interprets a medical privacy notice as a statement of taboo; she often feels like a lamb in front of her doctor: "As patients, there are many things we do not understand, nor are we given any choice" (63). Resisting "narrative surrender" to the authority of the modern medical story told by the physician, she tells her own illness story.[67] If knowledge is power, narrative is knowledge. As Rita Charon points out, it is within the reflective space created in the autobiographical gap between the I-narrator and the I-protagonist that "one beholds and considers the self in a heightened way, revealing fresh knowledge about its coherent existence."[68] In the process of transmitting previously neglected anthropotomical and medical knowledges through storytelling, Xi Xi discovers alternative knowledges of self and alternative modes of life. From the Imperial Medical Office of the Tang dynasty to the discourses of breast cancer (*ruyan* 乳岩) in medical books of the Song and Ming periods, from ancient Greek medicine to modern radiation oncology, the Hong Kong writer considers all medical systems to be "different readings of the human body as well as life" (239). Between traditional Chinese medical philosophy and modern Western medical science there lies a culturally hybrid Hong Kong body to be examined, diagnosed, defined, and redefined.

Anxious about the lack of an organ of sexual characteristics after a mammectomy, the woman writer puts herself side by side with "the eunuchs in the Forbidden City" (70) and the castrated historian Sima Qian 司马迁 (145-ca. 86 B.C.)—another "monster" writer. She realizes that her grotesque body as the vehicle of a health problem is inevitably objectified through the gaze, be it Foucault's "clinical gaze" or Lacan's self-gazing. The gaze represents a mechanism of social norms and self-evaluation. Public and private bathrooms, once the locales of leisure, have now become the "battlefields" of gaze and objectification that lay bare the emptiness on her chest:

> The entire breast is gone. The entire breast, including the nipple, the areola, the mammary gland, a large amount of fat and connective tissue....
>
> The peach treelike glandular tissue is certainly the main structure of the breast, but it only occupies a very small proportion of the entire breast's volume; the breast's contour is basically formed by a lot of fat and connective tissue, including the suspensory ligaments of Cooper. This peach tree on my body, with its nearby soil, is gone. If my right chest was

67 The term "narrative surrender" is coined by Arthur W. Frank in his *The Wounded Storyteller*, 6.

68 Charon, *Narrative Medicine*, 70.

> once a hill, it is now a sunken valley; if it was once a soft, tasty bun, what is left now is only an empty plate. [67–68]

Here the elegy is composed of a biologic breast anatomy of the body, a poetic portrait of the bodyscape, and an alimentary analogy of the mamma. It is the absence of this object—this tree or bun—that suddenly reminds her of her body:

> Discharged from the hospital, I felt like I have picked up my torso from the bed and brought it home. I should take care of this body now. I really had never been aware that I do have a body before. The books I read only call our attention to our souls; as a result, the body is simply put aside, and yet the soul apparently failed to make the slightest progress, while the body is deteriorating without notice.... Oh, I have a body. What happened to it? Why did it get a tumor? [77–78]

While White equates "objectification" with "thingification" as a means of social control of persons and their bodies, Xi Xi's "objectifying" is to rediscover the relationship between herself and her body.[69] In fact, her practice reminds us of Foucault's observation of "objectification which transform[s] human beings into subjects."[70] It is through knowing the body as an object that the subject comes into being. For Xi Xi, her subjectivity is gradually reconstructed by the illness experience with which she first feels detached from her corporeal self to observe and study herself, but then such "objectification" becomes a post-existential approach to accept, not to escape, her ailing self.[71] This necessitates "the corporeal gap," as Charon calls and defines it alongside of the autobiographical gap in the telling of the self: "The teller of the self tells of the body of the self.... This corporeal gap places distance between the person of the self and the self's body, especially when it must undergo humiliating or painful manipulations."[72] In terms of distancing, "objectification and alienation are not the same," as a Hong Kong critic distinguishes the two concepts,

69 White and Epston, *Narrative Means to Therapeutic Ends*, 24, 65.

70 Michel Foucault, "The Subject and Power" (1982), trans. R. Hurley et al., in *Michel Foucault: Power, the Essential Works of Michel Foucault 1954–1984*, ed. J.D. Faubion, vol. 3 (London: Penguin, 2001), 326.

71 For a study of post-existentialism with regards to wellbeing and psychoanalysis, see Del Loewenthal, "Introducing Post-Existential Practice: An Approach to Wellbeing in the 21st Century," *Philosophical Practice* 3.3 (Oct. 2008): 316–21.

72 Charon, *Narrative Medicine*, 90.

"objectification is the mind being distanced from the body and examining it; alienation is the body abandoning the mind and dominating over it."[73] Xi Xi is not subdued by her sick body; instead, she tries to textualize it, talk to it, feel it, heal it, and understand it, because it *is* me.

From her ailing body Xi Xi brings our attention to the textual form: "Since when did our art and literature, as well as philosophy separate the soul from the body, and oppose the form with the content?" (140) Tracing the divorce between the psyche and the soma in Chinese and Western philosophies, she laments "the content's discard of the form, the signified in loss of the signifier" (299). Early on in the narrative, while waiting for her first surgery and after being readmitted to the hospital, the author entertains herself and us twice with pages of comparative studies of Gustave Flaubert's *Madame Bovary* and François Rabelais' *Pantagruel and Gargantua*, both in the French original and their English and Chinese translations. Her scrutiny of the texts, typeface, and punctuations serves multiple ends: firstly, it is an effective means of distraction from the preoperational anxiety on the part of the patient; secondly, it is a self-prescription to maintain the preferred life of the writer amidst her surgeon's "disturbances"; thirdly, it is an attempt to transcend her own ill body's imperfection by seeking perfection in the written texts; fourthly, it is an alternation of styles played by the narrator; and fifthly, it is a metafictional reminder for the reader of their act of reading as highlighted in an endnote: "If you only want to learn about breast cancer treatments, don't waste your time, skip to page 115 and read 'Tamoxifen'." (18, 50)[74]

In his commentary on White's applied deconstruction theory, Karl Tomm points out his colleague's exoticizing use of familiar language in unfamiliar, even playful, ways: "Such linguistic novelty opens space for us to become more aware of certain nonconscious aspects of the familiar."[75] Xi Xi's ludic language is found throughout her narrative, such as a glossary of Chinese words under the "sickness" radical 疒 and an imagined letter of rejection from the hospital: "We are very sorry that your liver cannot be translated into readable ultrasound…" (196). When narrative therapy was introduced into Hong Kong in the 2000s, it was understood as "part of the linguistic shift within the humanities and social sciences, which focuses discussion on the language of representation rather

73 Xueying 雪萤, "Rufang ningdi—wo dang ai ziji 乳房凝睇——我当爱自己 [Gazing at the Breast: I Should Love Myself]," *Shun po*, Nov. 11, 1992, 6.

74 Besides *Madame Bovary* and *Pantagruel and Gargantua*, Xi Xi also briefly mentioned Susan Sontag's essay *Illness as Metaphor*, Aleksandr Solzhenitsyn's novel *Cancer Ward*, and Kurosawa Akira's film *To Live* (*Ikiru*).

75 Tomm, "The Courage to Protest," 74.

than the referents or objects themselves."[76] Xi Xi's dictionary of diseases, in particular, is reminiscent of what Foucault discusses about the nominalization of disease under the clinical gaze: in a sense "closer to a philosophy of language, since the form of composition of the being of the disease is of a linguistic type. In relation to the individual, concrete being, disease is merely a name; in relation to the isolated elements of which it is made up, it has all the rigorous architecture of a verbal designation."[77] Yet what most frustrates Xi Xi is her own ignorance about the language of her body:

> My body is getting more and more talkative, ...but the problem is, what is it saying? ... It is very difficult to communicate with people, and even harder to converse with our bodies. There are so many departments, each has its complaints, and the bodily language is divided into different dialects: the bone speech, the muscle speech, and the nerve speech. Ever since the human race built the Tower of Babel, we can no longer talk with each other easily.
>
> With the tumor, my body keeps sending out alarms, but even my doctor did not get them, and I had no idea how to read them. To my own body, I am "illiterate." [301]

Charon also suggests: "It is sometimes as if the body speaks a foreign language, relying on bilingual others to translate, interpret, or in some way make transparent what it means to say."[78] We depend on physicians and biologists, with the help of modern technologies, to translate the bodily language, but even

---

76 Chan, "Narrative Practice with Youth," 197. According to my July 2015 email correspondence with Angela On-kee Tsun 秦安琪, a narrative therapy pioneer in Hong Kong and Director of Center for Youth Research and Practice at Hong Kong Baptist University, Michael White gave his first public lecture there in 2001. It was not until recent years that the Dulwich Center co-directed by White began to send trainers from Adelaide, South Australia, to Beijing and other places in mainland China to conduct workshops.

77 Michel Foucault, *The Birth of the Clinic: An Archaeology of Medical Perception*, trans. A.M. Sheridan Smith (New York: Vintage Books, 1994), 118–19. In his "Framing Disease: Illness, Society, and History," Introduction to *Framing Disease: Studies in Cultural History*, ed. Charles E. Rosenberg and Janet Golden (New Brunswick, N.J.: Rutgers University Press, 1992), xiii, Rosenberg also asserts: "In some ways disease does not exist until we have agreed that it does, by perceiving, naming, and responding to it.... A disease does not exist as a social phenomenon until we agree that it does—until it is named."

78 Charon, *Narrative Medicine*, 87. The same statement also appears later in Charon, "Where Does Narrative Medicine Come From? Drives, Diseases, Attention, and the Body," in Rudnytsky and Charon, *Psychoanalysis and Narrative Medicine*, 30.

"scientific, objective" (302) methods may result in misreading or misinterpretation of symptoms and pains signaled from the body's "unknowable and ungovernable parts"[79] that need retranslation or multiple translations—just like the various renditions of *Madame Bovary* and *Pantagruel and Gargantua*. In a sense, the narrative is a therapeutic translation of the mamma trauma into a better understanding of the body and transition of its life.

Elegy for a Breast ends with a chapter consisting of thirteen masto-images around the world, from the Egyptian pyramids, a symbol of the birth of civilization in a vast desert, to I.M. Pei's 贝聿铭 Louvre Pyramid, a postmodern glass structure in the city of Paris. Contemplating the mamma-shape map of India and a Henry Moore sculpture of a female figure, Xi Xi extends the mourning of her breast humorously to the mastatrophy of the human body and civilization. She laments the commercial appropriation of the Vénus de Milo, in which the ancient Greek statue of Aphrodite's left breast is substituted by a long vertical scar to promote the sale of breast augmentation. It is intriguing to compare the goddess image, which also appears on the cover of the book, with Deena Metzger's postsurgical tattoo across her chest on Bi Shumin's *Save the Breast*: Where the beautified wound of Metzger is a celebration of cancer survival, the exploitive disfigurement of Vénus here is but an advertisement of artificial beauty.

From Bi Shumin's narrative therapy to Xi Xi's narrative *as* therapy, the fictionists play the role of a psycho-/socio-therapist and that of a patient, respectively. While Bi's third-person narrative penetrates the cancer patients' psyches to renew their sense of self in the society and necessitates them the right "to become storytellers in order to recover the voices that illness and its treatment often takes away," as well as the responsibility to become "witness[es] to the conditions that rob others of their voices,"[80] Xi Xi's first-person self-story is a healthy-minded effort that uses writing as medicine to redeem the self from a deadly disease. As the mainland Chinese writer uses group therapy to expand her own pain to social problems, her Hong Kong fellow retreats into herself and brings her literary imagination into play to seek personal relief. In effect, both *Save the Breast* and *Elegy for a Breast* give rise to an alternative narrative form, be it Bi's "new experience" or Xi Xi's experimentalism. When "narrative means to therapeutic ends," therapy also means to narrative ends: At the same time medicine utilizes the practical function of literature as a clinical instrument, it

79 Charon, *Narrative Medicine*, 77.

80 Frank, *The Wounded Storyteller*, xii, xiii.

too opens up the space of fiction—not only by providing the genre with contents but also by revisiting and revising the relation between reading and writing, because the forms of storytelling are our ways of living.[81]

References

Barthes, Roland. *S/Z*. 1970. Trans. Richard Miller. New York: Hill and Wang, 1974.

Besley, A.C. (Tina). "Foucault and the Turn to Narrative Therapy." *British Journal of Guidance and Counselling* 30.2 (2002): 125–43.

Bi Shumin 毕淑敏. *Nü xinlishi* 女心理师 [The Female Psychologist]. 2 vols. Chongqing: Chongqing chubanshe, 2007.

———. *Zhengjiu rufang* 拯救乳房 [Save the Breast]. Beijing: Renmin wenxue chubanshe, 2003.

Chan, Chitat 陈智达. "Narrative Practice with Youth: A Heuristic Case Study on a Youth-Centre Drama Workshop." *Journal of Social Work Practice* 26.2 (June 2012): 197–214.

Charon, Rita. *Narrative Medicine: Honoring the Stories of Illness*. Oxford: Oxford University Press, 2006.

Couser, G. Thomas. *Recovering Bodies: Illness, Disability, and Life Writing*. Madison: University of Wisconsin Press, 1997.

Deng Hanmei 邓寒梅. *Zhongguo xiandangdai wenxue zhong de jibing xushi yanjiu* 中国现当代文学中的疾病叙事研究 [A Study of Illness Narratives in Modern and Contemporary Chinese Literature]. Nanchang: Jiangxi renmin chubanshe, 2012.

Foucault, Michel. *The Birth of the Clinic: An Archaeology of Medical Perception*. Trans. A.M. Sheridan Smith. New York: Vintage Books, 1994.

———. "The Subject and Power." 1982. Trans. R. Hurley, et al. In *Michel Foucault: Power, the Essential Works of Michel Foucault 1954–1984*, vol. 3, ed. J.D. Faubion. London: Penguin, 2001.

Frank, Arthur W. *The Wounded Storyteller: Body, Illness, and Ethics*. Chicago: University of Chicago Press, 1995.

Freud, Sigmund. *Leonardo da Vinci and a Memory of His Childhood*. 1910. Trans. Alan Tyson. New York: W.W. Norton, 1964.

Fu Yonglin 傅用霖, ed. *Yuyue siwang* 预约死亡 [An Appointment with Death]. Beijing: Zuojia chubanshe, 1995.

81 In this sense, narrative as therapy comes close to Roland Barthes' idea and ideal of the "writerly text" (text scriptible) that invites the reader to actively re-author the story. For the concept of "writerly text" in contrast to the conventional "readerly text" (text lisible), see Barthes, *S/Z* (1970), trans. Richard Miller (New York: Hill and Wang, 1974), 4–6.

Gilligan, Stephen, and Reese Price, eds. *Therapeutic Conversations*. New York: W.W. Norton, 1993.

Hawkins, Anne Hunsaker. *Reconstructing Illness: Studies in Pathography*. West Lafayette, Ind.: Purdue University Press, 1993.

He Zhenbang. "Bi Shumin's Stories: Submersed in Reality." Trans. Chen Haiyan. *Chinese Literature* (Spring 1997): 59–62.

Herman, David, Manfred Jahn, and Marie-Laure Ryan, eds. *Routledge Encyclopedia of Narrative Theory*. London: Routledge, 2005.

Ho Fuk Yan 何福仁. "Shuxie de Ajian—du *Aidao rufang* 书写的阿坚——读《哀悼乳房》 [Ah Kien as a Writer: On *Elegy for a Breast*]." *Shun po* 信报 (Hong Kong Economic Journal), Nov. 11, 1992.

Jameson, Fredric. "Third-World Literature in the Era of Multinational Capitalism." *Social Text* 15 (1986): 65–88.

Kleinman, Arthur. *The Illness Narratives: Suffering, Healing, and the Human Condition*. New York: Harper Collins, 1988.

Knight, Sabina. "Cancer's Revelations: Malignancies and Therapies in a Recent Chinese Novel." *Literature and Medicine* 28.2 (Fall 2009): 351–70.

Leung, G.M., et al. "Trends in Breast Cancer Incidence in Hong Kong between 1973 and 1999: An Age-Period-Cohort Analysis." *British Journal of Cancer* 87.9 (Oct. 2002): 982–88. http://www.ncbi.nlm.nih.gov/pmc/articles/PMC2364319/ (accessed May 5, 2014).

Lin Xiu-rong 林秀蓉. *Zhong shen xianying: Taiwan xiaoshuo jibing xushi yihan zhi tanjiu (1929–2000)* 众身显影: 台湾小说疾病叙事意涵之探究 [Developing the Bodies: An Inquiry of the Implications of Illness Narratives in Taiwanese Fiction]. Kaohsiung: Chunhui chubanshe, 2013.

Liu Lili 刘俐俐. *Tuibai yu zhengjiu—Bi Shumin yu yi lei wenxue zhuti* 颓败与拯救——毕淑敏与一类文学主题 [Decline and Salvage: Bi Shumin and a Literary Theme]. Beijing: Huaxia chubanshe, 2000.

Loewenthal, Del. "Introducing Post-Existential Practice: An Approach to Wellbeing in the 21st Century." *Philosophical Practice* 3.3 (Oct. 2008): 316–21.

McDonald, Margaret, Robin P. Hertz, and Susan W. Pitman Lowenthal. "The Burden of Cancer in Asia." *Pfizer Facts*, Dec. 2008, 1–83. http://www.pfizer.com/files/products/cancer_in_asia.pdf (accessed May 5, 2014).

Payne, Martin. *Narrative Therapy: An Introduction for Counsellors*. London: SAGE, 2000.

Ren Xianghong 任向红. "Beimin yu jiudu [shu]—Bi Shumin xiaoshuo *Hong chufang* qianxi 悲悯与救渎[赎]——毕淑敏小说《红处方》浅析 [Sorrowful Sympathy and Rescue: Brief Discussion on *The Red Prescription* Written by Bi Shumin]." *Xibei minzu daxue xuebao (zhexue shehui kexue ban)* 西北民族大學學報 (哲學社會科學版) (Journal of Northwest University for Nationalities [Philosophy and Social Sciences]), 2007, no. 2:104–7.

Ricoeur, Paul. "Life: A Story in Search of a Narrator." Trans. J.N. Kraay and A.J. Scholten. In *Facts and Values: Philosophical Reflections from Western and Non-Western Perspectives*, ed. M.C. Doeser and J.N. Kraay, 121–32. Dordrecht: Martinus Nijhoff, 1986.

Rosenberg, Charles E. "Framing Disease: Illness, Society, and History." Introduction to *Framing Disease: Studies in Cultural History*, ed. Charles E Rosenberg and Janet Golden, xiii–xxvi. New Brunswick, N.J.: Rutgers University Press, 1992.

Rousseau, George Sebastian. Introduction to *Framing and Imagining Disease in Cultural History*, ed. George Sebastian Rousseau, et al., 1–48. New York: Palgrave Macmillan, 2003.

Rudnystsky, Peter L., and Rita Charon, eds. *Psychoanalysis and Narrative Medicine*. Albany: State University of New York Press, 2008.

Sontag, Susan. *Illness as Metaphor and AIDS and Its Metaphors*. New York: Anchor Books, 1990.

Soong, Stephen C. 宋淇. "Building a House: Introducing Xi Xi." 1985. Trans. Kwok-kan Tam 谭国根. In Xi Xi, *A Girl Like Me and Other Stories*, 127–34.

Tomm, Karl. "The Courage to Protest: A Commentary on Michael White's Work." In Gilligan and Price, *Therapeutic Conversations*, 62–80.

Waitzkin, Howard. *The Politics of Medical Encounters: How Patients and Doctors Deal with Social Problems*. New Haven: Yale University Press, 1991.

Wang Meng 王蒙. Preface to *Bi Shumin zixuan jingpin ji* (*xiaoshuo juan*) 毕淑敏自选精品集 (小说卷) [Self-selected Best Works of Bi Shumin: Fiction]. 1995. Beijing: Zhongguo shehui chubanshe, 2002.

Wells, Susan. Our Bodies, Ourselves *and the Work of Writing*. Stanford: Stanford University Press, 2010.

White, Michael. "Deconstruction and Therapy." In Gilligan and Price, *Therapeutic Conversations*, 22–61.

———. *Reflections on Narrative Practice: Essays and Interviews*. Adelaide: Dulwich Centre Publications, 2000.

——— and David Epston. *Narrative Means to Therapeutic Ends*. New York: W.W. Norton, 1990.

Wu Fei 吴菲. "Bi Shumin: Weishenme tuoxie, weishenme fangqi 毕淑敏:为什么妥协,为什么放弃 [Bi Shumin: To Compromise or to Give up]." *Beijing qingnian bao* 北京青年报 (Beijing Youth Daily), May 28, 2003.

Xi Xi 西西. *Aidao rufang* 哀悼乳房 [Elegy for a Breast]. Taipei: Hongfan shudian, 1992.

———. *A Girl Like Me and Other Stories*. 1986. Enlarged ed. Hong Kong: Chinese University of Hong Kong, 1996.

Xu Hong. "Epidemic Heralds Humanistic New Wave." *China Today*, Sept. 2003. http://vod.sxrtvu.edu/englishonline/bjzs/chinatoday/chinatoday2003/20039/9p34.asp (accessed Mar. 30, 2016).

Xueying 雪萤. “Rufang ningdi—wo dang ai ziji 乳房凝睇——我当爱自己 [Gazing at the Breast: I Should Love Myself].” *Shun po*, Nov. 11, 1992.

Yu Hong 于泓. “Qianyi ‘xin tiyan xiaoshuo’ 浅议 ‘新体验小说’ [Brief Remarks on ‘New Experience Fiction’].” *Liaoning shizhuan xuebao* (*shehui kexue ban*) 辽宁师专学报 (社会科学版) (Journal of Liaoning Teachers College [Social Sciences]), 2005, no. 3:41–42.

Zhao, Ping, et al. “Cancer Trends in China.” *Japanese Journal of Clinical Oncology* 40.4 (Jan. 2010): 281–85. http://jjco.oxfordjournals.org/content/40/4/281.full.pdf+html (accessed May 5, 2014).

Zhou Xiaoli 周晓丽. “Bi Shumin de zui xin changpian xiaoshuo *Zhengjiu rufang* 毕淑敏的最新长篇小说《拯救乳房》 [Bi Shumin’s Latest Novel *Save the Breast*].” Interview with Bi Shumin. Renminwang 人民网 (people), Aug. 1, 2003. http://www.people.com.cn/GB/14738/14754/21862/1995449.html (accessed May 27, 2012).

CHAPTER 6

Narrating Cancer, Disabilities, and AIDS: Yan Lianke's Trilogy of Disease*

Shelley W. Chan 陈颖

Since the establishment of the communist government in 1949, especially with the open-door policy that brings rapid economic growth after the Cultural Revolution (1966–76), China has developed tremendously over the past three to four decades. Its recent achievements, including the 2008 Olympic Games, the 2010 Shanghai Expo, China's overtaking Japan to become the second largest economic power, its docking of the nation's first manned spacecraft with a laboratory module in orbit, and its first moon landing, etc., have caught much attention from the rest of the world. As a result, many Chinese people believe that their country has shaken off its humiliating image as the "Sick Man of East Asia," which was the collective anxiety of the Chinese intellectuals in the late nineteenth and early twentieth centuries. Nevertheless, this anxiety is still troubling some Chinese who see present-day China as an unhealthy and even morbid world. Among them is Yan Lianke 阎连科, an award-winning but controversial writer, who is known for using illness to signify reality.[1] For instance, *The New York Times* published his article "On China's State-Sponsored Amnesia" on April 1, 2013, which aroused some socio-political debates.[2] Examining three novels of disease by Yan, namely, *Streams of Light and Time* (*Riguang liunian* 日光流年, 1998), *Pleasure* (*Shouhuo* 受活, 2004),[3] and *Dream of Ding Village* (*Dingzhuang meng* 丁庄梦, 2006), which are about cancer sufferers,

* [A shorter version of this essay was presented at the joint conference of the Association for Asian Studies & International Convention of Asia Scholars in Mar. 2011. Ed.]

1 Born in 1958, Yan Lianke has published important novels and stories and been the recipient of major awards in China and abroad, including the 2000 Lu Xun Literary Prize, 2004 Lao She Literature Award (3rd place novel category), 2011 Man Asian Literary Prize, and 2014 Franz Kafka Prize.

2 See Yan Lianke, "On China's State-Sponsored Amnesia," *The New York Times*, April 1, 2013, http://www.nytimes.com/2013/04/02/opinion/on-chinas-state-sponsored-amnesia.html?pagewanted=all&_r=0. (assessed June 27, 2014).

3 The title of *Shouhuo* is translated by Carlos Rojas as *Lenin's Kisses* (New York: Grove Press, 2012). I personally believe that "pleasure" is closer to the original meaning of the Chinese expression. Hereafter, I will use *Pleasure* in my discussion of the novel and *Lenin's Kisses* in footnotes when Rojas' translation is cited.

 | DOI 10.1163/9789004319219_008

physical disabilities, and HIV patients respectively, this essay investigates how Yan sees humans' hopeless struggle with fate as well as with absurd phenomena, including lust, greed and corruption, in the grotesque post-Mao China through writing about illnesses. These stories show how, according to the stern satirist, the nightmare of being a sick man is still haunting the nation.

Cancer: The Fate of Failure

Streams of Light and Time is about the inhabitants of Three-Surname Village (Sanxingcun 三姓村) who fight a fatal disease, throat block syndrome (*houdu zheng* 喉堵症) or, according to Chien-hsin Tsai, esophageal cancer that limits their lives to forty years of age.[4] The novel is a story about the Sisyphean efforts of four village heads to make their people outlive the age of forty: Du Sang 杜桑, Sima Xiaoxiao 司马笑笑, Lan Baisui 蓝百岁, and Sima Lan 司马蓝, with the last one being the protagonist. These efforts include encouraging birth to make new lives outnumber the dead; eating rape (*youcai* 油菜); and turning up the topsoil of the whole village, hoping that crops from the new soil will change their fate. Unfortunately, all these efforts prove to be in vain. When it comes to Sima Lan, he firmly believes that it is the water that has caused this lethal disease, and so he decides to dig a canal to lead water from about thirty miles away. Ironically, when the canal is completed, the supposedly life-saving water is seriously polluted and of no use at all. Eventually Sima Lan dies on his fortieth birthday.

Exemplifying the author's inheritance of medical narratives of the major May Fourth writers, such as Lu Xun 鲁迅 (1881–1936), Yu Dafu 郁达夫 (1896–1945), and Ba Jin 巴金 (1904–2005), who aim to bring the readers' attention to the collective social reality by writing about the individual biological reality, *Streams of Light and Time* makes itself a metaphor for disease, turning Three-Surname Village into a miniature of the society and revealing the negative side of human beings through displaying the poor health and miserable lives of the villagers.

Three-Surname Village, a remote rural community that can hardly be found on a map, is located in the barren Balou 耙耧 Mountains in Henan 河南 province of central China. Although this forgotten place is untouched by nationwide political turmoil, it is far from a utopia. Nobody from other villages is willing

4 Chien-hsin Tsai, "In Sickness or in Health: Yan Lianke and the Writing of Autoimmunity," *Modern Chinese Literature and Culture* 23.1 (Spring 2011): 91.

to marry anyone from Three-Surname Village for fear of cancer. Gradually it becomes a totally isolated place, and its inhabitants live in extreme poverty. In order to collect money for their fate-changing projects, the poor villagers sell their own bodies, the only properties they own, to buy necessary tools. While men sell their skins to a hospital specializing in healing burn patients, women engage in prostitution in the city. Here are how the men's legs look like:

> Scars covered them from the groin to the knees, where thin slices of skins had been cut off and sold, altogether over ten pieces. The big ones were the size of a palm, and the small ones about that of an oak leaf, one piece after another, full of bumps and holes like red tree tumors and watery bruises.[5]

When the villagers' legs look like tree trunks and their skins are similar to barks, they cease to be humans; instead, they are turned into things, objectified and degraded. Yet selling their skins is just a routine activity in their lives; at times it is even joyful as they would be a bit "rich" to keep a small amount of money for themselves. As a result, selling of skins becomes a carnival of celebrating pain and suffering, the only effective measures to defer the early appointment with death. They indeed should be celebrated as they can bring hope to people, even though this kind of celebration leads to a pathetically twisted and diseased reality.

While male villagers are obligated to make contributions, women make equal sacrifices to the life-prolonging projects, especially the female protagonist, Lan Sishi 蓝四十, the lover of Sima Lan. Lan Sishi is sacrificed when her father serves as the village head, in accordance with the belief that a virgin should be sent to sleep with a leader from the commune, so he will send manpower to the village to help with turning up the topsoil. Later when Sima Lan needs money to have surgery in a city hospital, Lan Sishi is sacrificed again by being asked to engage in prostitution in the city. Being forced to violate her body again and again, this woman, like the male villagers, is objectified and downgraded to a state of non-human. Eventually, not only does the violation harm her body, but it also destroys her desire to continue her life. When Sima Lan goes to her home one day, he finds her dead in her bed—in fact, she has killed herself:

5 Yan Lianke, *Riguang liunian* 日光流年 [Streams of Light and Time] (Shenyang: Chunfeng wenyi chubanshe, 2004), 240; my translation.

> ...he looked at the lower part of her body, between her legs that used to be powder-like white but now looked a dull green, at the thin and seductive light blue panties. Being stabbed five, six or seven times, or even ten or twenty times, with a pair of scissors that gleamed coldly, the front part of the panties had become a red honeycomb; flesh and blood brimming over from the honeycomb formed a withered yet blooming peony... he...started taking off her panties, ...blood had formed a kind of heavy blackness on the light blue underpants. When the blackish underpants were peeled off from her body, ...he looked at her private parts carefully and saw white particulate matter as if there were a pot of flourishing but crumbled white flowers. He stared at the flower and finally understood—
>
> She was infected with venereal disease from the business of selling her body.[6]

This graphic and disturbing scene as well as the description of the scar-covered legs mentioned above demonstrate the damaged bodies of the villagers. Paradoxically, when they are trying very hard to prolong their lives, they are actually harming their bodies. The Confucian teaching does not seem to be remembered in this poverty-stricken village: "Our bodies—from a single hair to a bit of skin—are derived from our parents, we must not in the least injure or wound them. This is the beginning of filial piety."[7] To impair one's body would be considered unfilial, a very serious misconduct according to the Chinese tradition. Nevertheless, the strong will of longevity motivates the villagers to do anything to fight the disease, including hurting their bodies, enduring pains, even losing chastity and life. Consequently, it seems that to outlive the age of forty becomes an ultimate yet empty and abstract goal, which is in lack of spiritual and corporeal supports. When living is for the sake of living only, it is no longer living but merely existing.

The most primitive concern of basic existence is the antithetical pair, life and death, which is powerfully described by the author. In the last chapter of the novel, under the leadership of Du, villagers are encouraged to have as many children as possible. Therefore, the entire village is busy at night when

---

6 Ibid., 120–21.

7 Liu Ruixiang 刘瑞祥 and Lin Zhihe 林之鹤, trans., *The Classic of Filial Piety* (Ji'nan: Shangdong Friendship Press, 1993), 3. This Confucian teaching is also quoted while discussing Yan Lianke's fiction of disease in Deng Hanmei 邓寒梅, *Zhongguo xiandangdai wenxue zhong de jibing xushi yanjiu* 中国现当代文学中的疾病叙事研究 [A Study of Illness Narratives in Modern and Contemporary Chinese Literature] (Nanchang: Jiangxi renmin chubanshe, 2012), 292.

every married man is trying to make his wife pregnant. A few months later, almost all married women are pregnant, and the scene of so many bulging bellies forms a unique landscape in the village. Before long all these women are in labor almost at the same time, and the whole village is filled with the smell of amniotic fluid. Sima Lan leads his hungry child-followers to go after the smell to get milk from the new mothers. The author's descriptions of the bedroom noise from different houses, the image of a large group of pregnant women's big bellies, the strong smells of sex, amniotic fluid and milk, and the army formed by starving children looking for milk paint a surrealistic yet lively picture that demonstrates the determination of the villagers to compete with death and to sustain the survival of their community.

As a major part of the villagers' lives, death is depicted in all five chapters. While the reader is astonished by how lightly death is treated due to its frequent occurrence, the death scene is particularly unforgettable in Chapter Four, which is about the story of Sima Xiaoxiao, the second village head. A big famine forces him to make a very cruel decision: to sacrifice the lives of handicapped children, so as to save food for the rest of the families. In order to set an example for his villagers, he takes the lead to abandon his three dwarf sons. Following his example, other families also give up their unhealthy kids, and altogether twenty-four disabled or just physically deformed children, including a boy suffering from polio, a mute child, and a harelip and single-eyed boy, are dumped into a valley far away from the village. While most of them die of starvation there and their corpses are eaten by crows, some are actually pecked to death.

This episode reminds the reader of Imamura Shōhei's 今村昌平 *The Ballad of Narayama* (*Narayama bushikō* 楢山节考, 1983), a film about a nineteenth-century remote Japanese village in which there is a rule that every person reaching the age of seventy must be sent to Mountain Narayama, where they are starved to death. This way they save food for the rest of the village to survive the extremely harsh living conditions. Both Yan's novel and Imamura's film showcase how human life can be degraded to the most primal existence or animal instinct and invite the reader/audience to ponder the fundamental concern of humankind, except that the death scene in Yan's novel is more disturbing because of its vivid depiction of the process of starvation and how the abandoned children's bodies are destroyed by crows. If the rule to sacrifice the aged in the Japanese film could be justified by the argument that elderly people are close to the end of their lives anyway, the abandonment of children in the Chinese fiction is an even more unacceptable destruction of the young. It lays bare the brutality behind the decision of who should live and who should die: it is all right for a group of "normal" people to live at the cost of a "less valuable" group or children of a lesser god.

When Sima Lan and his little friends found their handicapped siblings and playmates in the valley, most of them are already long dead. The children kill some crows and bring home the dead birds for food. So the adults also rush to the valley to get the crows that are eating their abandoned children, and crow meat enables the village to live on for some time before they once again lack food. While explicit cannibalism occurs in the village, this crow-eating behavior is in fact implicit cannibalism. The reader is hinted that the food shortage in the village is part of the large-scale famine attacking the whole country during the Great Leap Forward period (1958–60). Eventually, Sima Xiaoxiao makes another unbelievable decision: he kills himself in the valley to attract crows, so his villagers can have some more meat. The given name of this village chief is an irony: Xiao 笑 means "to smile/laugh," yet nothing in his life worthy of a smile or laugh about.

When Chinese people talk about the lot common to all people, four problems are always mentioned, namely, birth, agedness, illness, and death (*sheng lao bing si* 生老病死), but for the people of the Three-Surname Village, old age is missing from their life cycle. A piece of long, white beard left by an old passer-by becomes the motivation and a totemic item for Sima Xiaoxiao and his successors, symbolizing their dream and mission of leading the villagers to counteract cancer and reach an old age. Interestingly, while cancer serves to push the development of the story, the efforts they make are analogous to human bodily treatments; in other words, the whole story is in fact a medical discourse. While eating rape can be regarded as taking herbal medicine, the discarding of the topsoil—the first layer of the earth—is like the male villagers selling their skins. At last, when water is believed to be the key element for the villagers' health, the importation of new water is similar to blood transfusion or dialysis. When these efforts all fail, the disease is incurable and the villagers fall into an irredeemable predicament.

Diseases are traditionally believed to be punishments from the Heaven to the unhealthily ruled society, and the incurability of cancer will finally cause the village to be eliminated by the law of survival of the fittest. At this point the narrative on the surface level, i.e., the plots of disease, bears moral judgments that lead to an in-depth narrative level: a metaphor for the diseased community signifying the suffering of the villagers as well as the defects of the leaders, such as their selfishness and dishonesty in their strong desire for power, especially when they obtain power at the cost of the happiness, health, and chastity of their women. Ironically, they believe that once they have power they will be able to carry out an effective project to save the community, yet their passion or love for power itself is morbid. As a result, despite their determination to fight cancer, their flaws in morality make everything they do—all the symbolic medical treatments—undependable and ineffective.

As for the structure of the novel, the story of *Streams of Light and Time* is told in a reverse style. It is, however, not a simple flashback; instead, the entire structure is reversed. It is still in a linear order, but the order is regressive rather than progressive. It is a return—returning from the end to the beginning, from the effect to the cause, and from death to birth. Of the five chapters, the first one tells the story of the last village head, Sima Lan. The opening sentence of the book announces that Sima Lan is going to die; then the story goes on to relate his efforts of getting water from outside, his romance with Lan Sishi, and eventually their deaths. Chapters Two, Three, and Four return to the stories of the previous leaders, including Sima Lan as an ambitious young man who aims to become the village leader, then as a teenager, and finally as a child. In Chapter Five, both Sima Lan and Lan Sishi are newborn babies. The novel ends with Sima Lan in his mother's womb getting ready to come out to see the world and hearing people outside looking for his father to welcome his birth. Following the reversed flow of the story is like watching a rewinding video. By telling the end of the story in the beginning, the pessimistic attitude of the novelist is revealed by this special structure: Sima Lan's efforts as well as those of the other village leaders are doomed to failure, and Sima Lan himself is unable to outlive the age of forty. Keeping this result in mind, readers have no hope at all when reading on. The more one reads, the more depressed one gets, as one only reads on to find out how they fail, never experiencing the suspense of wondering whether they will be successful or not. By using this narrative method, the writer offers neither hope nor future for the characters; rather, they always live in the shadow of yesterday, in fear of cancer and death.

Furthermore, some carefully arranged details are very sophisticated. For instance, the name of Lan Baisui is as ironic as that of Sima Xiaoxiao discussed above, and the names of Sima Lan and Lan Sishi have rich meanings.[8] That the given name of the boy and the surname of the girl are the same character *lan* 蓝 implies the close connection between them: their lives, love, and death. The personal name of the woman is Sishi 四十, meaning "forty." It sounds like a curse as this is the ultimate age limit of the villagers, and Sima Lan, the man she loves, dies on the day he reaches forty no matter how much he wishes to transgress this limit. Another example is the underpants Lan Sishi wears when she is engaged in prostitution. There is a purely white lotus flower on the garment, symbolizing her purity and her strong love of Sima Lan though she is sleeping with other men. This white blossom is echoed by the "withered yet blooming peony" and the "flourished but crumbled white flowers" on her private parts in her death scene quoted above, creating a thrilling image of

8 Baisui literally means "hundred-year-old," suggesting a wish for longevity.

disease. Finally, the ending and the beginning of the novel echo each other very skillfully. At the end of the last chapter, as Sima Lan is about to be born, Yan writes: "In the tea-like womb, Sima Lan smiles a crispy and sparkling smile like a silver needle dropping to the ground, and then he squeezes his head and face out to join this world."[9] The first sentence of the book reads: "Bang! Sima Lan is going to die."[10] In the ordinary world, a newborn baby should be the symbol of hope; yet Yan uses the new life not to give a hopeful, happy ending, but to let this new life be predestinated to get a deadly disease—esophageal cancer—and the hopelessness of this new life is foretold in the very beginning. Consequently, death and life form a powerful dialogue, with death in absolute control in such a deftly fabricated story, a story that can be read as an allegory of modern China, a sick man who is fated to die if no right medicine is found for him. In fact, that the attempted salvation of this sick man is narrated in a grand narrative where absurd occurrences such as the Great Leap Forward and the astonishingly large-scale pollution exist gives the reader hints of the novelist's pessimistic view.

Disabilities: The Displayability of Deformity

Pleasure is set in Pleasure Village, another poor village in the Balou Mountains.[11] This is a highly marginalized rural community due to its remote location and the particularity of its population: most of the villagers are either physically or mentally handicapped. Because of its isolation and inaccessibility, this village remains an autonomous utopia until it falls victim to the daydreams of a local leader. Liu Yingque 柳鷹雀, the County Chief and a man driven by an extreme political fever, has an absurd plan to purchase the corpse of Lenin from Russia, and he collects money from local people to build a Lenin Memorial Hall similar to the Chairman Mao Memorial Hall in Beijing. He believes that this will attract tourists to the area and help its development, so he will gain favor with his boss and guarantee his career. Liu is an orphan raised by a schoolteacher who teaches him how to read and write. Due to his humble background, Liu is particularly hungry for power that will help him climb to the top of the hierarchy. What he desires is not only fame but also the submission of and worship

9 Yan, *Riguang liunian*, 551.

10 Ibid., 3.

11 Pleasure Village is translated as Liven in Rojas' English rendition, *Lenin's Kisses*. For the sake of maintaining the irony in the dual dimension of utopia and dystopia in its original meaning, I use Pleasure Village in my discussion of this novel.

from his people, or to be precise, his subordinates. After promising each family a new house and almost everything for free, including children's education, he naturally becomes the local people's god, and they post his picture next to those of Buddha, the Kitchen God, and Chairman Mao.

With the aim of collecting money to realize his farcical dream, Liu organizes two special-skill troupes consisting of disabled villagers from Pleasure Village and starts performing tours of the city. Pleasure Village has a population of one hundred and ninety-seven people, and the majority are disabled. Among them thirty-five are blind, forty-seven are deaf and dumb, more than fifty are lacking either a leg or an arm, and about a dozen are mentally challenged; in other words, the traditionally so-called "healthy" people, or *yuanquanren* 圆全人 'wholers' in the local dialect, are less than one seventh of the population. Ironically, such a special village, supposedly less productive due to its limited labor force, becomes the major source of Chief Liu's fund raising because of the villagers' "special skills," which actually differentiate and marginalize them from the "normal" people. For instance, a one-legged young man races with a healthy person, a single-eyed man threads eight to ten needles at one time, and a paralyzed woman does beautiful embroidery on a small leaf, etc. In this way, they are making money by displaying their disabilities.

Physical disability is not like illnesses such as tuberculosis (TB) or cancer that, according to Susan Sontag, are "understood as diseases of passion," and are mostly internal.[12] Sontag points out that "fever in TB was a sign of an inward burning," and that "according to the mythology of cancer, it is generally a steady repression of feeling that causes the disease."[13] The internality of TB and cancer often leads to a death sentence, especially in the past. Physical disability, however, no matter what it is caused by, is external and usually not life threatening. As a result, unlike the sensational and romantic TB, physical disability is more practical: since it is not life threatening, the patients must develop viability that allows them to maintain their dignity as independent human beings. However, the outward nature of their disabilities increases its displayability, and to demonstrate their skills is to highlight their deformity. In effect, special skills that they use to defend their self-respect are turned into measures that offend it. Moreover, some of the performances are not about their special skills but something merely for the purpose of singling out their disabilities to please the audience. For example, a polio boy squeezes his undeveloped and deformed foot into a bottle, and a deaf man lights a big firecracker by his ear.

12 Susan Sontag, *Illness as Metaphor and AIDS and Its Metaphors* (New York: Anchor Books, 1990), 20.

13 Ibid., 20, 22.

By so doing, the performers of the special-skill troupes are actually no more than trained monkeys in human clothes. Their bodies are grotesque, but not in the sense of the Bakhtinian carnivalesque disruption of social hierarchies. Instead, this is the modern Chinese version of the nineteenth-century American freak shows. The first "freak," Joice Heth, a "black, old, toothless, blind, crippled slave woman," was displayed in Philadelphia in 1853.[14] Freaks exhibited in other shows include dwarfs, giants, and the handicapped. One of the illustrations of the Circus World Museum in Baraboo, Wisconsin reads thus: "The freak show stage brought together people whose bodies could signify the enormous, the miniature, the exotic, the excessive, the lacking, the profuse, the indeterminate, or the alien to produce a motley chorus line of physical difference that made the onlookers' bodies seem ordinary and banal by comparison."[15] Another illustration from the same museum tells us that "freaks made from people with congenital disabilities usually performed mundane tasks in alternative modes choreographed to amaze audiences."[16]

Mary Klages has pointed out: "Disability in various forms has always existed both as a particular physical condition for individuals and as a cultural sign or signifier, a condition operating within a semiotic system and having reference or meaning to ideas beyond the existence of the individual."[17] In both the nineteenth-century American freak shows and the special-skill troupes of *Pleasure*, disability in different forms can be interpreted as a reference to understand and highlight the meaning of healthiness. The performers and audiences are in a binary opposition between normality and abnormality. Scholars believe that freak "exhibits challenged audiences not only to classify and explain what they saw, but to relate the performance to themselves, to American individual and collective identity," and "to the masses what science was to the emerging elite: an opportunity to formulate the self in terms of what it was not."[18] The Chinese word for "disabled" is *canfei* 残废, literally meaning "incomplete and useless." However, these "incomplete and useless" performers of the special-skill troupes show great abilities, which are beyond the imagination of the "complete and useful" audiences. To see how dis-abled abnormality is more capable than normality must be something very exciting:

---

14 See Rosemarie Garland Thomson, *Extraordinary Bodies: Figuring, Physical, Disability in American Culture and Literature* (New York: Columbia University Press, 1997), 59.

15 Ibid.

16 Ibid.

17 Mary Klages, *Woeful Afflictions: Disability and Sentimentality in Victorian America* (Philadelphia: University of Pennsylvania Press, 1999), 10.

18 Thomson, *Extraordinary Bodies*, 58–59.

> Everyone went crazy.
>
> No one could believe there was a performance troupe consisting entirely of blind and deaf people, cripples and mutes, together with people who were missing a limb or had an extra finger, and little nins less than three feet tall....
>
> There was not a single event in the entire performance that people could believe.
>
> The more unbelievable the performances seemed, the more audiences flocked to see them, to the point that every home, factory, and office closed its doors and its inhabitants or workers went to watch. The price of an admission ticket rose from three hundred to five hundred yuan....[19]

In order to further impress the audience so as to make more money, the performers even intentionally hurt their own bodies. For instance, the one-legged young man performs long jumps over a fire so his limb gets burned and big blisters emerge; the polio boy wearing a glass bottle as his shoe purposely breaks the bottle so the glass cuts his foot and it bleeds; the deaf man lights an especially big firecracker by his ear so that his face is burned. Seeing blood on the bodies of the performers, the urban audience, crazy about the exotic performance, is willing to pay more. After the polio boy broke the bottle, "the audience could clearly see the blood flowing out from under his foot. The audience would break into loud applause. The Polio Boy became even less concerned with the pain in his foot. He subsequently began to earn more and more money each month."[20] The relationship between the audience and the performers is in fact that between consumers and goods. Consuming the deformity of these handicapped people, Yan's audience not only shares the numbness of Lu Xun's spectators of decapitation, who stand around the Chinese man to be executed by the Japanese as seen in a slideshow, but also joins the spectators in "The True Story of Ah Q" ("A Q zhengzhuan" 阿Q正传) who cheer about other people's misfortune. Unfortunately, being exploited and consumed, the disabled do not have the consciousness to defend their dignity as human beings. On the contrary, their dignity gives way to their desire for wealth. They are all ill: Chief Liu, his performers, and their audience. While Liu is suffering from an obsessive lust for power, the villagers internalize their physical, outward imperfection and turn it into feverish money worship. In the meantime, by enjoying and consuming the misshapenness and pain of others, the audience

19 Yan, *Lenin's Kisses*, 257.

20 Ibid., 259.

becomes the target of Yan's criticism, echoing Lu Xun's condemnation of a physically healthy but spiritually ill people.

Eventually, the absurdity develops to an extreme when Liu's illusionary bubble breaks: the handicapped performers are robbed of all the money they have made in the city, and some young girls are raped. Liu is regarded as a madman who suffers from "political insanity" by the provincial governor and loses all he has gained.[21] At the end he intentionally gets hit by a car and cripples himself, so as to be allowed to reside in Pleasure Village as a member of the community. The "becoming disabled" of Liu is both ironic and paradoxical. As the local leader and an "able-bodied wholer,"[22] Liu used the physically handicapped people as a tool to satisfy his fantasy, which finally made him a mentally disabled madman. Not until he becomes one of the handicapped and loses the wholeness of his body does he regain his mental wholeness; in other words, by becoming physically incomplete Liu regains his mental completeness. What is equally paradoxical is that Pleasure Village is employed as a metaphor for the sick society first, and later, when it returns to the previous utopian state, it becomes a symbol of hope. The villagers are first victims to and later saviors of their god, Chief Liu.

The structure of the book also indicates a paradox of wholeness and incompleteness, just as the structure of *Streams of Light and Time* embodies the tension between life and death. The novel consists of eight odd-numbered books (*juan* 卷) and each book has several chapters (*zhang* 章). On the one hand, except for two books, the main story is supplemented by "further readings" (*xuyan* 絮言). Serving as notes, these further readings either explain certain dialectal terms or add history to the story to make it more complete. On the other hand, the author uses only odd numbers for all the books, chapters, and notes, and intentionally skips the even numbers. In addition, the original Chinese novel was published in a way that only odd page numbers appear in the book. According to the English translator of the novel, Yan "explains that the work's discontinuous numbering expresses the tragic sentiment of the novel as a whole (since in China odd numbers are considered inauspicious)."[23] The tragic sentiment indeed adds a heavy tone of irony to the title of the novel as well as the name of the village: Pleasure.

21 Ibid., 444.

22 Ibid., 470.

23 Carlos Rojas, "Translator's Note," in Yan, *Lenin's Kisses*, viii.

AIDS: The Epidemic of Economy

Adding to *Pleasure* and *Streams of Light and Time*, in 2006 Yan Lianke published an equally, if not more, disturbing novel, *Dream of Ding Village*, to complete what I would call his trilogy of illness. If *Pleasure* is like a Van Gogh painting full of grotesque insanity, *Dream of Ding Village*, like *Streams of Light and Time*, is another macabre story filled with depictions of death:

> *They died like falling leaves.*
>
> *Their light extinguished, gone from this world.*
>
> ...for the past two years, people in the village had been dying. Not a month went by without at least one death, and nearly every family had lost someone. After more than forty deaths in the space of two years, the graves in the village cemetery were as dense as sheaves of wheat in a farmer's field.... *Died like falling leaves, their light gone from the world....*[24]

Similar to Three-Surname Village and Pleasure Village, Ding Village is another poor community in Henan. The story is about how villagers engage in the infamous "blood economy" (*xuejiang jingji* 血浆经济) and get infected with AIDS. The first-person narrator is a twelve-year-old dead boy, who was poisoned by the angry villagers. His father, Ding Hui 丁辉, is a blood head, who collects blood from his fellow villagers and sells it to blood stations.

Despite the title, the story of *Dream of Ding Village* is a realistic reflection of the tragedy that occurred in China. In the mid-1990s, the local government promoted a policy to "shake off poverty and attain prosperity" (*tuo pin zhi fu* 脱贫致富) and urged poor people to make money by selling their blood. They called this the "blood economy" and believed that this policy would make "the people rich and the nation strong" (*min fu guo qiang* 民富国强). However, the blood economy proved to be the most absurd joke and the main reason of a terrible outbreak. According to Dr. Gao Yaojie 高耀洁, China's most outspoken AIDS activist, this "blood economy" was a "blood disaster" (*xuehuo* 血祸) and "national calamity" (*guonan* 国难).[25] With the increase of donors, more and more public and private blood stations mushroomed, and the hygienic

24 Yan Lianke, *Dream of Ding Village*, trans. Cindy Carter (New York: Grove Press, 2009), 9; original italics.

25 See Gao Yaojie, *Gaojie de linghun: Gao Yaojie huiyilu* 高洁的灵魂:高耀洁回忆录 [A Noble and Unsullied Soul: Gao Yaojie's Memoirs], revised and enlarged ed. (Hong Kong: Ming Pao, 2010), 177.

standards in the process of blood drawing and plasma production were not strictly controlled, leading to the outbreak of an AIDS epidemic, exactly the same situation as described in *Dream of Ding Village*.[26]

People in the West usually believe that AIDS often comes from homosexual communities. As Susan Sontag points out,

> Indeed, to get AIDS is precisely to be revealed…as a member of certain "risk group," a community of pariahs. The illness flushes out an identity that might have remained hidden from neighbors, job-mates, family, friends. It also confirms an identity and, among the risk group in the United States most severely affected in the beginning, homosexual men, has been a creator of community as well as an experience that isolates the ill and exposes them to harassment and persecution.[27]

However, the identity is different in Yan's writing of AIDS in the Chinese context, though gay people in China are also treated as a "risk group." Yan's novel discloses a fact that the authorities would rather not face, and that is why *Dream of Ding Village* was once banned in China. Scholars believe that "not only is AIDS writing a literary act involving conscious decisions about what to say or what not to say and how to couch what is said, but that writing about that writing is also a political act."[28] The novelist visited the AIDS village in his hometown in Henan seven times, and he also communicated with Dr. Gao. He was driven by an impulse to write something for the victims of the "blood economy," in spite of the fact that many Chinese are misled to think that AIDS is always related to homosexuality and sexual promiscuity; in other words, AIDS has been turned into a metaphor for (im)morality. As Gao points out, "people generally believe that AIDS is one kind of 'moral disease' (*daodebing* 道德病) as a result of the immoral life style of the patients. They [believe that AIDS sufferers] have only themselves to blame; other people, including the government, have no responsibility for it."[29] Yan's literary writing, however,

---

26 See Wang Jinping 王晋平, "Chongwen xuejiang jingji he aizibing de hunluan shidai—yi shi wei jian 重温血浆经济和爱滋病的混乱时代—以史为鉴 [A Review of the Chaotic Times of the Blood Economy and AIDS: Benefit from History]," *Huanqiu shibao* 环球时报 (Global Times), Oct. 31, 2008, http://www.haodf.com/zhuanjiaguandian/wangjinping_22943.htm (accessed June 28, 2014).

27 Sontag, *Illness as Metaphor and AIDS and Its Metaphors*, 112–13.

28 Suzanne Poirier, Introduction to *Writing AIDS: Gay Literature, Language, and Analysis*, ed. Timothy F. Murphy and Suzanne Poirier (New York: Columbia University Press, 1993), 5.

29 Gao, *Gaojie de linghun*, 342.

boldly discloses the fact that in China many HIV patients are victims of the "blood economy," for which the government must take responsibility.

Some critics compare *Dream of Ding Village* with Camus' *The Plague*. Yet Yan's work is darker than that of Camus, because Camus' characters are not as hopeless as those created by Yan. Ding Hui is an out and out bloodsucker. He makes big money by collecting and selling his fellow villagers' blood, including that of his own brother, who is unfortunately later infected and dies. Then Ding Hui makes a fortune by selling coffins provided by the government, which are meant to be distributed to the dead for free. Even worse, this blood head who will do anything to make money starts a new business—arranging marriages, not between living people but between the dead. He even sells the remains of his own son—the twelve-year-old boy—to the dead daughter of a local leader. This way he becomes a relative of the leader, directly connecting himself to the authority and power. Eventually, this greedy and evil man is killed by his own father, who wants to avenge the victims. This can be read as a victory of morality that Ding Hui's father wishes to uphold over the father-son bond, an important Confucian family ethic.[30] If AIDS is regarded as a moral disease implying the immoral behavior of the patients, the killing of Ding Hui by his own father is an attempt to eliminate the cause of immorality and give the reputation back to the victims of the blood economy. When it comes to the characters inside the quarantine (all AIDS patients live in a deserted school of the village), the patients are equally hopeless, displaying the dark side of human nature: they steal, they cheat, they lie, they fight for power, and they publicly humiliate adulterers. It is not so much the illness as their evil human nature that makes these people ugly and repulsive. Like Pleasure Village, the entire Ding Village is also physically and spiritually ill. While the quarantined town in Camus' *The Plague* is finally opened again and people are able to reunite with their loved ones, Ding Village becomes a dead world, and the neighboring villages are also deserted; no humans or animals are seen, and no trees or wooden furniture are left—all are used for making coffins. Interestingly, the word AIDS (*aizibing* 爱滋病) is not as frequently mentioned as the term "fever disease" (*rebing* 热病) throughout the novel. *Rebing* not only refers to the fever associated with AIDS, but also signifies people's irrational and crazy materialistic desire, hence an absurd and ill-practiced modernization. One of the basic goals of the Chinese Communist Party was to overthrow bureaucratic capitalism. Ironically, the postrevolutionary ruling party continues the unfinished cause of capitalism in

30 Deng Hanmei believes that Ding Hui's father has transcended the affection between father and son when he kills his son with the "stick of justice" (*zhengyi de gunbang* 正义的棍棒). See Deng, *Zhongguo xiandangdai wenxue zhong de jibing xushi yanjiu*, 224.

China in the high fever of materialistic modernization through a market blood economy.

As noted above, *Dream of Ding Village* is narrated by a twelve-year-old boy whose omnipresent child's point of view should have served to reduce the heaviness of the narrative. To the contrary, however, the facts that he is a dead boy, who was poisoned by the villagers out of hatred toward his father, and that later he falls victim of the death marriage arranged by his own father make the narrative rather disturbing. At the same time, the narrator's grandfather, an important character contributing to the experimental structure of the book, deserves some discussion. The structure of the novel is a mixture of reality and dreams, the dreams of the narrator's grandfather who can foretell life and death. "Dream" appears in the title and is also the full content of Volume 1, which consists of three short dreams: "The Cupbearer's Dream," "The Baker's Dream," and "The Pharaoh's Dream."[31] In fact, the dreams are part of and yet more eye-catching than reality when they are printed in boldface and in a different font. To be precise, the narrative is often boldfaced and set in a special font throughout the entire book, mostly for Grandpa's dreams, and sometimes for something else, such as the lyrics of songs an AIDS patient sings to entertain the villagers, the regulations set for the patients by two men who take over power from Grandpa, and the notes indicating Grandpa has lost position. In addition, it also includes the whole section of how the twelve-year-old first-person narrator is arranged to marry the County Governor's dead daughter and his screams: "**Save me, Grandpa, save me...**," "**Grandpa, don't let them take me**,"[32] and how eventually Grandpa kills his own son to end the latter's sinful businesses. The most noticeable boldfaced sentences that are repeated several times in the novel are: "**They died like falling leaves. Their light extinguished, gone from this world**." This way the message of death is conveyed with the utmost gravity. By making parts of the real illusory and imaginary, the author adds an artistic dimension to the story, creating a wider and deeper blurred space between reality and unreality, and highlighting the absurdity of the blood economy and human greediness.

Paralleled to the evil force represented by Ding Hui, the image of Grandpa who always has a sense of guilt embodies a sober force to counteract the shocking irrationality. From the beginning, Grandpa constantly urges his son to apologize to the villagers for selling their blood and causing the "fever disease." When Ding Hui keeps refusing to apologize, Grandpa mobilizes all AIDS

31 Ibid., 3.
32 Ibid., 321.

victims to move into the village school as quarantine and volunteers to take care of them. Everything he does is an attempt to redeem his son. Grandpa's act to end Ding Hui's life suggests that evil will not prevail over the good. An ultimate hope is revealed at the end in the last dream of Grandpa, in which he sees

> *a woman, digging in the mud with the branch of a willow tree. With each flick of the branch, each stroke of the willow she raised a small army of tiny mud people from the soil. Soon there were hundreds upon thousands of them, thousands upon millions, millions upon millions of tiny mud people leaping from the soil, dancing on the earth, blistering the plain like so many raindrops from the sky.*
>
> *Grandpa found himself gazing at a new and teeming plain.*
>
> *A new world danced before his eyes.*[33]

After the death of the old world, a freshly created new world emerges with new people dancing before the eyes of Grandpa, the representative of the positive force. Undoubtedly, such an ending brings some hope to the reader to compensate for the heaviness and darkness of the story.

Narrating: The Strategy of Self-censorship

Sontag believes: "Plagues are invariably regarded as judgments on society, ...to be described as punishments not just of individuals but of a group...."[34] Yan's trilogy is what Sontag might call "interpret[ation of a]...catastrophic epidemic as a sign of moral laxity or political decline."[35] As Yan claims in an interview: "When I wrote about AIDS, I did not write so much about the physical

---

33 Ibid., 341; italics in the English rendition. The woman can be related to Nüwa 女娲, the legendary Chinese goddess who created human beings. Here I would like to point out a discrepancy between my reading and that of the translator. While the dreams are printed in boldface and a different font in the Chinese text, they are printed in italics in the translation. The very last one-sentence paragraph is not boldfaced in the original Chinese text, but in the same font as the non-dream parts of the novel. This indicates the author's belief in the certainty that a brand new world will be created by Nǚwa. In the translation, however, this last paragraph is also italicized, treating it as part of the dream and conveying a totally different message.

34 Sontag, *Illness as Metaphor and AIDS and Its Metaphors*, 142.

35 Ibid.

body as about the epidemic in people's minds."[36] One commonality in these three novels makes them cross-referential to one another: they are all about selling—skin, blood, and bodies. AIDS in *Dream of Ding Village* and disabilities in *Pleasure* are not used so much as markers of judgment but as metaphors for the society in which people are lost in the pursuit of quick success and instant profits, as well as their extreme hunger for power, while cancer in *Streams of Light and Time* is a contrasting metaphor for the hopelessness of people's existence. By driving the imperial forces away and modernizing the nation, modern China seems to have gotten rid of the humiliating nickname of the "Sick Man of East Asia." Yet Yan's narratives, with their biting satires of contemporary Chinese society where moral decline has driven it to morbidity, reveal that the malpractices of materialistic modernization is driving people to self-destruction, and that the image of a sick man is still haunting the nation in another form: now modern China has grown into a strong madman.

Nevertheless, when put together, a change in the author's pessimistic attitude in the trilogy is found within the narrative of illness and gender/sex in each story, especially in the endings of each novel. Let us first examine male–female relationships in each work. *Streams of Light and Time*, the earliest novel among the three, depicts a most desperate relationship. As demonstrated above, the romance between Sima Lan and Lan Sishi has such a tragic conclusion: the tragedy lies not only in the death of the lovers but also in the victimization of Lan Sishi, whose true love toward Sima Lan is taken advantage of repeatedly. In order to satisfy the male desires for sex by the commune leader and for power and longevity by Sima Lan, she sacrifices her virginity, her marriage, and her health. Eventually, when she discovers that she has caught venereal disease, she chooses to end her own life. This woman finishes her life as a complete victim, leaving the reader with unfathomable disappointment and heartache. Lan Sishi's body has become, to borrow the words of Taiwanese scholar Lin Xiu-rong 林秀蓉, a "sexually passive body" (*xing beidong shenti* 性被动身体), though her body is not that of a wife.[37]

---

36 Li Bing 李冰, "Yan Lianke: You san zhong ren bu shihe kan *Dingzhuang meng* 阎连科:有三种人不适合看《丁庄梦》 [Yan Lianke: *Dingzhuang meng* Does Not Suit Three Types of People]," Zhongguowang 中国网 (China), Jan. 23, 2006, http://www.china.com.cn/chinese/RS/1101469.htm (accessed July 9, 2014).

37 Lin Xiu-rong, in her *Zhong shen xianying: Taiwan xiaoshuo jibing xushi yihan zhi tanjiu (1929–2000)* 众身显影:台湾小说疾病叙事意涵之探究 [Developing the Bodies: An Inquiry of the Implications of Illness Narratives in Taiwanese Fiction] (Kaohsiung: Chunhui chubanshe, 2013), 221, divides the female body into four categories in her analysis of illness narratives in Taiwan fiction, the second category being "the sexually passive body as wives" (*zuowei qizi de xing beidong shenti* 作为妻子的性被动身体).

When we look at *Pleasure*, the story of Liu Yingque's abandonment of a young woman is less miserable. The young Liu was in love with a girl, a rarely "complete" person in Pleasure Village, before he became the County Chief. After he left the village, she gave birth to girl quadruplets—a set of dwarf daughters—but he never came back to marry her. Many years later, Chief Liu returns to the village to collect money for his unusual project, and his daughters also joined a special-skill troupe. However, he does not intend to reunite with his daughters and their mother. The body of the abandoned woman first becomes what Lin Xiu-rong calls "the productive body of a mother" (*zuowei muqin de shengzhi shenti* 作为母亲的生殖身体) and then a forgotten body.[38] Yet such a story of abandonment ends with Liu's decision to disable his own legs and become a resident of Pleasure Village. Whether his "becoming incomplete" will bring him and his woman as well as their daughters together to "complete" the family remains unknown, but at least this story is not as hopeless as that of Sima and Lan.

Finally, the episode of two HIV patients falling for each other in *Dream of Ding Village* is a touching love story. There is no doubt that they commit adultery in the quarantine as they are both married, but it is the unsympathetic attitude of their own spouses that drives them together. They are fellow sufferers, both suffering from the same illness and the indifference or even rejection of their other halves after they are infected. They sincerely value the brief time they can be together and eventually die for each other. Their moral misconduct is erased by their true love. The fact that after much hardship they finally obtain a marriage certificate, which is a termination of their illicitness, discloses the novelist's sympathy toward their relationship. Furthermore, when the woman chills her own body with icy water to help cool down her husband, who is having a high fever, and eventually dies before him, she transforms her body from one that carries out sexual/moral misbehavior into an agent that conveys love.[39]

Not only do the author's writings of love gets more and more merciful, but the ending of each story also becomes increasingly positive. *Streams of Light and Time* can be read metaphorically as the efforts to prolong people's lives and can be regarded as prescriptions to heal the sick society, but the society is so incurably ill that it is beyond any redemption after all attempts failed. When it comes to *Pleasure*, the author gives the novel a little hope by healing the

38 Ibid.

39 The adultery episode was taken out from the book and developed into a full-length story in Gu Changwei's 顾长卫 2011 film *Love for Life* (*Zui ai* 最爱). For a detailed analysis of the film, see Chapters 7 and 8 in this volume, by Kun Qian and Li Li respectively.

insanity of Chief Liu even though the character's "wholeness" is taken away by being disabled. Yet being disabled is not a bad thing in Pleasure Village, particularly when the novelist paints a rosy picture of the paradise in the last "further reading" of the novel. Finally, we see a completely fresh and new world created by the presumed goddess Nüwa dancing before Grandpa's eyes in *Dream of Ding Village*, suggesting a hopeful future.

What brings such a change to the novelist? In a review article, the issues of censorship and self-censorship are discussed:

> Just in case, Yan said with a twinkle, he is writing two versions at once, watering down the controversial sections for Chinese readers—and party watchdogs—while keeping the full flavor of his provocative imagination for editions to be published abroad, outside the censor's grasp. "Of course, this will affect the quality of the book," he acknowledged in an interview, smiling softly as if sharing a dark family secret.[40]

The above quotation was not a comment on *Dream of Ding Village* but something else Yan was writing. Then we have this from another interview: Yan "admitted to a certain degree of self-censorship when trying to get some of his works, including *Dream of Ding Village*, into the daylight."[41] The following is from yet another interview on how he wrote *Dream of Ding Village*:

> In a rare insight, the author told the Guardian how he attempted [to] forestall a ban by doing the censors' work for them. Out went the novel's most ambitious features: the blood pipeline, the global trade angle and direct criticism of national politics. Instead he narrowed the focus to a single village, where blood is bought and sold with horrific consequences. "This is not the book I originally wanted to write," says Yan, who has won China's top two literary awards. "I censored myself very rigorously. I didn't mention senior leaders. I reduced the scale. I thought my self-censorship was perfect."[42]

---

40 Edward Cody, "Persistent Censorship in China Produces Art of Compromise," *The Washington Post*, July 9, 2007, http://www.washingtonpost.com/wp-dyn/content/article/2007/07/08/AR2007070801063.html (accessed June 28, 2014).

41 Jaycee Lui, "A Rendezvous with China's Satirical Writer Yan Lianke," *gbtimes*, May 7, 2014, http://gbtimes.com/life/rendezvous-chinas-satirical-writer-yan-lianke (accessed July 9, 2014).

42 Jonathan Watts, "Censor Sees through Writer's Guile in Tale of China's Blood-Selling Scandal," *The Guardian*, Oct. 8, 2006, http://www.theguardian.com/world/2006/oct/09/books.china (accessed June 28, 2014).

Although Yan calculated much to conduct self-censorship so he could get his book published, he was not happy about it. He also told the Guardian that

> he still regrets self-censoring when he wrote *Dream of Ding Village*, which deals with the blood-selling scandal that led to mass HIV infections in Henan province. He wanted to ensure it was published, he said; but now his priority was reaching the highest literary standard.[43]

A skillful strategy to compose the trilogy in a progressive way, Yan's change of attitude is probably a practice of self-censorship, an "internalization of external censorious impulses and practices" on the part of the author.[44] Nevertheless, it would be encouraging to imagine that the writer is becoming more optimistic and now sees China as a curable sick man. From a feminist point of view, it would also be inspiring to believe that the change in the pessimistic stance of the author is reflected by the increasing awareness of female subjectivity throughout the trilogy: from a completely sacrificial victim in *Streams of Light and Time* to a woman who willingly becomes a mother to fulfill the feminine function of her body in *Pleasure*, then to a woman who actively chooses her lover and boldly pursues true love in *Dream of Ding Village*, the final installment of the trilogy in which a brave new world is created by a legendary female immortal.

References

Branigan, Tania. "Chinese Intellectuals Avoid Key Issues amid Censorship Fears, Says Author: Award-Winning Satirist Yan Lianke Says Chinese Intellectuals and Writers Must Push Leaders to Embrace Social Reform." *The Guardian*, Feb. 6, 2013. http://www.theguardian.com/world/2013/feb/06/chinese-writers-failing-censorship-concerns (accessed July 9, 2014).

Cody, Edward. "Persistent Censorship in China Produces Art of Compromise." *The Washington Post*, July 9, 2007. http://www.washingtonpost.com/wp-dyn/content/article/2007/07/08/AR2007070801063.html (accessed June 28, 2014).

---

43 Tania Branigan, "Chinese Intellectuals Avoid Key Issues Amid Censorship Fears, Says Author: Award-Winning Satirist Yan Lianke Says Chinese Intellectuals and Writers Must Push Leaders to Embrace Social Reform," *The Guardian*, Feb. 6, 2013, http://www.theguardian.com/world/2013/feb/06/chinese-writers-failing-censorship-concerns (accessed July 9, 2014).

44 Tsai, "In Sickness or in Health," 77.

Deng Hanmei 邓寒梅. Zhongguo xiandangdai wenxue zhong de jibing xushi yanjiu 中国现当代文学中的疾病叙事研究 [A Study of Illness Narratives in Modern and Contemporary Chinese Literature]. Nanchang: Jiangxi renmin chubanshe, 2012.

Gao Yaojie 高耀洁. *Gaojie de linghun: Gao Yaojie huiyilu* 高洁的灵魂—高耀洁回忆录 [A Noble and Unsullied Soul: Gao Yaojie's Memoirs]. 2008. Revised and enlarged ed. Hong Kong: Ming Pao, 2010.

Klages, Mary. *Woeful Afflictions: Disability and Sentimentality in Victorian America*. Philadelphia: University of Pennsylvania Press, 1999.

Li Bing 李冰. "Yan Lianke: You san zhong ren bu shihe kan *Dingzhuang meng* 阎连科:有三种人不适合看《丁庄梦》[Yan Lianke: *Dream of Ding Village* Does Not Suit Three Types of People]." Zhongguowang 中国网 (China), Jan. 23, 2006. http://www.china.com.cn/chinese/RS/1101469.htm (accessed July 9, 2014).

Lin Xiu-rong 林秀蓉. *Zhong shen xianying: Taiwan xiaoshuo jibing xushi yihan zhi tanjiu (1929–2000)* 众身显影:台湾小说疾病叙事意涵之探究 [Developing the Bodies: An Inquiry of the Implications of Illness Narratives in Taiwanese Fiction]. Kaohsiung: Chunhui chubanshe, 2013.

Liu Ruixiang 刘瑞祥 and Lin Zhihe 林之鹤, trans. *The Classic of Filial Piety*. Ji'nan: Shangdong Friendship Press, 1993.

Lui, Jaycee. "A Rendezvous with China's Satirical Writer Yan Lianke." *gbtimes*, May 7, 2014. http://gbtimes.com/life/rendezvous-chinas-satirical-writer-yan-lianke (accessed July 9, 2014).

Murphy, Timothy F., and Suzanne Poirier, eds. *Writing AIDS: Gay Literature, Language, and Analysis*. New York: Columbia University Press, 1993.

Sontag, Susan. *Illness as Metaphor and AIDS and Its Metaphors*. New York: Anchor Books, 1990.

Thomson, Rosemarie Garland. *Extraordinary Bodies: Figuring, Physical, Disability in American Culture and Literature*. New York: Columbia University Press, 1997.

Tsai, Chien-hsin. "In Sickness or in Health: Yan Lianke and the Writing of Autoimmunity." *Modern Chinese Literature and Culture* 23.1 (Spring 2011): 77–104.

Wang Jinping 王晋平. "Chongwen xuejiang jingji he aizibing de hunluan shidai—yi shi wei jian 重温血浆经济和爱滋病的混乱时代—以史为鉴 [A Review of the Chaotic Times of the Blood Economy and AIDS: Benefit from History]." *Huanqiu shibao* 环球时报 (Global Times), Oct. 31, 2008. http://www.haodf.com/zhuanjiaguandian/wangjinping_22943.htm (accessed July 10, 2014).

Watts, Jonathan. "Censor Sees through Writer's Guile in Tale of China's Blood-Selling Scandal." *The Guardian*, Oct. 8, 2006. http://www.theguardian.com/world/2006/oct/09/books.china (accessed June 28, 2014).

Yan Lianke 阎连科. *Dingzhuang meng* 丁庄梦 [Dream of Ding Village]. Shanghai: Shanghai wenyi chubanshe, 2006.

———. *Dream of Ding Village*. Trans. Cindy Carter. New York: Grove Press, 2009.

———. *Lenin's Kisses*. Trans. Carlos Rojas. New York: Grove Press, 2012.

———. "On China's State-Sponsored Amnesia." *The New York Times*, April 1, 2013. http://www.nytimes.com/2013/04/02/opinion/on-chinas-state-sponsored-amnesia.html?pagewanted=all&_r=2& (assessed July 10, 2014).

———. *Riguang liunian* 日光流年 [Streams of Light and Time]. Shenyang: Chunfeng wenyi chubanshe, 2004.

———. *Shouhuo* 受活 [Pleasure]. Shenyang: Chunfeng wenyi chubanshe, 2004.

PART 3

AIDS and Virus: From Film to Forum

CHAPTER 7

Reluctant Transcendence: AIDS and the Catastrophic Condition in Gu Changwei's Film *Love for Life*

Kun Qian 钱坤

> Cinema is like a cancer. No, it is infectious, it is more like AIDS.
>
> ALAIN TANNER, *La Vallée Fantôme* (1987)

Ever since an unknown, threatening disease was identified as Acquired Immunodeficiency Syndrome (AIDS) in the 1980s, AIDS has been a subject of filmmaking in Western cinemas. Directors usually capture the alienation and suffering of the AIDS patients—mostly urban, marginal individuals such as gays, drug addicts, and prostitutes who are portrayed as having a deviant lifestyle, and for whom the disease is a stigma for which they are held responsible. Often seen as a threat to the community, they serve as warnings and "bad" examples for the general public.[1] Gu Changwei's 顾长卫 recent film, *Love for Life* (*Zui ai* 最爱, 2011), on the contrary, portrays a group of AIDS bearers in a rural environment in China as innocent peasants conforming a conventional life, whose biggest mistake lies in having followed the rhetoric of "getting rich quickly" by means of selling blood; in other words, the collective nature of this Chinese "tainted community" sets Gu's film apart from other AIDS narratives and, to a large extent, appears as a social criticism of national characteristics and contemporary economic development. As such, AIDS in the film is rid of the common stigma associated with gay sex and drug abuse, but is quintessentially tied to blood transfusion—the most direct way to depict the communicativeness and infectiousness of viruses which, as will be shown below, are not limited to HIV.

Moreover, beyond capturing the horizontal, spatial pandemic of this formidable catastrophe, Gu Changwei attempts to deliver a sense of vertical, spiritual transcendence by highlighting a passionate love story between two young AIDS patients who, performed by the internationally known actors Zhang Ziyi 章子怡 and Aaron Kwok Fu-shing 郭富城, aestheticize the disease and probe the more universalistic questions regarding identity and subjectivity.

1 António Pais de Lacerda, "Cinema as an Historical Document: AIDS in 25 Years of Cinema," *Journal of Medicine and Movies* 2 (2006): 102–13.

 | DOI 10.1163/9789004319219_009

This obviously has to do with censorship and commercial concerns,[2] yet it also reflects the director's ambivalent attitude—both engaged and detached—toward love and disease, life and death, which differs from Yan Lianke's 阎连科 novel on which the film is based.[3]

In fact, even before its official appearance in May 2011, *Love for Life* attracted substantial attention from all kinds of potential audiences. For its pioneering portrayal of the AIDS patients in rural China, a void and taboo in public discourse, the film was from its beginning destined to generate politically conscious sensations. Critics have mostly been drawn to the issues revolving around the film's release and its potential function as social criticism: how much the film diverges from Yan Lianke's banned novel *Dream of Ding Village*; how the film has managed to strategically pass censorship; how a director-cut version will differ from the version publicly shown in cinemas; and how the drama of changing titles helps understand China's film censorship process. Excitement, aspiration, caution, and relief seem to be the common sentiments that accompany the film's production and initial reception. After applause mixed with slight disappointment with the shorter version available in the market, the audience then immediately moved their expectation to the director-cut version, hoping that the longer version would fulfill the full potential of what such a topic promised. Yet from what is available to us now, we could still see an imperative of catastrophe at work, a dark theme prevalent throughout Yan's novel, one that not only determines the fate of the individual characters in the film, but also brings to light the inverse perspective of the "catastrophic condition" of the society. The difference between the film and the novel, then, resides in Gu's paradoxical attempt to make AIDS a metaphor for the collapse of the social immune system and at the same time to aestheticize it by proposing love as a way of transcendence.[4] On the surface, *Love for Life* seems not so much different from other rebellious tales of forbidden love in an oppressive social environment, a topic that has been explored by many modern and contemporary filmmakers.[5] What distinguishes this film from others is that AIDS as an overpowering existence *conditions* the community

---

2 "*Zuiai*: Juewang he huangmiu de yuyan 《最爱》：绝望和荒谬的寓言 [*Love for Life*: An Allegory of Despair and Absurdity]," *Xin Jing bao* 新京报 (Beijing News), May 11, 2011, http://www.bjnews.com.cn/ent/2011/05/11/123371.html (accessed Feb. 23, 2013).

3 [For a detailed discussion of Yan Lianke's novel, see Chapter 6, by Shelley W. Chan, in this volume. Ed.]

4 Using disease as a metaphor for social ills has been an enduring topic for modern Chinese writers. The most discussed example is Lu Xun's "A Madman's Diary."

5 For example, Ling Zi's 凌子 *Yuanye* 原野 [Wilderness] (1986), Ling Zifeng's 凌子风 *Chuntao* 春桃 (1988) and *Kuang* 狂 [Madness] (1992), and Zhang Yimou's 张艺谋 *Ju Dou* 菊豆

and *fosters* love. Gu employs AIDS to explore the problems both of individual subjectivity against disciplinary social norms and of other social ills. This multi-layered task brings about a fundamental paradox, the question whether the AIDS pandemic or the contagious, self-destructive behavior of the society is more disastrous. The film celebrates (forbidden) love while the destiny of the lovers is death. As a way out, Gu's film seems to suggest that love eventually redeems the tainted characters, for through AIDS, they gain an enlightened perspective overcoming death. Whereas Yan's novel ends with a violent act of filicide and the obliteration of the village, Gu's film projects a heavenly utopia that breaks out of the vicious circle of the catastrophe.

This article addresses the double sides of the catastrophe: the contagious disease AIDS and its inverse image—postsocialist economic development in *Love for Life* to approach Gu's ambivalent transcendence. AIDS in the film serves as a real catastrophe as much as an instrument that helps illuminate the "catastrophic condition" of the society. In particular, the love story evolving out of this catastrophe demonstrates a frenzied life drive encountering death. The desire to love overcomes the desire to profit, indicating an enlightened, and equally "contagious," perspective that points to the future.

Insofar as the film is an ambitious, multi-task endeavor that resists simple generalization, the following sections will be devoted to several independent yet related questions. The primary narrative is a love story through which Gu presents the age-old question of the individual versus society, the formation of subjectivity that can be best approached through Gilles Deleuze's and Félix Guattari's notion of "the-body-without-organs." Exploring the delicate relationship between the body and the subject, illness and desire, the film dramatizes the lovers' return to humanity in the face of death. Celebrating love as a redeeming force that transcends death, this narrative also suggests, through the adulterous lovers' eventual marriage, the social legitimization of what has been another stigmatized identity—the AIDS patients. A second narrative presents a group of self-exiled patients as a microcosm of contemporary social transition. Capturing the socialist afterlife in a quasi-communist "patient commune," the film suggests that AIDS offers a privileged perspective about life, constitutes the characters as active subjects to transform their lives (as in the lovers), and at the same time mirrors the failure of socialist practice and its grotesque afterimage in the market economy. In a third narrative AIDS offers a privileged perspective on the postsocialist catastrophe, the market economy that fosters a social disease that is disastrously contagious. Finally, enveloping

---

(1990) all depict illicit love affairs to legitimize the female characters' search for the self and free love.

the critical elements discussed above, the last narrative attempts to convey a reluctant transcendence. By giving voice and subjective position to the AIDS patients and framing the story in a dead boy's uncertain, mythic narrative, the film blurs the boundary between life and death. Along with its accompanying documentary film *Together* (*Zaiyiqi* 在一起), which could be seen as its double in real life, *Love for Life* seems to present a gesture of "becoming-patients" to look at contemporary China as a pathological society.

Self vs. Society: Body-without-Organs

The released version of *Love for Life* features a touching love story between two AIDS patients: Deyi 得意 and Qinqin 琴琴, whose forbidden love highlights the film's inquiry about life and death, illness and health. Insofar as their love affair is saturated with physical pain, emotional abuse, social alienation, and spiritual quest for subjectivity and identity, it evokes Gilles Deleuze's and Félix Guattari's idea of "body-without-organs" in describing their search for a meaningful life and redefinition of their identity.

"Body-without-organs" is a term invented by Deleuze and Guattari to denote their understanding of an embodied subjectivity.[6] Neither an essentialist, anatomical body separated from social discourses, nor a Foucauldian symbolic body as a site of power, a node contested between forces of discipline and resistance, a "body-without-organs" is both material and spiritual. For Deleuze and Guattari, the lived physical body and the self that "experiences" itself as being "inside" the body are both consequences of reflexive, normative ways of thinking about embodiment and individuality. The lived body-self is the "body-without-organs," as opposed to the anatomical, physical body—"the body with organs," and reflects the dynamic between psyche and the forces of the social. The formation of subjectivity is a continuous process of negotiations between the body and the disciplinary forces impinging on it. Here, Deleuze agrees with Foucault that the body-self is a product of social construction, but the "body-without-organs" emphasizes the active, constructive agency of the body enacting and engaging social forces to construct its subjectivity.[7]

In our case, Deyi and Qinqin appear to be two examples struggling with their bodies and minds. From the beginning they have been infected with

6 Gilles Deleuze and Félix Guattari, *Anti-Oedipus: Capitalism and Schizophrenia*, trans. Robert Hurley, Mark Seem, and Helen Lane (London and New York: Penguin, 1977).

7 Gilles Deleuze, *Foucault*, trans. S. Hand (Minneapolis: University of Minnesota Press, 1988), 99.

AIDS—as both physical suffering and emotional burden, a death sentence that is also seen as their being stigmatized with a filthy plague. Yet rather than passively accepting this social inscription, one that Susan Sontag has described as the "metaphorical uses of illness,"[8] and waiting to die in pain and anguish, they choose to rebel, actively pursuing a passionate life through love. Their sick bodies unexpectedly unleash a powerful life force, a desire to live a normal life that eventually redefines their identity. This embodied subjectivity, this "body-without-organs," as will be discussed below, finally brings them back to the un-alienable humanity of life.

Masterfully performed by Aaron Kwok and Zhang Ziyi, Deyi and Qinqin at first appear as two lost, marginal young people, still having difficulty coming to terms with their newly-inscribed identity as AIDS patients. Seduced by monetary desire and infected with AIDS, they are both shunned by their healthy spouses and come to live in the unoccupied village school with other AIDS patients. The territory of their previous marital relations has been shattered because of the disease, yet they still hold onto the nominal identity as others' spouses. Deyi is unsettled and unsure about his wife, obviously disturbed by a battle between libido and reason: on the one hand, he asks his wife to remarry after his death; on the other hand, he secretly hopes that she will stay in the marriage and agonizes over her not coming to see him. Always a bit irresolute and mischievous, Deyi at this point only starts to taste the bitterness of the "social inscription" implied by his wife's silent estrangement. While Deyi is tormented by irreconcilable feelings of desire and rejection, tossing and turning in bed at night, Qinqin emerges in his desiring gaze. Wearing a bright red padded jacket and an otherworldly look, Qinqin stands out among the gray-colored village folk. Needless to say, Zhang's distinguished beauty and fame endow the character with tremendous charm, which reflects Gu's intention that she transcends the role of a peasant woman.[9] Unlike the portrayal in the novel where the prototype of Qinqin's character should show unpleasant marks of advanced AIDS on her face,[10] Zhang's flawless complexion in the film makes Qinqin an instant object of desire. Seeing Qinqin as his companion

---

8 Susan Sontag, *Illness as Metaphor and AIDS and Its Metaphors* (New York: Picador, 1988), 3.

9 In an interview, Gu admitted that he tried to present a universal theme about love and life, and it was his design that Zhang Ziyi does not completely look like a girl from the countryside. See "Zhuanfang Gu Changwei, Jiang Wenli: *Zuiai* bushi yibu nongcun pian 专访顾长卫、蒋雯丽：《最爱》不是一部农村片 [Interview with Gu Changwei and Jiang Wenli: *Love for Life* Is Not a Film about Countryside]," *Tengxun yule* 腾讯娱乐 (Tencent Entertainment), Mar. 22, 2011, http://ent.qq.com/a/20110322/000451.htm (accessed Feb. 23, 2013).

10 See Yan Lianke, *Dream of Ding Village*, trans. Cindy Carter (New York: Grove Press, 2009), 77.

on the same boat, Deyi immediately ventures his aggressive seduction, with the convincing reasoning that since they cannot sleep with their spouses (and their spouses don't care about them anyway), they'd better sleep together to fulfill their youth, a rationale that effectively resonates with Qinqin, whose recent memory about her husband is only his abuse of her. The physical fever they endure seems only to fuel their desire for each other, and the visual beauty of their coupling in the grip of a fatal disease undermines the erotic connotation of their sexual adventure, while emphasizing suffering, rebellion, and later freedom and hope. It seems that Gu intentionally attempts to present this ongoing transformation of the body-mediated subjectivity, accentuating the pain, desire, and degradation the body suffers as leading to the characters' spiritual liberation.[11] Sex is thus imbued with a temporal, spiritual quality that eventually turns the seemingly light-hearted escapade into serious commitment that ties life and death together.

In an early spring scene, the camera captures the couple's newly found emancipation in life. When Qinqin says: "It is meaningless to live," Deyi responds: "Then we should create something to live for!" The scene that follows presents the alternate images of their making love and their running in the field, off-screen moaning overlapping with the interchanging images. The disembodied, joyous sound, and the soaring images together create an imaginary space, as if to imply that the vigorous free spirits have conquered the shadow of death. Deyi then runs onto the railroad tracks, racing ahead of a coming train loaded with coal, playfully teasing the driver to brake the train. Laughing, shouting, and singing, his blatant exhibition of energy and vitality annoys the driver and makes Qinqin laugh and cry (Fig. 7.1–7.3).[12]

In this sequence, besides the brightly colored *mise-en-scene* that incorporates ebullient movements of the lovers and the train, the non-diegetic music also presents an upbeat emotive texture that contributes to the overall spirit-lifting effect. Along with other on- and off-screen sounds, the blaring of the train air horn included, the music creates a lively "*mise-en-bande*," a term coined to capture the relationships among sound components.[13] Synchronized

11 Gu explained in an interview that the film in the beginning portrays Deyi as a non-serious country lad in order to give room for character development. See "*Zuiai*: Juewang he huangmiu de yuyan."

12 Still images in this chapter are snapshots from the online version of the film on *Aiqiyi* 爱奇艺 (IQIYI), http://www.iqiyi.com/dianying/20110627/ede303b69df4ea66.html (accessed Feb. 24, 2013).

13 Rick Altman, "Inventing the Cinema Soundtrack: Hollywood's Multiplane Sound System," in *Music and Cinema*, ed. James Buhler, Carly Flinn, and David Neumeyer (Hanover: Wesleyan University Press, 2000): 341.

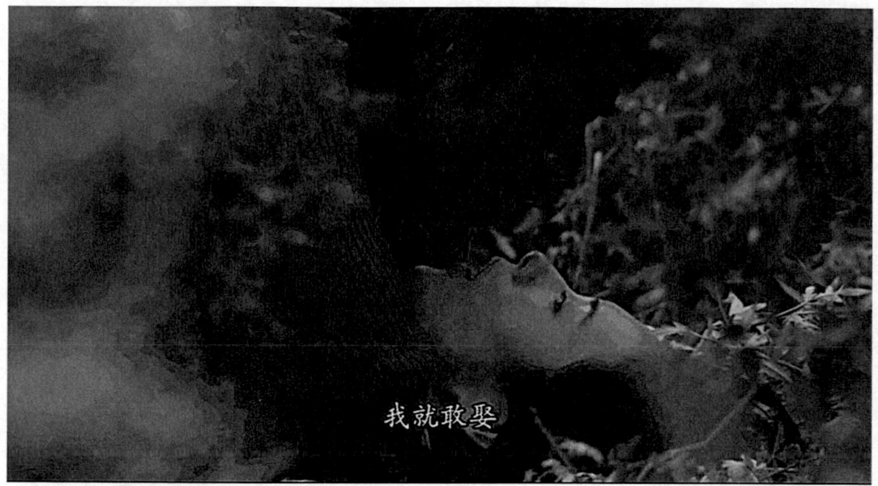

FIGURE 7.1 *Deyi and Qinqin make love in the spring field.*

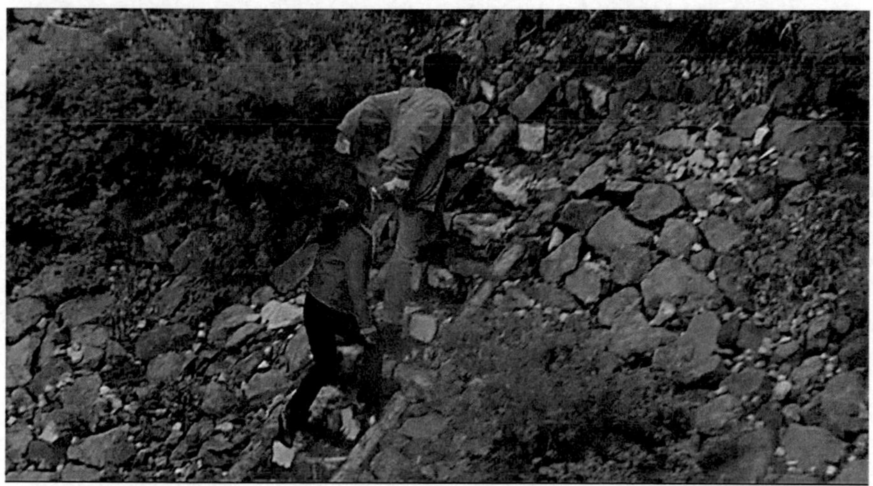

FIGURE 7.2 *Deyi and Qinqin run toward the railway.*

with the images, the relative music volume vis-à-vis other sounds from piano to forte, and finally to fortissimo directly addresses the viewer's psychoacoustic interest,[14] constructing an atmosphere that sonically "enrolls the spectators

14 See Harry F. Olson and Frank Massa, "On the Realistic Reproduction of Sound with Particular Reference to Sound Motion Pictures," *Journal of the Society of Motion Picture Engineers* 23.2 (Aug. 1934): 63–81; quoted in Altman, "Inventing the Cinema Soundtrack," 352–53.

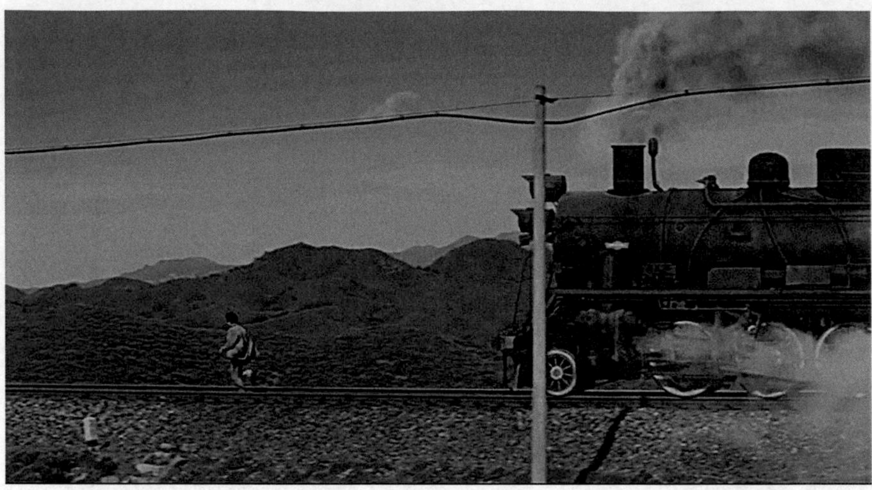

FIGURE 7.3 *Deyi teases the train driver.*

in the film's space" to identify with the characters. This atmospheric effect of the music is in stark contrast to that of a previous scene where, after uncle Silun's 四伦 death at school, Deyi and his father go back home to celebrate New Year. The sad, gloomy background music carries over the cuts from the deserted schoolyard to Deyi's home. Even the loud cracking of the firecrackers cannot subdue the melancholic music. The continuous music assures the unity of time and space, extending the shadow of death to Deyi's family. However, in the spring scene, the episodic *mise-en-bande* intermittently breaks the continuous mood of sadness, delivering a cheerful atmosphere that celebrates love and life. Here, sex is presented as a natural, innate life force that entails not so much pleasure as desire for life, generates less guilt than legitimacy to live, and produces more strength to safeguard dignity. Deleuze once characterized desire as a positive force and a creative power that should be favored over the notion of pleasure. "The idea of pleasure is a completely rotten idea," Deleuze claimed, for it is a notion spoiled by the Platonic-Schopenhauerian tradition with its negative ontology of lack.[15] Pleasure is always burdened with anxiety and loss. Desire, on the contrary, lacks nothing and is tormented by no vain aspiration or melancholy impasse. It is constructive, affirmative, and transformative, engendering movement of multiple flows and becomings. The rejection of finitude in Deleuze's characterization of desire fits snuggly with Deyi and Qinqin. Insofar as their sexual desire combines with the right to live,

15 Gilles Deleuze, "Dualism, Monism, and Multiplicities (Desire-Pleasure-Jouissance)," seminar on Mar. 26, 1973, trans. Daniel W. Smith, *Contretemps* 2 (May 2001): 96.

which is overshadowed by death, the pleasure that comes with it has to be put in the framework of life and death. The sexual pleasure is therefore not just guilty pleasure constrained by forbidding social norms, but is more productive, generating more desire, a stronger life force confronting death. In light of this, Deyi's and Qinqin's love affair is more constitutive than transgressive. It does not stop at the clichéd formula of "body-rebelling-against-mind" to achieve sexual liberation, but opens new possibilities to define one's identity, making them turn inward to look for human nature that is more intrinsic for life. This inverse turn manifests itself not only in their decision to live together, despite other people's disapproval, but also in their determination to get married, to defend their right to create and be incorporated in a community.

Deyi's and Qinqin's decision to marry is triggered by both the rejection of their families and the desire to defend their basic rights of life. After Qinqin's husband, Xiaohai 小海, gets wind of the affair, he publicly beats, humiliates, and verbally attacks Qinqin and drags her away; both Deyi's and Qinqin's empty marriages come to an end. They are despised by family members and alienated by fellow AIDS patients. Qinqin, in particular, feels more than ever lonely and helpless. Negativity creates identity. The looks of contempt from others serve as a mirror that reflects their unfavorable image. Yet instead of identifying with this negative image as social transgressor, Deyi and Qinqin choose what Carlos Rojas called "*dis*identification," a self-motivated act triggered by a "psycho-immune response."[16] It seems that it is in this moment of *dis*identification—rejection of social inscription—that the characters start redefining their new identity, one that negates conventional social norms and follows their desire to live like dignified human beings. Deyi announces his declaration of rebellion like this: "We will live together, let Xiaohai and his family see it! Let Hao Yan 郝艳 [Deyi's wife] and other villagers see it!" "We live together, not just for dignity in life, but also for having company after death." For Deyi and Qinqin, both dignity and companionship are inalienable needs of life. By defending these needs, they finally embrace their fundamental humanity, without vanity and material pursuit.

Later in the film, when they discover that the other fellow AIDS patients have quietly died one after another, Qinqin despondently utters the most memorable line: "Let's get married, now that we are alive." The approaching shadow of death has reinforced the desire to live with dignity and to be incorporated into the community. One may argue that Qinqin's desire to marry is another "inscription" of the social order that the self-body cannot resist. But it

16 Carlos Rojas, "Of Canons and Cannibalism: A Psycho-Immunological Reading of 'Diary of a Madman'," *Modern Chinese Literature and Culture* 23.1 (Spring 2011): 57.

should be clear that this demand is full of subjectivity and agency, reflecting the constant negotiations between the self and the society to construct the body-mediated subjectivity, the "body-without-organs."

Indeed, Qinqin's decision to marry is genuinely rooted in her defense of the legitimacy and dignity of their relationship. When she kneels down to Old Zhuzhu 老柱柱 (Deyi's father) to ask his help for her divorce with Xiaohai, she declares her reasoning and will to live: "… I AM shameless, but I am not dead. I must live. Getting married to Deyi, even though only for half a year, half a month, we will still be legitimate husband and wife, then when we die we can be justifiably buried together." This little speech, not only brings Deyi to his knees to kneel together with her in front of his father, but also moves Old Zhuzhu to petition with Xiaohai on their behalf. For Qinqin, *tangtang zhengzheng* 堂堂正正 "uprightness" and *ming zheng yan shun* 名正言顺 "justifiableness" are inalienable rights for life, and the approaching of death only reinforces the desire to defend such rights. At the end of the film, following the death of both Qinqin and Deyi, a flashback of their "wedding day" appears on the screen. After obtaining the marriage certificate, Deyi and Qinqin dress up as groom and bride to deliver wedding candies to their neighbors in the village. In the empty village valley where people close doors before them in order to avoid accepting the candies, Qinqin loudly and passionately repeats the words on the marriage certificate, words that give approval and legitimization of their marriage from the government. Particularly, she stresses the term "marry voluntarily" (*ziyuan jiehun* 自愿结婚) many times, revealing their consciousness of self and strong will to change their lives (Fig. 7.4). Her voice penetrates the walls of the village

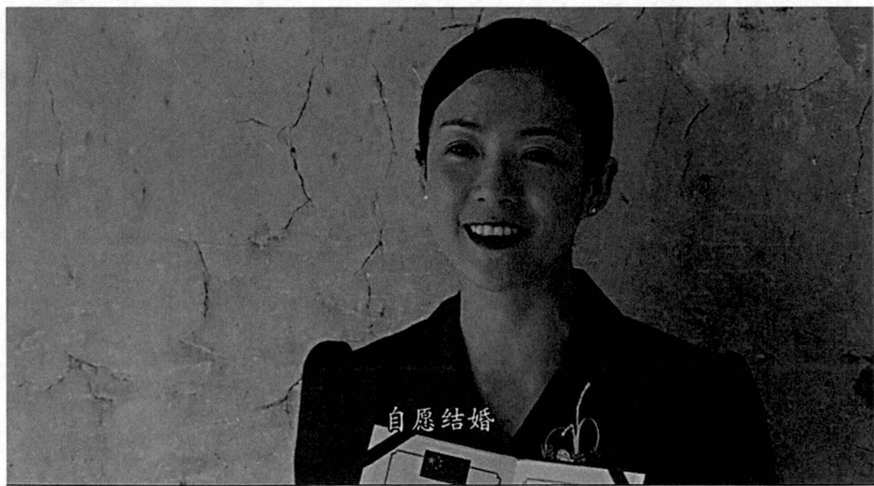

FIGURE 7.4 *Qinqin repeats the words on the marriage certificate.*

houses, demonstrating the triumph in redefining their identity against the grain of conventional "inscription."

It deserves attention that life and death at this point exhibit a dialectical relationship. It is the shadow of death that intensifies the desire to love and to live. Confucius once responded to his disciple's question on death this way: "Without knowing about life, how can one know about death?"[17] He meant to teach the disciple to treasure life instead of wasting time on imagining death. However, if we inverse the order, a dialectical relationship emerges from the saying: "Without knowing about death, how can one know about life?" Death is instrumental to life. Only after understanding death could one realize the real transience of life. Perhaps, this is the point of departure that inspires Gu Changwei to portray such a "love story of life and death" (*shengsi juelian* 生死绝恋).[18] The film visualizes this dialectic by highlighting the shadow of death at the doorstep while proposing life as simple, bare, without material embellishment. The effort to obtain the marriage certificate costs Deyi his property—he has to bequeath the house to Xiaohai in his will in order to free Qinqin from her original marriage. This decision angers Deyi's brother Qiquan 齐全 for being reckless and irresponsible with his property. However, for Deyi, the house shouldn't be in the way for his pursuit of a loving, bare life. Deyi and Qinqin call each other "Mom" and "Dad," suggesting not only the primordial bond between people that cannot separate from life, but also that they have figuratively given birth to each other and to themselves (Fig. 7.5).

The rebirth of Deyi and Qinqin, nurtured by unconditional love and unyielding dignity, soon becomes an object of envy. As the narrator Xiaoxin 小鑫 says, their love is like the Himalayas in the textbook, something everybody can see. Their vigorous sex life evokes other healthy young men's envy. One of them even sighs that he should have contracted AIDS. When Deyi and Qinqin send out candies to celebrate their marriage, Huang Shulang 黄鼠狼, a fellow AIDS patient who, out of jealousy, has reported their love affair to Xiaohai in order to seize power among the patients, weeps in front of a picture of his deceased wife (Fig. 7.6–7.7). The exuberance on the new couple's faces mirrors his loneliness, despair, and bitterness.

---

17 *Lun yu* 论语 (The Analects) 11.11.

18 During his publicity trip to Nanjing, the director admitted that he intended to present a warmer theme in the film. See Shu Ke 舒克, "Gu Changwei Nanjing shuo *Zuiai* 顾长卫南京说《最爱》 [Gu Changwei Talks about *Love for Life* in Nanjing]," *Shiguang wang* 时光网 (Mtime), May 11, 2011, http://i.mtime.com/shuke/blog/5958665/(accessed Feb. 24, 2013).

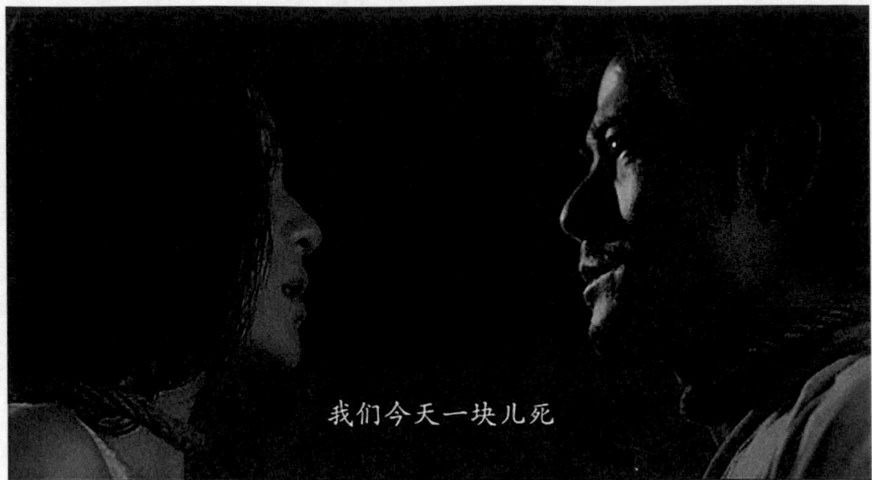

FIGURE 7.5 *In a half-serious manner, Deyi and Qinqin attempt to hang themselves together to make sure they will stay together forever.*

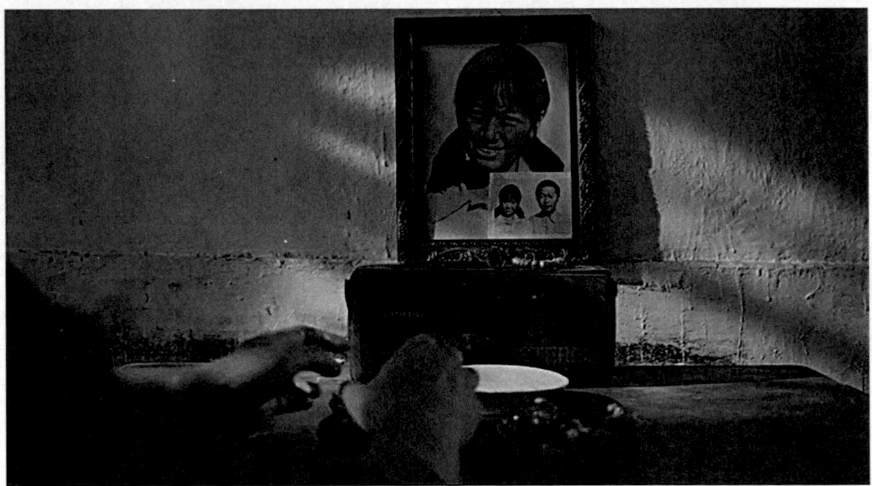

FIGURE 7.6 *Huang Shulang puts the wedding candy in front of his wife's shrine.*

The contrast between Deyi's and Qinqin's intense love and other villagers' pale life exhibits an interesting twist in the film: AIDS has transported Deyi and Qinqin back to inborn humanity, one that inversely mirrors the emptiness of their previous and other people's current lives. In a sense, AIDS has offered a privileged perspective to look at life (and death), a mirror to create intersubjective relationship with oneself and each other, and a constructive element that reflects the real catastrophic condition of life.

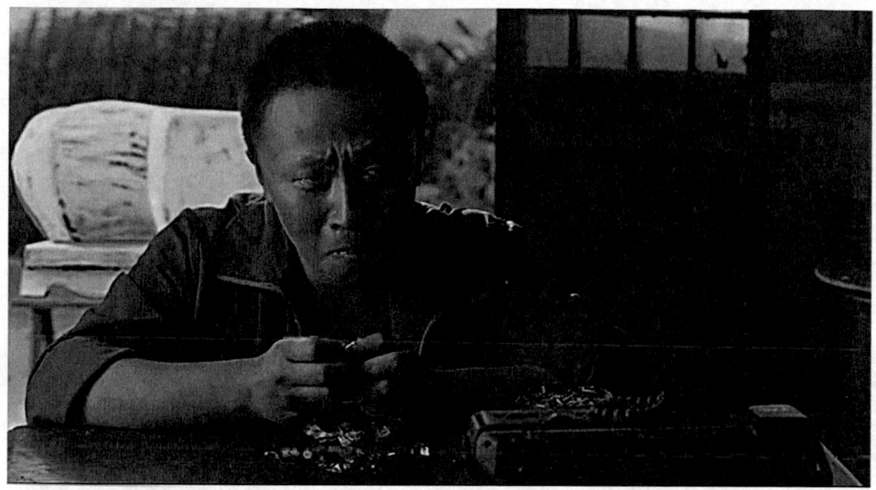

FIGURE 7.7 *Huang Shulang weeps while eating the wedding candy.*

The Exiled Community: National Characteristics and Disease as a Privileged Perspective

Deleuze once stated that illness could provide a "privilege" for people. In talking about his infection with tuberculosis in 1968 at an interview, Deleuze maintained that this particular illness was in some ways "a privilege." It allowed him to come to contact with "life," to perceive a wider sense of life that went beyond his illness. "Illness sharpened one's perceptions and provides a privileged perspective on life. Even though illness is debilitating, it still offers possibilities for realizing one's 'forces'."[19] As we have discussed, this statement remains true for Deyi and Qinqin—AIDS stimulates their desire for life, giving them a privileged perspective to experience love, life, freedom, and death, while other people are constrained, "territorialized" in their established, alienating social patterning. To push it further, we could see that AIDS offers a privileged situation, whereby not only an *inversion of perspective* has taken place as reflected on Deyi's and Qinqin's self-realization for life, but also a *fracture of perspective* has been evoked, which is manifested in the construction and collapse of a marginal, microcosmic "patient commune" wherein other social illnesses are revealed.

Out of tremendous guilt for his son Qiquan's exploitation of villagers' blood, Old Zhuzhu helps the AIDS patients to stay in a deserted school to create a self-reliant commune similar to that in the Maoist era. People put their rice

19 John Marks, *Gilles Deleuze: Vitalism and Multiplicity* (London: Pluto Press, 1998), 10.

together and eat at the public kitchen. However, soon a variety of problems emerge in this seemingly peaceful "socialist community." First is the theft of Qinqin's red jacket, the investigation of which reveals that Sister Liangfang 粮房, the voluntary cook, has stolen rice from the public kitchen (Fig. 7.8). More seriously, Uncle Silun, suggestively the previous head of the Production Team in the Maoist period, has been terrified by the loss of his "red notebook" in which he has documented all the secrets in the past that he has never dared to tell anyone (Fig. 7.9). Jacket, rice, and the "red notebook" remind one of the

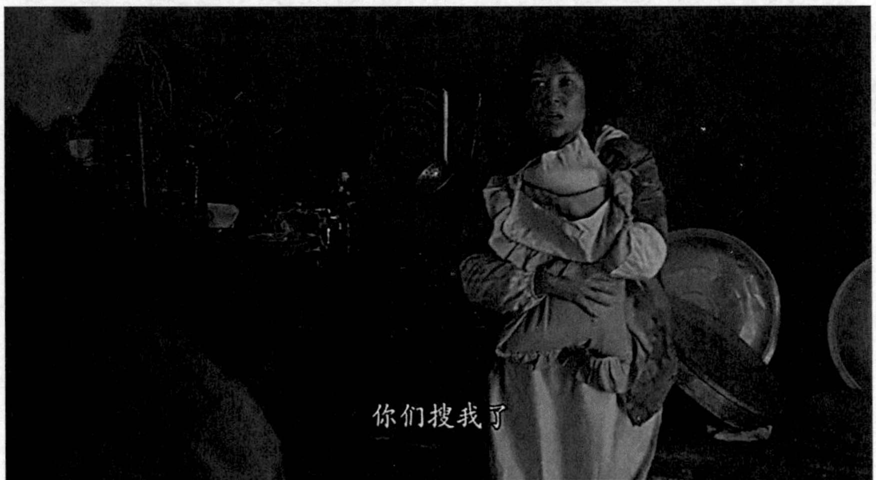

FIGURE 7.8 *Sister Liangfang is caught stealing rice from the public kitchen.*

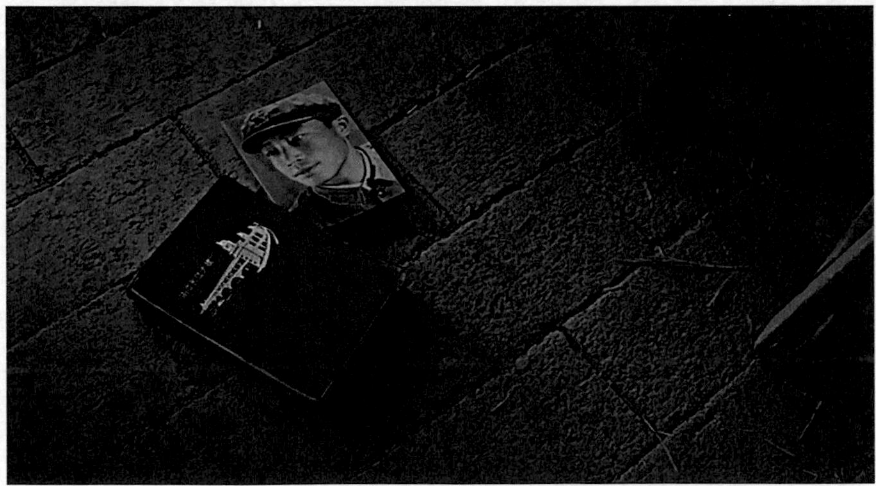

FIGURE 7.9 *The loss of his red notebook prompts Uncle Silun's death.*

materially deprived and spiritually controlled conditions in the Maoist socialist period. The theft of Qinqin's jacket makes it explicit that people still live in material poverty that both the Maoist era and the postsocialist period have failed to improve. We are told later that the thief is in fact an honest man whose stealing is meant to fulfill a long-expired promise to his wife, a promise he made many years ago when they got married. The inability to buy a red jacket for his aged wife costs a good man his dignity and reputation before death. Similarly, the behavior of Sister Liangfang (literally "food and house") reanimates the grotesque memory of hunger that lingers to dominate one's life. Rice represents the fundamental need of life, the vehement attachment to which makes Liangfang a sympathetic character. Her death prompted by her battle with a pig for rice leaves an unsettling reminder about the bygone era of hunger. In Uncle Silun's case, it is the political terror of blackmail and abuse symbolized by the "red notebook" that exacerbates his illness and invites the early arrival of death. Silun is introduced as a man who is still haunted by the military lifestyle and spirit of the revolutionary past. The loss of the "red notebook," indicative of Mao's "little red book" that defines the time period of the Cultural Revolution characterized by political terror, physical abuse, and emotional control, undoubtedly accelerates his death. The lack of clothes and food mixed with the heightened political discipline of one's mind represents the deprived condition of Maoist socialist community. The afterlife of it, manifested in the "patient commune," not only exhibits the lasting influence of that period, but also foregrounds the collapse of the community from within in a postsocialist context.

In fact, the quasi "patient commune" offers a mirror image of the social transition from the socialist past to the postsocialist society. Out of jealousy and desire for power, Huang Shulang and another guy stage the exposure of Deyi's and Qinqin's affair. After Qinqin got dragged away by her husband from the commune, they blackmail Old Zhuzhu, for the sake of Deyi, to give leadership position to them in the commune, and subsequently make rules of their own, rules written on the "big-character poster" (*dazibao* 大字报) and broadcast over a loudspeaker. The language they use and the manner they deliver the rules make a vivid mimicry of the political scene during the Cultural Revolution. Establishing their authoritarian power through terror and blackmail, they later expel Old Zhuzhu in order to sell the school property to make money. This Maoist style of collective dictatorship and its marriage with market force quickly crumple the "patient commune," an allegorical microcosm of contemporary social conditions.

It is ironic that the self-exiled community favors collectivism as a counterforce to deal with their ostracism, a return to the socialist past to evade capitalist alienation, very much like the enclosed early Maoist PRC countering the outside capitalist world. Yet what they experience is the failure and downfall of collective practice from both within and without. It is as if history repeats itself in a smaller scale and, without offering much hope, drives the characters to eternal banishment. Except for Deyi and Qinqin, who have found their enlightened identity, most people are neither able to diachronically sever with the memory of the past, nor synchronically detach from the contamination of the market.

On another level, the trajectory of the "patient commune" also evokes the lasting discussion of Chinese national character that has plagued Chinese intellectuals since the late Qing period. From Liang Qichao 梁启超 (1873–1929) and Lu Xun 鲁迅 (1881–1936) to Su Xiaokang 苏晓康 and others, intellectuals have been obsessed with finding the shortcomings embedded in Chinese culture that are responsible for China's failure in the modern world arena. Mediating the discourse of national character that the European nations first used to claim their own racial superiority, Chinese intellectuals employed the same discourse, albeit fixated on the negative side, to diagnose China's social ills.[20] Dependence, cowardliness, laziness, and selfishness are among the common characteristics that intellectuals found responsible for preventing China from achieving modernity, which are mostly embodied in Chinese peasants who are resistant to change.[21] For instance, Liang asserted that the Chinese have a clannish character and village mentality that lack national consciousness and self-discipline.[22] In a number of articles published at the turn of the twentieth century, he saw a huge gap between Chinese and a modern citizenry.[23] Lu Xun continued the discussion to stress the "slavish character" of the Chinese masses, suggesting that Chinese people hereditarily indulge in self-delusions of a happy ending while being slaves.[24] His "The True Story of Ah Q" ("Ah Q zhengzhuan" 阿Q正传, 1921) creates a quintessential image of the Chinese peasant who is ignorant, delusional, shortsighted, and pathetic. The debate on national

---

20 See Lydia H. Liu, *Translingual Practice: Literature, National Culture, and Translated Modernity—China, 1900–1937* (Stanford: Stanford University Press, 1995), 49.

21 See Sun Lung-kee, *The Chinese National Character: From Nationhood to Individuality* (Armonk, N.Y.: M.E. Sharpe, 2002), 21, 85–86, 102–3.

22 Liang Qichao, "Liang Qichao on His Trip to America" (1903), trans. R. David Arkush and Leo O. Lee, in Patricia Buckley Ebrey, ed., *Chinese Civilization: A Sourcebook*, 2nd ed. (New York: The Free Press, 1993), 335–40.

23 See Liu, *Translingual Practice*, 48.

24 Lu Xun, "Deng xia manbi 灯下漫笔 [Discursive Writing under the Lamp]" (1925), in *Lu Xun quanji* 鲁迅全集 [Complete Works of Lu Xun] (Beijing: Renmin wenxue chubanshe, 2005), 1:222–32.

character was central to the enlightenment movement during the May Fourth period and was revived in the postsocialist era. In 1986, Su Xiaokang in the six-part TV documentary *River Elegy* (*He shang* 河殇) re-broached the question of national character, criticizing a peasant mentality that has kept China from boarding the fast train of advanced industrialization.[25]

Needless to say, for almost a century, modern Chinese intellectuals have been engaged in reforming Chinese national character to transform the masses from "a plate of loose sand" into enlightened, disciplined, independent, and responsible citizens who are devoted to national salvation and modern nation building. Mao's construction of *renmin* 人民 'the People' carried on this legacy, and the practice of the People's Commune during the Great Leap Forward campaign was the peak of the effort to build a nationwide collective community, transcendent over the clans and villages, so as to maximize productivity, equality, and transparency among the people. The people were expected to be organized and selfless, suppressing private desires in favor of public good. Yet what happened during the Great Leap Forward and the Cultural Revolution only evokes a chicken-egg question regarding the failure—we don't know what transpired first: Does the failure result from the flawed national character that was not suited for the collective endeavor (as people were still seeking private interests) or from the glorified communist movement that further alienated people and drew out the worst of human nature (stealing, lying, and victimizing other people)? In any case, the microcosm of the "patient commune" relives this failure and, once again, exposes the ugliness of the Chinese national character, which is only reinforced by the postsocialist market initiatives.

It is no coincidence that for intellectuals, disease has always been a favored parable for flawed national characters in modern Chinese literature. Lu Xun's madman cries out against the cannibalism embedded in Chinese culture.[26] Yu Dafu made use of hypochondria to explore the schizophrenic condition that Chinese youths suffered.[27] In our case, AIDS is employed as a metaphor of illness to reveal other social ills. The catastrophe of AIDS, by the same token, represents the collapse of the community and the demise of the individuals brought about not by AIDS, but by other serious social illnesses. These diseases, consist of not only the capital-related fever that is epidemic in the postsocialist

25 Stephen Field, "*He Shang* and the Plateau of the Ultrastability," *Bulletin of Concerned Asian Scholars* 23.3 (1991): 4–13.

26 Lu Xun, "A Madman's Diary" (1918), trans. Yang Xianyi and Gladys Yang, in *The Columbia Anthology of Modern Chinese Literature*, ed. Joseph S.M. Lau and Howard Goldblatt (New York: Colombia University Press, 2007), 8–16.

27 Yu Dafu, "Sinking" (1921), trans. Joseph S.M. Lau and C.T. Hsia, ibid., 31–55.

village, but also the terror and abuse of power rampant in the previous socialist era. The combination of political power and economic capital mirrors the fundamental catastrophic condition in postsocialist China.

The Catastrophic Condition: Capital and Power as Contagious Disease

In a recent essay on the writings of Yan Lianke, Chien-hsin Tsai evokes a phonetic pun, *aizi* 爱滋—the transliteration of AIDS in Chinese—and *aizi* 爱资 "love for capital," to illustrate the intrinsic connection between the spread of AIDS and capitalist development in China.[28] The juxtaposition of the two words in a remote country setting, as in the film, thus reveals a dangerous cause and effect relation between capital and AIDS and the catastrophic spatial movement of the disease. Indeed, since the beginning of the film, we have been told that a catastrophe has invaded an otherwise peaceful and unknown village. The film opens with an empty shot slowly panning from the cloudy sky to the faraway mountains where a village becomes progressively visible as a boy's voiceover lingers off screen:

> Let's say our village is called Goddess Temple,
> High up in the mountains.
> Don't know from when,
> A Fever that the world called AIDS,
> Snuck into our village quietly from outside.
> With the Fever, life perishes like the fallen leaves.

Then the camera focuses on a boy, clothed in common school uniform with a backpack on his back. Walking on the country road, he holds a magnifying glass right in front of his eyes. The voice over suggests the boy is the narrator himself, Xiaoxin, a twelve-year-old, whose attention is obviously fixed on this new toy and, as the camera shows, immediately seized by a fresh tomato appearing enlarged in his magnifying glass. Lying on a piece of clean napkin paper on the road, the golden red tomato covered with sparkling water-drops seems to tempt Xiaoxin to eat it, which Xiaoxin does, as indicated in the film. The camera follows Xiaoxin's back in an extreme long shot as he is gradually immersed in the enveloping landscape, when he begins to stagger and his

28 Chien-hsin Tsai, "In Sickness or in Health: Yan Lianke and the Writing of Autoimmunity," *Modern Chinese Literature and Culture* 23.1 (Spring 2011): 77–104.

small torso bends forward, hands on stomach, then quietly disappears below the frame. Next an extreme long shot shows Xiaoxin's doubled over and eventually collapsing on the road, a minute figure against large silent mountain landscape that fills the frame (Fig. 7.10). At this moment we as audience are probably confused as what is going on with Xiaoxin, until the next shot introducing Xiaoxin's father Qiquan and uncle Deyi. Carrying knives in their hands, Qiquan and Deyi furiously search the empty village alleys, shouting: "Who did it?" This easily omitted scene implies that Xiaoxin has been poisoned to death by someone in the village. Unable to find the murderer, the saddened and defeated Qiquan and Deyi, squatting on the steps, gaze emotionlessly into space while Old Zhuzhu, Xiaoxin's grandpa, bitter beyond description, looks despairingly at Xiaoxin's body, now in a well decorated little coffin where a Xinhua 新华 Chinese dictionary and a magnifying glass sit comfortably by each side of his head. In contrast to the haggard faces of the family members, Xiaoxin's face remains peaceful, and his voice calm: "People say it is Dad's fault that villagers got the Fever disease, and that Uncle had it coming." Then a bird's-eye view cuts to the house, a newly built, spacious courtyard, one that makes the people inside and the coffin once again disproportionately small (Fig. 7.11).

Such is the opening sequence of the film, a mythical account about an encroaching catastrophe that has overshadowed a seemingly enclosed community. The catastrophe is introduced as AIDS, Fever, and revenge, destroying human lives and shattering community relations. Perhaps, for strategic reasons, Gu Changwei deliberately detached his film from Yan Lianke's novel and obscured the specific location of the village. The boy's voice indicates an accent

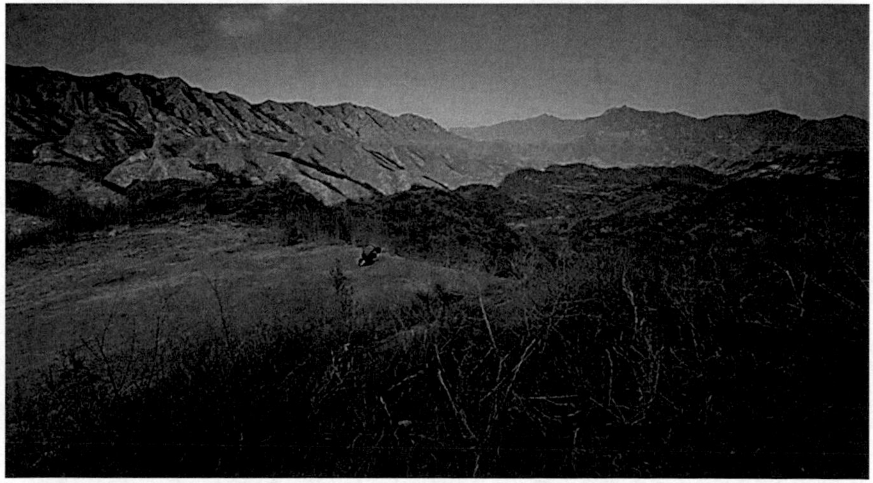

FIGURE 7.10 *Xiaoxin collapses on his way home.*

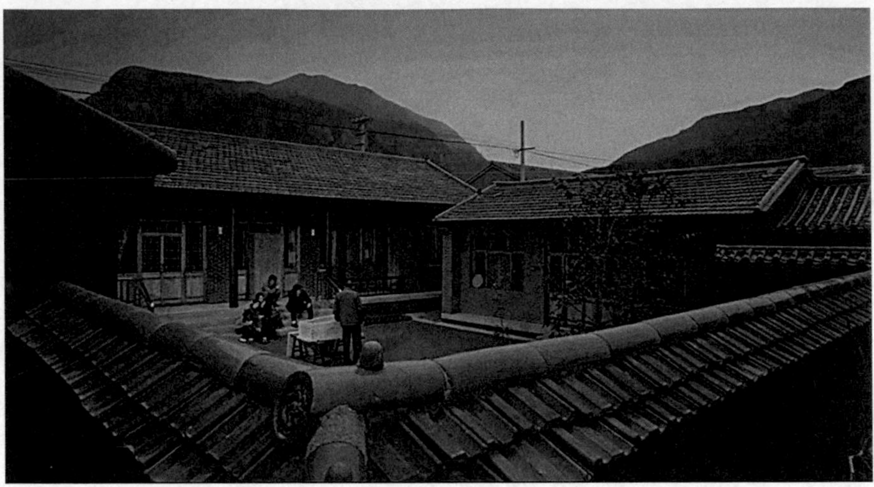

FIGURE 7.11 *Xiaoxin's coffin in his courtyard house.*

closer to that of Shaanxi province, but there is no way to tell the exact geographic location of the village. The unspecified space, mythically portrayed, could be employed to evade government censorship; however, it is also geared toward a sense of national allegory, one that reveals a universal condition of catastrophe of the society. The empty shot presents a distant, peaceful, isolated place where it seems nothing will ever happen; yet AIDS has intruded and transformed human lives into "fallen leaves." This monstrous disease brings fever with it, both as a symptom and a drive, or in other words, it is the drive for monetary gain that results in the physical fever, AIDS. We soon know that villagers contracted the disease because they have been persuaded by Qiquan to sell blood. The idea of a bodily fluid suddenly turning into a regenerative capital that could be transformed into big houses and luxurious commodities has motivated people to fulfill their material desires. Indeed, desire is far from being uni-directionally positive or negative. It could be life-destroying as much as life-affirming. For Deyi and Qinqin, it is also desire that has brought them the disease. They contract AIDS because they have sold blood in exchange of commodities. Qinqin once confesses that she sold blood in order to buy an expensive brand of shampoo advertised on TV. The image on TV heightens the vanity of a young woman, motivating her to cash in on the most convenient capital she has—blood. Images of commodities are contagious, and so is desire. The epidemic of desire for commodities suggests, no doubt, the classical Marxist notion of "alienation," the estrangement of human beings from human nature for the pursuit of commodities. The desire to "consume" commodity in effect brings about the commodification of the body that is being "consumed" by the market and eventually, by AIDS. Seen in this light, desire becomes a double-edged sword, pointing to both life drive and death drive, the death drive that privileges "capital," taking blood as a form of capital, circulatable and exchangeable in the commodity market. Capital dwarfs and swallows human beings, visually represented in Qiquan's courtyard where Xiaoxin's coffin is placed. As Chien-hsin Tsai observes, when one turns to one's own body (blood) for commodity exchange, one contracts a self-destructive autoimmunity in the society.[29] The result is disastrous—blood is contaminated, and AIDS comes along. Needless to say, selling blood itself should not cause AIDS. The real cause latent in the film is the shared needles used to draw blood, which is driven by the urge to make maximum profit on the blood collector's part. The film is synecdochic of the huge AIDS scandal that took place in Henan 河南 province in the 1990s. The rampant blood-selling was particularly encouraged by the local government that advocated a "plasma economy" in the countryside in order to catch up with the high-speed train of Chinese economic development. The cheaply collected plasma then was sold to drug companies to make more profit.[30] Thus emerges a figurative equation in the film: blood=capital=AIDS. Once AIDS drives blood out of the capital market, the commodity circulation stops, and with that collapses the capitalist logic. Such is the autoimmune consequence of the postsocialist market economy.

Equally disturbing and fatal is another autoimmune consequence—Xiaoxin's death. Innocent Xiaoxin dies of villagers' revenge against his father. His sudden demise as a small figure against the disproportionately large landscape is no different from that of an AIDS patient: "life perishes like the fallen leaves." The insignificance of life in front of capital-related disease and desire is the heightened expression of "alienation," most tellingly, Qiquan's alienation. It is as if Qiquan invites this event on himself—because of his aggressively exploiting other people's blood, his own son, that is, his flesh-and-blood, is taken away from him. Meanwhile, Deyi, Qiquan's younger brother, has also

29 Tsai, "In Sickness or in Health," 97.

30 Gao Yaojie 高耀洁, *Xuehuo: Zhongguo aizibing diaocha* 血祸：中国爱滋病调查 [Blood Disaster: An Investigation on Chinese AIDS Condition] (Nanning: Guangxi shifan daxue chubanshe, 2005), 3–4. In the book, Gao points out that under the rubric of developing "plasma economy," people were given misleading information on blood-drawing: Since drug companies only needed plasma and the red blood cells were transfused back to the seller's body after blood is collected, people were told that this way of selling blood would not harm one's body; instead, it will benefit one's health. Available online at http://vip.book.sina.com.cn/book/chapter_39055_23184.html (accessed Feb. 20, 2012).

contracted AIDS despite Qiquan's warning, which the villagers perceive as a sort of cosmic retribution against Qiquan. Both events signify the catastrophic condition of the postsocialist society where the capitalist logic fights against itself, eroding from within. Once blood becomes a commodity, family lineage and kinship relations not only risk being shattered, but also face the possibility of being discontinued. In this regard, it is "love for capital" rather than AIDS that is the death drive that brings forth the suicidal activity in the lure of capital. AIDS, ironically, as discussed above, delivers life force to transport the subjects back to humanity.

Moreover, implicitly, this catastrophic condition is exacerbated by the underlying marriage between capital and political power. Just as the selling of the school property in the "patient commune" signifies the abuse of power driven by capitalist impulse, Qiquan's material success suggests corruption and "rent seeking activity" from government officials. In fact, Qiquan literally marries the deceased Xiaoxin to a much older dead woman—a marriage in afterlife—to secure a beneficial relationship with a county official (Fig. 7.12). He has obtained a large piece of land from the government (presumably at a low price) to build an upscale cemetery. When he tells Old Zhuzhu about his grand plan, he cannot conceal his excitement: "It is impossible for everybody to be born in Suzhou 苏州 and Hangzhou 杭州, but I will make it a reality that everybody can be buried in paradise."[31] The paradise he envisions has been foreshadowed in a previous scene when he lures the power-and-material-obsessed leaders of the "patient commune" to chop trees in exchange for luxurious coffins. Trying out the comfortable coffin lined with genuine leather, Huang Shulang has "contracted" the vision of an afterlife living in paradise. Both power and capital are contagious. The desire to own a luxurious coffin motivates Shulang to be Qiquan's accomplice to steal public property, despite Qiquan's bringing him AIDS. The grotesque image of Qiquan sitting in the dark to observe Shulang putting himself in the coffin most vividly symbolizes the relationship between the exploiter and the exploited, between the hunter and his prey. Heavenly cemetery and luxurious coffin, for Qiquan, are both sources of capital. While people's blood has brought him wealth, their dead bodies will continue enriching his wallet. With the marriage of capital and power, Qiquan is able to transform public property into private capital and turn death into a business of huge profit.

31 In Chinese culture, the cities of Suzhou in Jiangsu 江苏 province and Hangzhou in Zhejiang 浙江 province have traditionally been described as "paradise on earth" to elaborate their material abundance, scenic beauty, and cultural maturity.

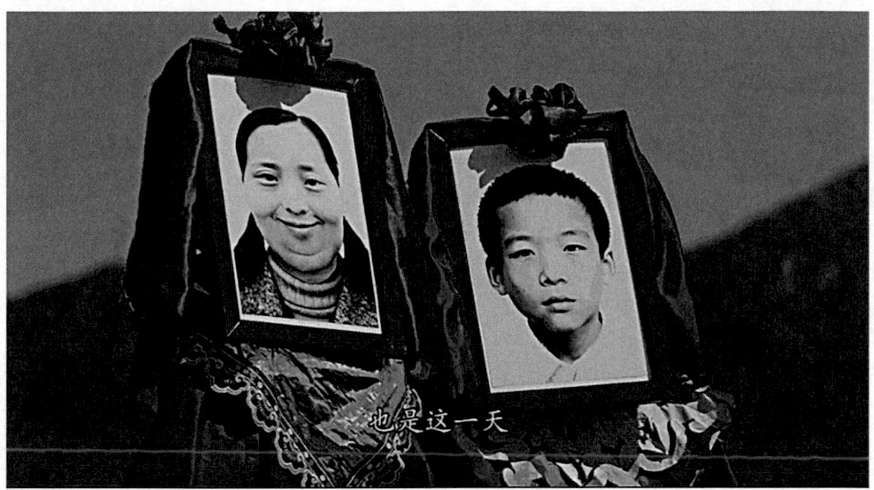

FIGURE 7.12 *Xiaoxin is married by his father to an older woman in afterlife.*

Reluctant Transcendence: "Becoming-Patients" with *Together*

One of the significant differences between the film and the novel resides in the ending. Whereas the novel ends with a chilling event of filicide—the boy-narrator's Grandpa killing Father, signifying the total collapse of the sociopolitical immune system and the perishing of the entire village, the film portrays a heavenly utopia in afterlife, suggesting a transcendent view for the future. As discussed above, AIDS in the film is depicted as something deadly, yet not frightening. It unleashes life forces and facilitates love, and is instrumental in uncovering the catastrophic condition of postsocialist society. This unthreatening side of AIDS is partly achieved by the aestheticization of Deyi's and Qinqin's love, partly achieved by the narrative of the dead boy Xiaoxin. To some extent, the unique narrative voice adds a fantastic, surrealistic flavor to the film. Xiaoxin's voice is peaceful, even delightful, in unfolding the events happening in the village. He describes "his" world—the underworld—as lively as the life in the village. At the end of the film, when both Deyi and Qinqin have died, Xiaoxin's voiceover sounds again, lingering over the images of Deyi and Qinqin who, after passing around candies and citing the words on the marriage certificate, passionately gaze at each other in their wedding clothes:

> My uncle finds me a beautiful aunt named Shang Qinqin. I also like her. Because of the red marriage certificate, they can stay together, enjoying themselves whenever and however they wish. In your world, villagers live

> together. On our side, Uncle, Aunt, and I still remain a family, together with other villagers who came here. We also eat, cultivate the land, live a life, and when we have time, we also laugh, watch operas, and tell stories.

While Xiaoxin's voice describes "his world," the camera cuts from Deyi and Qinqin to the vast landscape, panning upward toward the empty sky while the village gradually disappears from the frame (Fig. 7.13). This empty shot echoes the opening scene of the film in which Xiaoxin's voice accompanies a shot tilting downwards that progressively captures the image of a village on the horizon. The framing of the story in a dead boy's narrative and in two matching empty shots imbues the film with a sense of dreaminess and a fantastic quality. It suggests a utopian afterlife in contrast to the catastrophe of mundane life. Once again, death is not the end of life, but the extension of life, the mirror image of life that provides a privileged perspective to look at life. This cosmic vision of life undermines the threatening consequence of AIDS, while at the same time revealing the catastrophic condition of the society.

Herein lies Gu Changwei's fundamental paradox and deepest ambivalence: simultaneously revealing the inhuman nature of AIDS and humanizing it, engaged in criticizing the pathological society and detached from it. It seems that Gu had a hard time defining his film as social criticism or a redeeming piece of art. The drama of changing titles reflects his wavering intention. The film's title changed several times, from *Time of Magic* (*Moshu shidai* 魔术时代), *Tale of Magic* (*Moshu waizhuan* 魔术外传), to *Guilty Love* (*Zui ai* 罪爱), until it

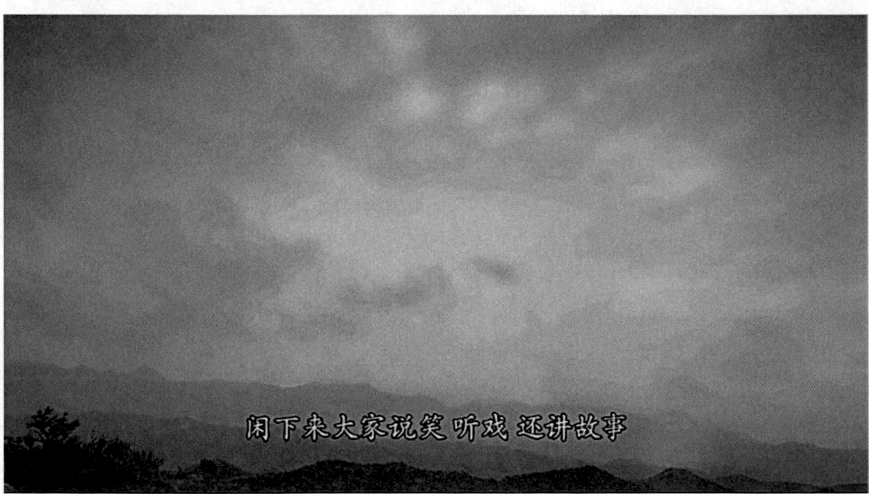

FIGURE 7.13 *The closing shot of the film.*

settles for *Love for Life* (*Zui ai* 最爱).[32] The transformation of the title betrays the trajectory of the film from a surrealistic, critical national allegory to a more upbeat, positive account of love and life.[33] Perhaps, it was the negotiation with social obligation, commercial concern, and political censorship that altogether resulted in the current film, one that reluctantly projects a transcendent vision of love and hope that points to the future in a magical, phantasmagorical manner.[34]

In their *Social Construction of Reality*, Berger and Luckmann suggest that the specific ways of talking about something help people construct a socially shared understanding, hence institutionalized knowledge, of what is reality and how best to approach it.[35] Our communication puts us into a particular way of thinking and acting. In terms of fighting medical conditions such as syphilis, cancer, AIDS, and recently SARS, different rhetorical devices and media coverage result in different public understandings and responses to them.[36] As a medium of mass communication, film has since the beginning played an important role in constructing a "reality" of AIDS. Whereas Western films tend to associate AIDS with what are perceived as unhealthy lifestyles and socially disapproved conduct such as prostitution and homosexuality,[37] Gu's film at once highlights and downplays the cause of the disease. Through the cinematic framing in Xiaoxin's narrative and the glorification of love, Gu's film exhibits a sense of "becoming patients" from the filmmakers to provide a privileged perspective. Gu is obviously motivated to make the film both by an artist's sensibility to portray AIDS as a social metaphor and an activist's obligation to represent AIDS as just a fatal disease. Informed by his wife Jiang Wenli, a volunteer AIDS educator associated with the Ministry of Health who is also the actress who plays Sister Liangfang, Gu attempted to raise social awareness for AIDS through his film, and this may also be one of the important reasons that

---

32 Yang Weiwei 杨薇薇, Zuiai *dianying shouji* 《最爱》电影手记 [*Love for Life*: A Handbook] (Nanchang: Jiangxi jiaoyu chubanshe, 2011), 20. See also the film's database on *Shiguang wang*, http://movie.mtime.com/107438/(accessed Feb. 18, 2012).

33 Shu Ke, "Gu Changwei Nanjing shuo *Zuiai*."

34 Gu explains that the earlier version of the film does not emphasize the love story between Deyi and Qinqin; instead, it is one of two parallel plots. Yet for the reasons of marketing and censorship, the released version only highlights the theme of love. See "*Zuiai*: Juewang he huangmiu de yuyan."

35 P.L. Berger and T. Luckmann, *The Social Construction of Reality: A Treatise in the Sociology of Knowledge* (Garden City, N.Y.: Doubleday, 1967), 1–3.

36 John H. Powers and Xiaosui Xiao, *The Social Construction of SARS: Studies of Health Communication Crisis* (Amsterdam: John Benjamins Publishing, 2008), 2.

37 De Lacerda, "Cinema as an Historical Document," 102–13.

helped the film pass censorship.[38] He deliberately cast AIDS patients and volunteer AIDS educators (including Jiang) in the film,[39] melding the otherwise contradictory roles of a critical individual thinker and a passionate social activist. While the critical thinker in him desires to expose the catastrophic condition of society, the social activist needs to obscure the danger of the cause and instead focus on AIDS patients as "normal" human beings who deserve to be loved and cared for. The resulting product, then, is paradoxical, both realistic and magical—the emotionally charged tale that is *Love for Life*.

The emotional investment of the filmmakers best manifests itself in the accompanying documentary film *Together*. In order to improve general understanding of AIDS among Chinese audiences, Gu invited real HIV-positive people to stay with the film cast and crew and asked director Zhao Liang 赵亮 to shoot a documentary film about HIV-positive patients in China. In fact, the boy actor who plays Xiaoxin is HIV-positive. His name is Hu Zetao 胡泽涛, from Shanxi 山西 province, whose disease was transmitted from his mother by birth. *Together* captures the life experiences of Hu and several other patients, including those who were reluctant to come forward and remained anonymous in the online chat room, to raise awareness of AIDS and eliminate social discrimination against HIV-positive patients. By foregrounding the patients' narratives and showing their friendly interactions with the film crew, the documentary displays a loving atmosphere that indicates hope and change in the future. If we put *Love for Life* together with this documentary film, we will see a dialogic relationship between fiction and reality, between life and death, and between filmmakers and the patients. Hu Zetao is the real life double of Xiaoxin. They share the same innocence and misfortune. The future for the boy, the documentary suggests, must depend on love, the universal love that transcends the narrowly defined romance. It is the "love for life" in general and the love for AIDS patients in particular that injects a fresh dose of hope into the deadly infected community. In this sense, the surrealistic transcendence in *Love for Life* finds its empirical placeholder in reality—the message

---

38 Shenzhen tequ bao 深圳特区报, "Gu Changwei: Haoxi bushi kao 'zhidao' de, Jiang Wenli dui wo hen zhongyao 顾长卫：好戏不是靠'指导'的，蒋雯丽对我很重要 [Gu Changwei: A Good Film Does Not Result from 'Directing'; Jiang Wenli Is Important to Me]," *Zhongguo xinwen wang* 中国新闻网 (China News Service), May 6, 2011, http://www.chinanews.com/yl/2011/05-06/3021874.shtml (accessed Feb. 24, 2013).

39 Besides Jiang, there are other volunteer AIDS educators in the film. In fact, two professional singers joined the team to promote awareness for AIDS. One is Cai Guoqing 蔡国庆 who plays Xiaohai, Qinqin's husband; the other is Li Danyang 李丹阳 who plays Hao Yan, Deyi's wife. Moreover, the actor Pu Cunxin 濮存昕 who plays Qiquan is also an AIDS educator.

of "becoming patients" more tellingly conveyed in *Together*. Beyond raising awareness for AIDS, Gu also directs us to the catastrophic condition of the postsocialist society and indicates that, just as love redeems Deyi and Qinqin from their abjection, "becoming patients" will redeem the nation from the illness of postsocialist development.

References

Altman, Rick. "Inventing the Cinema Soundtrack: Hollywood's Multiplane Sound System." In *Music and Cinema*, ed. James Buhler, Carly Flinn, and David Neumeyer, 339–59. Hanover: Wesleyan University Press, 2000.

Anon. "Zhuanfang Gu Changwei, Jiang Wenli: *Zuiai* bushi yibu nongcun pian 专访顾长卫、蒋雯丽：《最爱》不是一部农村片 [Interview with Gu Changwei and Jiang Wenli: *Love for Life* Is Not a Film about Countryside]." *Tengxun yule* 腾讯娱乐 (Tencent Entertainment), Mar. 22, 2011. http://ent.qq.com/a/20110322/000451.htm (accessed Feb. 23, 2013).

———. "*Zuiai*: Juewang he huangmiu de yuyan 《最爱》：绝望和荒谬的寓言 [*Love for Life*: An Allegory of Despair and Absurdity]." *Xin Jing bao* 新京报 (Beijing News), May 11, 2011. http://www.bjnews.com.cn/ent/2011/05/11/123371.html (accessed Feb. 23, 2013).

Berger, P.L., and T. Luckmann. *The Social Construction of Reality: A Treatise in the Sociology of Knowledge*. Garden City, N.Y.: Doubleday, 1967.

De Lacerda, António Pais. "Cinema as an Historical Document: AIDS in 25 Years of Cinema." *Journal of Medicine and Movies* 2 (2006): 102–13.

Deleuze, Gilles. *Foucault*. Trans. S. Hand. Minneapolis: University of Minnesota Press, 1988.

———. "Dualism, Monism, and Multiplicities (Desire-Pleasure-Jouissance)." Seminar on Mar. 26, 1973. Trans. Daniel W. Smith. *Contretemps* 2 (May 2001).

——— and Félix Guattari. *Anti-Oedipus: Capitalism and Schizophrenia*. Trans. Robert Hurley, Mark Seem, and Helen Lane. London and New York: Penguin, 1977.

Field, Stephen. "*He Shang* and the Plateau of the Ultrastability." *Bulletin of Concerned Asian Scholars* 23.3 (1991): 4–13.

Gao Yaojie 高耀洁. *Xuehuo: Zhongguo aizibing diaocha* 血祸：中国爱滋病调查 [Blood Disaster: An Investigation on Chinese AIDS Condition]. Nanning: Guangxi shifan daxue chubanshe, 2005. http://vip.book.sina.com.cn/book/index_39055.html (accessed Feb. 20, 2012).

Liang Qichao. "Liang Qichao on His Trip to America." 1903. Trans. R. David Arkush and Leo O Lee. In *Chinese Civilization: A Sourcebook*, ed. Patricia Buckley Ebrey, 2nd ed., 335–40. New York: Free Press, 1993.

Liu, Lydia H. *Translingual Practice: Literature, National Culture, and Translated Modernity—China, 1900–1937*. Stanford: Stanford University Press, 1995.

Lu Xun. "Deng xia manbi" 灯下漫笔 [Discursive Writing under the Lamp]. 1925. In *Lu Xun quanji* 鲁迅全集 [Complete Works of Lu Xun]. Beijing: Renmin wenxue chubanshe, 2005. Vol. 1:222–32.

———. "A Madman's Diary." 1918. Trans. Yang Xianyi and Gladys Yang. In *The Columbia Anthology of Modern Chinese Literature*, ed. Joseph S.M. Lau and Howard Goldblatt, 8–16. New York: Colombia University Press, 2007.

Marks, John. *Gilles Deleuze: Vitalism and Multiplicity*. London: Pluto Press, 1998.

Powers, John H., and Xiaosui Xiao. *The Social Construction of SARS: Studies of Health Communication Crisis*. Amsterdam: John Benjamins Publishing, 2008.

Rojas, Carlos. "Of Canons and Cannibalism: A Psycho-Immunological Reading of 'Diary of a Madman'." *Modern Chinese Literature and Culture* 23.1 (Spring 2011): 47–76.

Shenzhen tequ bao 深圳特区报. "Gu Changwei: Haoxi bushi kao 'zhidao' de, Jiang Wenli dui wo hen zhongyao 顾长卫：好戏不是靠'指导'的，蒋雯丽对我很重要 [Gu Changwei: A Good Film Does Not Result from 'Directing'; Jiang Wenli Is Important to Me]." *Zhongguo xinwen wang* 中国新闻网 (China News Service), May 6, 2011. http://www.chinanews.com/yl/2011/05-06/3021874.shtml (accessed Feb. 24, 2013).

Shu Ke 舒克. "Gu Changwei Nanjing shuo *Zuiai* 顾长卫南京说《最爱》 [Gu Changwei Talks about *Love for Life* in Nanjing]." *Shiguang wang* 时光网 (Mtime), May 11, 2011. http://i.mtime.com/shuke/blog/5958665/(accessed Feb. 24, 2013).

Sontag, Susan. *Illness as Metaphor and AIDS and Its Metaphors*. New York: Picador, 1988.

Sun, Lung-kee. *The Chinese National Character: From Nationhood to Individuality*. Armonk, N.Y.: M. E. Sharpe, 2002.

Tsai, Chien-hsin. "In Sickness or in Health: Yan Lianke and the Writing of Autoimmunity." *Modern Chinese Literature and Culture* 23.1 (Spring 2011): 77–104.

Yan Lianke. *Dream of Ding Village*. Trans. Cindy Carter. New York: Grove Press, 2009.

Yang Weiwei 杨薇薇. Zuiai *dianying shouji* 《最爱》电影手记 [*Love for Life*: A Handbook]. Nanchang: Jiangxi jiaoyu chubanshe, 2011.

Yu Dafu. "Sinking." 1921. Trans. Joseph S.M. Lau and C.T. Hsia. In *The Columbia Anthology of Modern Chinese Literature*, 31–55.

CHAPTER 8

Alone Together: Contagion, Stigmatization and Utopia as Therapy in Zhao Liang's AIDS Documentary *Together*

Li Li 李力

> Infectious diseases to which sexual faults are attached always inspire fears of easy contagion and bizarre fantasies of transmission by non-venereal means in public places.
>
> —SUSAN SONTAG[1]

Introduction

In 2009, when the distinguished cinematographer-turned-director Gu Changwei 顾长卫 was preparing to shoot his high-profile feature film *Love for Life* (*Zui ai* 最爱),[2] he made a public announcement to invite members of the HIV infected and Persons With AIDS (PWA) communities to participate in making a film about the AIDS epidemic, loosely adapted from Yan Lianke's 阎连科 banned novel *Dream of Ding Village* (*Dingzhuang meng* 丁庄梦).[3] In order to allow the general audience to see the interactions between the crew and a group of the HIV positive volunteers who might be willing to work on the screen or behind the scenes, Gu conceived of a documentary film as a companion piece and invited Zhao Liang 赵亮 to direct this documentary, later entitled *Together* (*Zai yiqi* 在一起). Trained at the Beijing Film Academy as a photographer and media visual artist, Zhao had established himself in the rapidly expanding circle of independent documentary filmmakers as "one of China's most prolific

---

1 Susan Sontag, *Illness as Metaphor and AIDS and Its Metaphors* (New York: Anchor Books, 1990), 115.

2 The title of this film was changed multiple times, from *Moshu shidai* 魔术时代 [Time of Magic], *Moshu waizhuan* 魔术外传 [Tale of Magic] *to Zui ai* 罪爱 [Guilty Love]. The additional English renditions also include *Life is a Miracle* and *Til Death Do Us Part.* Kun Qian suggests in her chapter in this volume that these changes reflected director Gu Changwei's "fundamental paradox and deepest ambivalence" in configuring the theme of this film.

3 [For a detailed discussion of Yan Lianke's novel, see Chapter 6, by Shelley W. Chan, in this volume. Ed.]

 | DOI 10.1163/9789004319219_010

and respected indie directors."[4] His *Petition* (*Xinfang* 信访) and *Crime and Punishment* (*Zui yu fa* 罪与罚) are internationally well acclaimed for the director's "fearless" speaking out for powerless people, but banned from public exhibition within the country. Zhao accepted Gu's invitation to make the documentary without much hesitation. This agreement, however, took Zhao's career in an unexpected direction later when the Chinese Ministry of Health decided to fund half of the production cost of the projected documentary, and, subsequently sponsored the finished product for approval for public exhibition by the infamous Film Bureau.[5] This news has provoked worldwide discussions over whether Zhao has switched paths "from rebel to insider," as the title of a major report in *The New York Times* suggests. In a broader sense, this dispute over Zhao's engagement with a state-sanctioned project is more about changes in the nature of independent film making in present-day China.[6] Though there

---

4 Cindy Carter, English translator of Yan Lianke's *Dream of Ding Village*, offers this comment in her recent interview with *Ethnic ChinaLit*. Carter has closely worked with Zhao Liang in the past decade and translated the subtitles of four out of five documentaries Zhao made. See Bruce Humes, "The Transparent Translator: Cindy Carter on 'Dream of Ding Village'," *Ethnic ChinaLit*, http://www.bruce-humes.com/?p=6871 (accessed Aug. 23, 2012).

5 The film, completed in November 2010, was shown in seventeen Chinese cities on World AIDS Day (Dec. 1). It was selected to participate in the 61st Berlin International Film Festival in the following February and nominated for the 25th Teddy Award, a lesbian-gay film award officially recognized by the film festival. Then, it also screened in the 35th Hong Kong International Festival in Mar. 2011.

6 In the Aug. 14, 2011 edition of *The New York Times*, Edward Wong contributed a lengthy report featuring Zhao Liang, titled "Chinese Director's Path from Rebel to Insider," commenting that Zhao "has made several independent documentaries and now a state-sanctioned one [*Together*], a move that has cost him some friends." One such lost friend is the high-profile fulminator Ai Weiwei 艾未未. Ai furiously criticized Zhao for accepting government funding, and associated this fact with Zhao's decision, following Jia Zhangke 贾樟柯, to withdrew his work from the 2009 Melbourne Film Festival. Critic Richard Brody of *The New Yorker*, however, argued in his blog on the *New Yorker* website that although Ai's fury is justified, because of "his horrific ordeals in order to live freely under a tyrannical régime,...he is entitled to view those who make common cause with [that régime] of any sort, as being on the wrong side of morality. But...those of us who write and make art without fear of arrest should pause before accusing Zhao of collaboration or cowardice." Brody further argued, using Jia's *I Wish I Knew* (*Haishang chuanqi* 海上传奇), a government-approved documentary made for the 2009 Shanghai Expo, that Jia's work is a rich, symbolic art which is "ingeniously conceived to say exactly what is on his mind regardless of external constraints." Despite his apparent effort to save Jia's and Zhao's works from Ai's self-righteous attack, Brody's comments perpetuate a lasting and simplistic binary between the "State" and the "independent" filmmakers. In fact the boundaries between old categories, such as the official, the intellectual, the underground, the dissident, the mainstream, the popular, are constantly changing, either re-dividing or

have appeared sizable debates in newspapers and on the Internet about the funding of *Together* and whether this had changed the way Zhao makes documentaries, few in-depth investigations have been made into the thematic and stylistic experiments in which Zhao engaged while making *Together*, exploring such aspects as how those experiments contribute to the existing Chinese narratives of the AIDS epidemic, and what kinds of cultural work these narratives do in changing or enhancing public understanding of the AIDS epidemic.

This chapter aims at a close examination of Zhao Liang's making of *Together* through investigation of such matters as how the disease of AIDS is constructed in *Together*, as a medical problem, a social issue, an individual agony, and a collective socio-psychological crisis, and how the disease is texturized to become "the spectacle" through language, visual images, sounds, or silence. It demonstrates that, whether entrenched in medical or social rhetorical realms, the fear and fantasy of AIDS contagion in China is always closely associated with the "risk group" considered prone to spread the disease as well as pollute public morality. The complex, often paradoxical, nature of AIDS seems to be perfectly captured by the oxymoronic "alone together." Indeed, AIDS (Acquired Immune Deficiency Syndrome) is believed to be "acquired" from "the other," suggesting human contact, relatedness, interconnectedness, that is, intimate "togetherness." This disease, however, has been so threatening to the sense of protection that it has forced the carriers of the HIV virus into a stigmatized and insular life—the desperate "aloneness," as this essay demonstrates from

merging, in postsocialist China. In this regard, Paul Pickowicz and Yinjing Zhang shed important new light on our understanding. In the Preface to their co-edited *From Underground to Independent: Alternative Film Culture in Contemporary China* (Lanham: Rowman & Littlefield, 2006), ix–x, Pickowicz and Zhang call our attention to two important points about Chinese "independent" films and filmmakers: first, "independent means a cinematic project's independence from the state system of production, distribution, and exhibition, rather than from its sources of financial support…," not necessarily due to censorship pressures; second, Chinese directors are "divided as to their self-positioning to postsocialist politics. While some may thrive on political controversy by astutely acquiring and cashing in on their 'political capital' overseas…, others insist on the 'apolitical' nature of their work, strategically distancing themselves from previously cherished roles of intellectual spokespersons for the nation and the party." This is probably why Zhao claimed that, though he "did not directly oppose the party," "his subjects, from oppressed peasants to drug-addicted rock musicians, live on China's margins," as Edward Wong mentioned in his report. Indeed, to rigorously search marginal issues and bring out the voices of the underrepresented communities and the innovative aesthetics are the essential characteristics of Zhao's documentaries, including *Together*. For Richard Brody's comments cited here, see Kevin Lee, "The New Yorker's Richard Brody on Zhao Liang, Jia Zhangke, Ai Weiwei," *dGenerate Films*, Aug. 23, 2011, *dgeneratefilms*.com./page/24 (accessed Aug. 1, 2012).

place to place. Whereas "the terrible accident of the HIV epidemic and the terrifying social threats constructed around it gave new virulence to the category of 'deviance',"[7] Zhao's faith on being "together" as a "family" supplies a wishful, utopian therapy for a psychological release of social threats, however ambivalent and imaginary.

Means of AIDS Contagion, Types of Moral Story

The emergence of certain diseases is often conceived by historians as conditioned by modern times. For instance, sexually transmitted diseases are often imagined as a side effect of increased physical mobility, social interconnectedness in the historical contexts of industrialization, urbanization, colonialism, and globalization with their consequent transgression of old social norms, individual boundaries, and inspiration of unconventional ways of living. This imagination is often enhanced by the ever-evolving metaphors of circulation, mutation, and contagion. Since the first case of AIDS as such was detected in 1981, HIV, the underlying virus, is believed to spread exclusively through two means: corporeal and non-corporeal, and in two stages. In the first stage, at least in the West, the epidemic is believed to have spread via bodily fluids primarily in homosexual intercourse, as the syndrome was first called the "gay plague." The controversial gay culture and AIDS in the United States and Europe is also seen as "the perfect emblem of the postmodern era."[8] The second stage of AIDS contagion is "disembodied and nonsexual," spread through "tainted blood" that invades one's healthy body via anonymous blood donations, contaminated invasive medical instrument, or intravenous drug injection. Vertical infection, that is, the infection a mother passes through the placenta or through breastfeeding of a baby is also related to the second type.[9]

What makes the HIV/AIDS epidemic more difficult to grasp than many other diseases as a conceptual and a practical challenge is that it is fundamentally cultural rather than merely a set of biomedical facts. It is simultaneously an "epidemic of transmissible lethal disease and an epidemic of meanings of

7 Sarah Brophy, *Witnessing AIDS: Writing, Testimony, and the Work of Morning* (Toronto: University of Toronto Press, 2004), 5.

8 Paula A. Treichler, *How to Have Theory in an Epidemic: Cultural Chronicles of AIDS* (Durham: Duke University Press, 1990), 33.

9 See Kevin A. Clark, "The Archetype of Blood and Pool of Infinite Contagion," in *Power in the Blood: A Handbook on AIDS, Politics, and Communication*, ed. William N. Elwood (Mahwah, N.J.: Lawrence Erlbaum Associates, 1999), 10.

signification," as Paula Treichler famously comments with the support of a list of thirty-eight social significations of AIDS collected from printed sources published since 1981.[10] Many of those significations, Sarah Brophy further notes, are arranged in a series of seemingly natural dichotomies, such as "homosexual and heterosexual," "passive and active," "homophobic and open," "innocence and guilt," attempting to reassure a notional general, healthy public while connecting infection with moral corruption, deviance, retribution and doom.[11] In line with these dichotomies of socio-moral significations, patients with HIV/AIDS in general public discourse are also divided into two kinds: the "straight"—those who got AIDS from blood transfusion or mother-to-baby transmission, and the "deviant"—those who became infected via homosexual or bisexual intercourse or illicit drug abuse.

Interestingly, in Western AIDS literature, most protagonists are either counter-cultural, faithful lesbian, gay, and bisexual lovers, or to a lesser degree social outcasts who are involved in unprotected sex or drug use and allegedly responsible for contracting HIV/AIDS due to their consciously chosen life styles. The literature of AIDS in those countries is a powerful means of debating gay culture and negotiating gay rights in public discourse. In China, it is much more difficult for the AIDS story to surface in the public discussion space. The "non-straight" stories, always containing "bizarre fantasies of transmission by non-venereal means" in the popular imagination, rarely find expression in the Chinese public media. Meanwhile, the "straight" stories have been forbidden by officials in order to cover up their responsibilities for a series of blood donation campaigns for money in the early 1990s, which caused thousands of new HIV infections in central China.[12] Yan Lianke's fiction *Dream*

10 Treichler, *How to Have Theory in an Epidemic*, 33.

11 Brophy, *Witnessing AIDS*, 3–4.

12 Beginning in the early 1990s local officials in the resource-strapped and impoverished Henan 河南 province promoted a "blood economy"—to procure and resell blood—as a rural development scheme to lift the local farmers from poverty. The government-run blood collection centers and private collectors, known as "blood heads," would pool blood, extract plasma, and inject the leftover blood back into donors in order to increase donation frequency. To reduce the cost, needles and un-sanitized equipment were often reused. These practices resulted in the HIV infection of tens and perhaps hundreds of thousands of local farmers. The uses of contaminated blood product in hospital and virus transmissions through sexual activities and child bearing of the infected rapidly produced an HIV pandemic not only in Henan, but also in its neighboring provinces Hebei 河北, Shanxi and Hubei 湖北. Dr. Gao Yaojie 高耀洁 at the China Center for Disease Control first identified and called the attention of the central government and society about this crisis. See her research *Zhongguo aizibing diaocha* 中国爱滋病调查

of Ding Village first brought the incident to the attention of the reading public though printed copies of it were banned from public distribution. This novel tells how the rural farmers got involved in government-sanctioned, unsanitary blood procurement conducted by organizers known as "blood heads" and were consequently infected with HIV. Ai Xiaoming's 艾晓明 documentary *Care and Love* (*Guanai* 关爱, 2007) recorded the HIV-infected villagers fighting for state compensation. Gu Changwei's star-studded *Love for Life* is the first publicly screened AIDS film in China. Gu's melodramatic visual presentation of the culpability of the "blood heads" in this film essentially moralizes the innocent victims, and thus makes possible his radical romanticization of the film into "a passionate love story" between the two innocent victims Shang Qinqin 商琴琴 and Zhao Deyi 赵得意. Through the making of this film, Gu strives to illuminate the human being's fundamental desire for life, even while facing such an unimaginable catastrophe as AIDS.[13] As a set, these texts of "straight" AIDS stories launched, first and foremost, a rigorous social criticism of the state-sanctioned "blood economy" as a political crisis in postsocialist China. This political crisis refers to an illness viewed "not so much as a biological disease as a spiritual malady."[14]

The desperation of AIDS-ravaged villages in these narratives is no accident. The stories that impoverished individuals regard their blood as a commodity could be found in a range of narratives appeared much earlier than in texts of AIDS proper. For instance, the story about how now famed director Zhang Yimou's 张艺谋 "gave blood over a period of months to earn enough money to purchase his first camera" at the end of the Cultural Revolution had circulated in various contexts before Steven Spielberg made it known worldwide.[15] Zhou Xiaowen's 周晓文1994 award-winning film *Ermo* 二嫫 provides another engrossing tale about how a strong-willed peasant woman eventually purchased a 29-inch color television set, the biggest one at the time in her town, and

[The Investigation of the AIDS Epidemic in China] (Guilin: Guangxi shifan daxue chubanshe, 2005). This crisis has also garnered international media attention. Among many reports, the most well known are Elisabeth Rodenthal's two detailed reports in *The New York Times*: "AIDS Visits Rural China, while Many Look the Other Way" (Oct. 28, 2000) and "Silent Plague: Deadly Shadow Darkens Remote Chinese Village" (May 28, 2001).

13 [For a detailed discussion of Gu's film, see Chapter 7, by Kun Qian, in this volume. Ed.]

14 Chien-hsin Tsai, "In Sickness or in Health: Yan Lianke and the Writing of Autoimmunity," *Modern Chinese Literature and Culture* 23.1 (Spring 2011): 94–95.

15 For Spielberg's article, see *Time* 172.26 (2008): 96.

fulfilled her dream of being modern and competitive.[16] Acclaimed novelist Yu Hua's 余华 national bestseller *Chronicle of a Blood Merchant* (*Xu Sanguan maixue ji* 许三观卖血记) recounts how a poorly-paid factory worker supported his family by selling blood from the Great Leap Forward through the Cultural Revolution and to the economic reform era.[17] Though the protagonists in these "blood-as-commodity" tales might not yet find themselves being infected by the HIV virus, the extent to which they signed up for the lethal proposition suggests a high risk of becoming infected. It is against the broad background of "blood as commodity," in which life symbolized by blood is pathetically reduced to a commodity, as a last resource for exchange, that the spread of AIDS vastly increased, especially in China's poverty-stricken provinces in the Yellow River region.

It is apparent that the existing body of Chinese AIDS narratives is primarily written for an audience made of normal (read "straight") people in society to whom AIDS is presented to be primarily an accidental tragedy through official wrongdoings. In these stories, AIDS as a medical disease and its presence in a significant number of HIV carriers in the vast Chinese cities are still largely left untouched and unexamined. The danger of HIV contagion has not yet become a contingent reality that the entire society, both AIDS patients and the "general healthy public," have to deal with together. Furthermore, the claims made for "innocent victims" sometimes mark out the existence of other victims who are not, or not entirely, innocent (read: who are, through personal choices made, responsible for their contraction of the disease). In this sense, the existing AIDS narratives in mainland China still largely maintains its tendency of omission, non-naming, or denial of the "norm" of the AIDS epidemic—the existence of the gay and other "risk" communities which neither the official nor the members of "general, healthy society" want to confront. In the practice of treating AIDS as a signification of social ills, gay people and other "risk" groups are often reduced to the status of being "only a disease," worthy of attention merely for the purpose of "universalizing the AIDS crisis." Indeed, as Lee Edelman warns us about the indelibility of the dualistic and oppositional concepts and categories in AIDS discourse, "the logic and implications of some of the terms through which an 'AIDS activist' identity…is being formed—formed, to

16 See Ping Fu, "*Ermo*: (Tele)Visualizing Urban/Rural Transformation," in *Chinese Films in Focus II*, ed. Chris Berry (New York: Palgrave Macmillan, 2008), 98–105.

17 Andrew Jones, the translator of *Chronicle of a Blood Merchant* (New York: Pantheon), 261, noted in his Afterword that Yu Hua "seems eerily prescient" to the catastrophic incident happening only several years after the novel was published.

be sure, both for and by, but also, I think, in significant ways, at the expense of gay men."[18] To further pinpoint the problems of partial representation, Joseph Cady categorizes AIDS discourses as "immersive" or "counter-immersive," depending on the ways through which AIDS and the experiences of PWA are presented and represented. "Immersive" writings of AIDS "defy the dominant culture directly and fully and their faithfulness to the emotional and social anguish of people affected by AIDS, especially to the catastrophic texture of gay men's experience under the double denial directed at them during the crisis…." On the contrary, "counter-immersive" AIDS writings "make no compelling demands on the denying reader," because characters, speakers or writers in those literatures are "in various degrees of denial about AIDS themselves."[19] It is with this light of inclusiveness in "immersive" AIDS writing and representation that we can identify the unique social ethnic contributions and the coincidental formative and aesthetic innovations that *Together* makes to the existing body of AIDS discourse in present-day China.

HIV Transmission and Computer Viruses

Zhao Liang's *Together* represents a decisive new approach, not just reaffirming the existing topic AIDS is normally associated with, but bringing changes in many aspects of existing AIDS discourse, e.g., in expanding types of AIDS stories in mainstream media, employing new social media which could reach all kinds of AIDS patients, "straight" and "non-straight" alike, and bring out their much repressed voices. The film's "stylistic schizophrenia," as Dan Edwards puts it, was reflected in its dual missions of documenting the behind-the-scene shooting of Gu's feature and Zhao's own search for volunteers though his interactions with chat room users on the HIV/AIDS websites to identify candidates for Gu's production.[20] Though the former mission initially gave Zhao a chance to make this documentary, it is the latter that makes it alive.

The journey of *Together* started from a search for the HIV/AIDS infected who would volunteer to work on site for the feature film, a task that proved

18 Lee Edelman, "The Mirror and the Tank: 'AIDS', Subjectivity, and the Rhetoric of Activism," in *Writing AIDS: Gay Literature, Language, and Analysis*, ed. Timothy Murphy and Susanne Poirier (New York: Columbia University Press, 1993), 4.

19 Joseph Cady, "Immersive and Counter-immersive Writing about AIDS: The Achievement of Paul Monette's *Love Alone*," ibid., 245, 261.

20 Dan Edwards, "Zhao Liang on His New Documentary *Together*," *Screening China*, Dec. 11, 2010, http://screeningchina.blogspot.com/2010/12/zhao-liang-on-his-new-documentary.html (accessed Aug. 1, 2012).

quite challenging. As Zhao recalled in an interview, "the really difficult thing was finding AIDS sufferers—I looked for several months but couldn't find anyone willing to be interviewed on camera or to join the crew. They were very protective—they really didn't want other people to know."[21] Among his fellow independent documentarians, Zhao belongs to a younger, more Internet-savvy group. To identify potential candidates, he decided to take advantage of the online chat rooms set up by HIV patients and PWAs. The elasticity of this new form of social media allows the AIDS patients to tell their personal stories in a protected fashion. During the online conversations, Zhao first wrote questions to his interlocutors on the computer screen with text scrolling across the screen in real time. This invited the audience to experience the proximate connection between the interviewer and his interviewees. Among numerous HIV positive people and PWAs with whom Zhao and his crew chatted on QQ forums, they persuaded some sixty to receive longer interviews offline; and among these interviewees, some physically appeared in his documentary though most insisted on having their faces pixelated to hide their identity (Fig. 8.1). In the end, six joined the production as members of the cast and crew, of whom, three allowed Zhao to reveal their identities on screen.

The key member is a woman registered on QQ under the name AIDS Rose (Ai Meigui 艾玫瑰) who later revealed her true name Liu Liping 刘丽萍. At the time Liu worked for "Red Ribbon" primary school at Linfen 临汾, Shanxi 山西 province. With her help, Zhao secured an opportunity to interview some of the sixteen HIV infected students in this school. An eleven-year-old boy, Taotao 涛涛 (Hu Zetao 胡泽涛), was selected to play the twelve-year-old Xiaoxin 小鑫 in *Love of Life* (i.e., Ding Qiang 丁强 in Yan Lianke's original novel), son of the notorious "blood head" Zhao Qiquan 赵齐全 in the film (Ding Qiang 丁辉 in the novel). In the beginning of the film, Xiaoxin dies of poisoning by villagers who sought revenge for Zhao Qiquan's evil action of building the blood bank that caused many of his fellow villagers to die of the "illness of fever" (*rebing* 热病)—the local term for AIDS. The unquiet soul of the murdered Xiaoxin haunts the village as a clear-eyed observer, his omniscient narration serving to illuminate his father's culpability in the dissemination of the virus, in sharp contrast to his grandfather's concerns for the ill. When Taotao was invited to play Xiaoxin, Teacher Liu was hired to be an on-the-scene caretaker of her student during the time of filming. Both Liu and Taotao belong to the group of "innocent victims," the former contracted HIV via polluted blood transmission during the emergency of an ectopic pregnancy; the latter, by his

---

21 See Nicola Davison, "Zhao Liang on Gu Changwei's *Til Death Do Us Part*," *Satellite Voices*, May 3, 2011, http://www.dazeddigital.com/satellitevoices/shanghai/film/493/zhao-liang-on-gu-changweis-til-death-do-us-part (accessed Aug. 1, 2012).

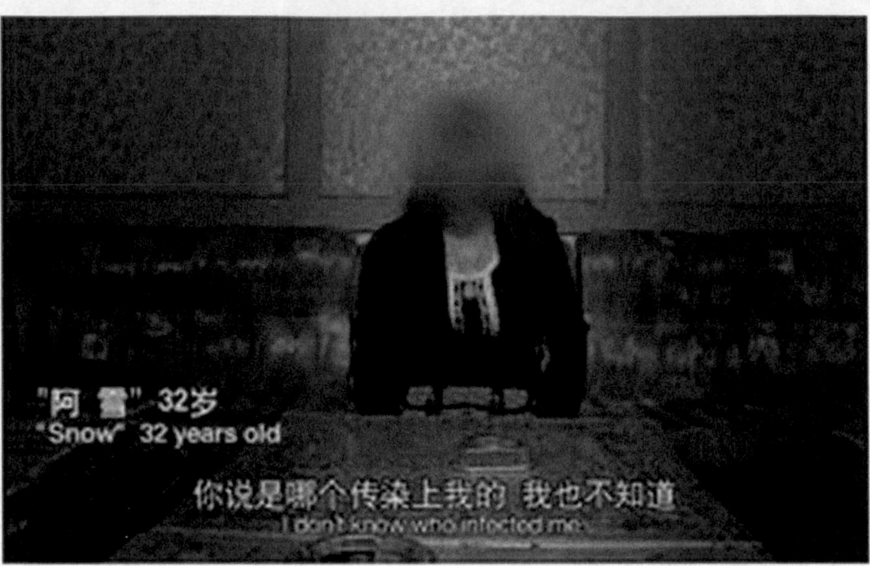
"阿 雪" 32岁
"Snow" 32 years old
你说是哪个传染上我的 我也不知道
I don't know who infected me.

FIGURE 8.1 *Pixelated face on screen.*

infected mother. The third HIV positive person who agreed to appear on screen is a middle-aged man surnamed Xia 夏. We know from his interview with the director back in 2000 that he was tested HIV positive "eight years ago" and, shortly after that, he was kicked out of the house by his wife. After his wife died in an accident "one year ago," he decided to abandon the earthly life, living as a lay practitioner in a local temple. Xia was invited to the crew as an extra and a lighting stand-in. Unlike Liu and Taotao, Xia didn't reveal what caused his infection in the documentary.

Zhao Liang's effort goes far beyond to identifying the cast members, encouraging the hidden members of the "risk groups" with a broad-range of social backgrounds to "come out." In addition to documenting the process of shooting of the film in rural China, the lens of his camera penetrates the opaque darkness surrounding the HIV/AIDS communities in China's vast cities via searching for and maintaining interactions with the HIV infected in chat forums. As Zhao usually conducted interviews indoors, he projected the indoor scene against a backdrop of a panoramic cityscape: endless streams of cars, crowds on the street, and especially, lights from the myriad windows framed by the dark contour of apartment buildings. It is against this mysterious and opaque urban background that Zhao explored, through his camera, the hidden world of the infected communities. Audiences were first let into the world of the "risk groups" through the names the PWAs and HIV carriers chose to use in the chat forum, most telling of each patient's self-perception of their situations and identities. Names such as Down-and-Out (Tianya Lunluo Ren 天涯沦落人), Duckweed (Fuping 浮萍), Quietly Living (Jingjing de Huo 静静地活) tell their situation as social outcasts. Invisible Angel (Yinxing Tianshi 隐形天使), Gold (Jinzi 金子) and Snow (Ah Xue 阿雪) speak out the ironies of their conceived self-identity as pure or valuable, though they knew that society would think otherwise.[22] Some self-labels exhibit a strong tone of social-defiance, such as AIDS Rose (Ai Meigui 艾玫瑰) and Endless Love (Ai Buwan 爱不完). As the real names of these people have been erased in normal society, their fabricated online names vividly show their situations as well as their discontents.

The close-up shots of the documentary allow the audience to read the director's dialogues with the people whom he interviewed onscreen as scrolling text in real time, as if we were sitting with the filmmaker in front of his computer. This method could force the audience to have an intimate interaction with the infected people, because "the stripped back approach makes the pain of the interviewees woven into the simple lines on screen all the more heartbreaking."[23] True, as Susan Sontag observes, "in the description of AIDS the enemy is what causes the disease, an infectious agent that comes from the outside,"[24] because AIDS in the popular mythology is often coupled with what many in mainstream society view as deviant sexual behavior, moral decadence, danger of contagion and inexorable punishment. To answer this question of how their positive HIV status came to be is, for many infected people, to make public the deepest secret in their personal life which is normally concealed from public discourse. Duckweed told Zhao that she was infected by sharing with her husband needles of intravenous drug injection, passing her acquired virus to her then six-year-old son. Her husband left her and their son without any child support. She once attempted to kill her own son and herself by putting rat poison in rice hoping to end the physical agony and social stigmatization society imposed on them. Among those interviewed via chat forum and camera, many contracted HIV via sexual intercourse with their partners, and the most alarming thing is that when being asked if those alleged vectors of HIV knew if they had been infected, many answered "don't know whether he knew or not"; and

22 "Jingjing de huo" is original translated as "tranquility" in the film. "Tranquility," which has the connotation of peace and self-content, I argue, does not properly convey the despair from the silence imposed by the society that Jingjing de Huo had experienced. "Quietly Living" is more expressive of the true reality of many patients—hanging on biologically, but only silently, as if they were diseases.

23 Dan Edwards, "Fear, Loathing and HIV: Zhao Liang's *Together*," *Screening China*, Jan. 19, 2010, http://screeningchina.blogspot.com/2011/01/fear-loathing-and-hiv-zhao-liangs.html (accessed Aug. 1, 2012).

24 Sontag, *Illness as Metaphor and AIDS and Its Metaphors*, 105.

when asked whether "you plan to tell your partner that you are infected," the reply is frequently "no," with the excuses of protecting themselves from being stigmatized by their partners, families, communities and society in large.

This kind of cover-up, for Zhao Liang, has proved to be the greatest menace to public health. For instance, 23-year-old Quietly Living was certain that her only boyfriend passed her the virus, but wasn't sure whether her boyfriend had known about his own condition. She didn't plan to reveal her own infection to her boyfriend either, so she would not be abandoned by him. Lili contracted HIV from her husband and was abandoned once the symptoms started to show. Endless Love believed that the virus he contracted was from one of his gay partners, but he was uncertain whether he will confront him for fear of losing him. These stories demonstrate that in present-day society AIDS is not only spread via illicit intercourse but through normal sexual, even marital relationships; the real threat is not the virus itself, but the virulence of the fear for being left alone.

Computer-based Internet media are not only instrumental for Zhao's project, but also illustrative of the profound analogy between the HIV virus and a computer virus in popular imagination of the disease. Like HIV viruses that slowly infect a biological body, the circulation of information linked to the computer is exposed to and threatened by viral software. People who enjoy "promiscuous," unprotected computing, running programs of unknown provenance, or connecting with unknown sites in pursuit of perceived benefits (information, pirated materials, free online games, etc.) run a higher risk of computer virus infection, just as people who expose themselves to promiscuous, unprotected relationships in exchange for either sexual pleasures or monetary benefits are at a high risk of HIV viral infection. Informational and biological bodies exist and provide a medium for reproduction by communication or exchange of materials with another. What draws AIDS and computer viruses even closer, I argue, is their shared nature of latency. AIDS is often conceived of as insidious because of its characteristic latency, regarded as "a menace in waiting, as mutable, as furtive…," allowing undetected harboring and dissemination without knowledge. This attribution is probably best captured by a famous line in *The Early Frost* (1985), the first television-film on AIDS broadcast in the U.S. While the protagonist, Michael, was being informed of his seropositive diagnosis, he questioned his doctor in dismay and with seeming disbelief: "You mean you can pass it on without actually getting it?" Of course, this question is merely an indication of Michael's reluctance to face "the story behind the story." Paula Treichler explains in her study of this landmark media work on AIDS: "Since one does not transmit AIDS itself but rather a virus that destroys the immune system, and since one does not transmit the virus without carrying it oneself, this statement is accurate only if *it* in *pass it on* means the virus and *it* in *not getting it* means full-blown AIDS.... The message intended to be communicated here is no doubt that an infected person may not look sick or be sick but is still infectious to others."[25] Paralleling the behavior of biological viruses, software viruses often "won't produce immediate signs of damage to the computer's memory, which gives the newly 'infected' program or file time to spread to other computers."[26] The unexpectedness and insidiousness of the HIV virus, as the many cases of Zhao's interviewees show, prove to be one of the major reasons for making the old mythology of AIDS a real dread in popular imagination.

In short, *Together* should be credited with serving a number of cultural functions. It gives "disease a human face"—though, in many cases, only giving it a human voice, because many patients still felt compelled to have their faces hidden—and provides a rare example of non-selectively showing marginalized individuals, their stigma, and living situations. The innovative adoption of the form of new social media allows broader coverage of both AIDS stories and the kinds of damage public ignorance and prejudice have done. Most remarkably, it demonstrates a new effort to fully explore the epidemic through disassociating an AIDS patient from social stigma, so as to restore the identity of a PWA as simply a patient with whom the audience can share stories and discern common points, even if his/her biological life inevitably cannot be saved.

Polluted Blood and Imaginary Family as Therapy

Although both cancer and AIDS are deadly diseases, practicing physicians routinely use different approaches when communicating with patients and their families about the diagnoses of the patients. It has been noticed that when a patient is diagnosed with cancer, his physician usually first discloses the bad news to the family of a patient, allowing the family to inform the patient in an appropriate time and way. When a patient is found to be HIV positive, however, the doctor always tells the patient him/herself, leaving the patient alone to deal with family. After receiving the bad news, families of cancer patients are mostly supportive, while those of the AIDS patients typically act out either in rage or in denial. One of the reasons for this phenomenon is that cancer is understood as a disease of the individual—"cancerphobia teaching us the fear of a polluting environment," not the fear of being infected by the patient, whereas

25 Treichler, *How to Have Theory in an Epidemic*, 191.

26 Sontag, *Illness as Metaphor and AIDS and Its Metaphors*, 158.

AIDS is contagious and invasive, imposing on the general public "the fear of polluting people" with contaminated body fluid, whether the fluid is from a stranger, a neighbor, a lover, or one's kin.[27] It is the fear of polluted blood that imposes the worst threat in Chinese society.

In the Chinese understanding of biological and social reproduction, blood is a power that not only sustains individual life but also determines the continuity of kinship that is largely defined by consanguinity (*xueyuan* 血缘). Chinese society, as sociologist Fei Xiaotong 费孝通 suggests, is traditionally a consanguineous society which "maintains structural stability by using the biological process underlining reproduction as a medium to establish social continuity."[28] According to Fei's theory, a family sharing the same blood linkage forms the basic social unit. In this system, when the father dies the son succeeds, not only linking to the next circle of biological reproduction, but also keeping family wealth and social status within the clan. Clean, genuine blood is essential to both individual life and the continuity and expansion of family or clan. HIV, however, makes the blood-life itself a bearer of contamination that is not only lethal to individual life but, more seriously, disrupts the bloodline, the core of marriage, parenthood, continuity of kinship.[29] It also affects property consolidation and social status of a family/clan. This partially explains why cancer patients and AIDS patients are often treated differently by their families: a cancer patient is regarded as an unfortunate individual whose suffering is the result of a failure to act; AIDS, on the contrary, is often linked to a proscribed behavior which spreads degenerative disease and destroys genealogy. Moreover, the pervasive "epidemic of signification" evoked by AIDS not only stigmatizes the PWAs but also is often considered to bring social shame and threats to their families.

---

27 For the discussion, see Sontag, *Illness as Metaphor and AIDS and Its Metaphors*, 161.

28 Fei Xiaotong, *The Soil: The Foundations of Chinese Society*, trans. Gay Hamilton and Wang Zheng (Berkeley: University of California Press, 1992), 120.

29 This point is further confirmed by Didi Kirsten Tatlow in his article on Chinese people's responses to a hit story about CNN anchor Anderson Cooper's coming out. It points out that due to the fact that "familial and cultural pressures to be heterosexual, marry and produce an heir are simply too great," "more than 90 percent of China's gay men bow to pressure and marry women—without revealing their homosexuality." Zhang Beichuan, a leading researcher of homosexuality at Qingdao University, warns that China faces a new kind of AIDS epidemic "related to the non-acceptance of homosexuality, including AIDS transmission from gay men to their wives and unhappy marriage in which one partner is secretly gay." See Tatlow, "Anderson Cooper's Coming Out Rattles China's Closet," *The New York Times*, July 5, 2012, http://rendezvous.blogs.nytimes.com/2012/07/05/anderson-coopers-coming-out (accessed Sept. 13, 2012).

Because of these reasons, AIDS patients are often distanced and stigmatized in the first place by their own families. In *Together*, when Zhao asks Quietly Living, a twenty-two-year-old girl who claims to have been infected by her first and only boyfriend, whether she plans to tell her parents about her sickness, the reply is: "Absolutely not! They would jump out of the building." The reason for such an extreme potential action, as Quietly Living perfectly understands, is more because of her parent's fears for social humiliation than the eventual loss of their only daughter. Twenty-five-year-old Gold was diagnosed HIV positive in a physical examination for entering a police academy and has been struggling to keep jobs as the physical de-configuration of AIDS has become visible on him. When Zhao asks him on QQ whether he would consider joining the crew, Gold says he would should his family allow him to do so. Zhao encourages him to call his parents. Gold eventually reaches his mother and their conversation is recorded and played in the documentary. In the conversation, the mother exasperatedly blames Gold for bringing "such a shame and humiliation to our family—not only our direct family, but the extended family." She emphasizes: "Don't you know that we are a big family/clan (*da jiazu* 大家族)? The whole family, your own siblings and your cousins, everyone has been trying so hard to hide your sickness from people outside. How dare you even think about exposing your identity in public and bringing shame to everyone in our family?" Apparently, the concerns the angry mother voices here are more explicitly related to the reputation of the kinship connected by the same bloodline externalized by the same family name.

It is strange why the concern of the clan is so seriously voiced by the mother instead of the father, the head of the patriarchal family system. Is this merely a special case? As a matter of fact, the relationship between gay men and their families has long been a topic under examination among scholars of the AIDS discourse. For instance, Treichler points out in her study on *An Early Frost* that the real protagonists in this film are not the PWAs, but "the American nuclear family," mirroring a family's pains and concerns with its own future.[30] Another well-known early AIDS drama on network television is *Our Sons*, which exclusively deals with the relationship between PWAs and their mothers. John Clum argues that the omnipresent presence of the mother figure in *Our Sons* indicates "the image of the gay man has been woven through with some of the most terrifying representations of degenerative disease," borrowing British video artist Stuart Marshall's observation, and that the missing father figure in *Our Sons* is because "fathers shouldn't have to deal with gay sons or HIV-infected

30 Paula Treichler, "AIDS Narratives on Television: Whose Story?" in Murphy and Poirier, *Writing AIDS*, 169.

sons, who have obviously transgressed the Law of the Father."[31] In this light, Gold, with contaminated blood, is apparently regarded as a dysfunctional link in the familial reproduction chain, and therefore has to be hidden away from outsiders in order to keep the reputation of the clan. Still, a clan's fears of the infected member also stems from the sibling intimacy that is essentially built on the same blood linkage. Male siblings and cousins, who could cosign the same surname in claiming family property, are, in the case of AIDS, "joint inheritors of the family hurt"—"I might have died where he did," to borrow Ross Chambers' phrase; thus, in facing the crisis of an infected male member "the sense of danger and precipitousness coexists with the family's denial, its careful maintenance of a façade of happiness, order, and normalcy."[32]

The depth of the familial crisis evoked from blood pollution is also revealed in another example. Duckweed seemed to have a happy life with her husband and son. A son is highly valued in Chinese society particularly considering that the one-child policy, despite its high controversy, was then still implemented in China. Duckweed, unfortunately, later tested HIV positive due to sharing needles in drug injection, and worse of all, her six-old son is also touched. For the father, the son with contaminated blood is no more than a biological cell of disease. He consequently divorced Duckweed and, without much hesitation, abandoned his son, too. The biological needs of reproduction and the protection of family reputation from society are the two important reasons that have caused families of the PWAs to distance and abandon the infected members of their own. This, to some degree, can also be explained by the medical theory of "autoimmunity."

Indeed, in the case of AIDS, the very problematic nature of "family" seems to stand in as the very site of tragedy for the PWAs and the HIV infected rather than the anodyne of it. It is no wonder that in Zhao's attempt to make a conversion of popular homophobic ignorance to a more sympathetic understanding, he places much emphasis on the imaginary "family" or "family-like" community/society in a positivist sense. The three AIDS patients who are willing to be shown onscreen in the documentary give the audience an impression of a family: the gentleman-like Xia, a father figure, Taotao's care-taker teacher Liu, a mother figure, and Taotao, the child. In the process of their participating in shooting the film, Xia is seen frequently dropping by the cozy room of Liu and Taotao, chatting about various personal stories and sharing with them everyday concerns, such as weather, food, and medicine. Liu and Xia act as the

---

31 John M. Clum, "And Once I Had It All," ibid., 203.

32 Ross Chambers, *Untimely Interventions: AIDS Writing, Testimonial, & the Rhetoric of Hunting* (Ann Arbor: University of Michigan Press, 2004), 332.

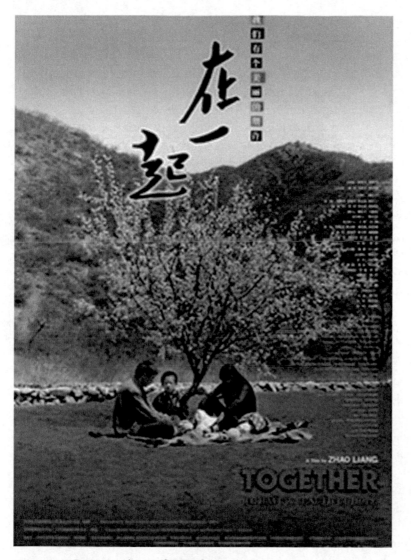

FIGURE 8.2 *Promotional poster for* Together.

surrogate parents of Taotao: while Liu is seen helping the boy to put on clothes and reminding him to take medicines, Xia is shown wrapping the boy with his cotton overcoat to keep him warm in the chilly evenings when they are watching the shooting of the feature film.

The most exemplary image is the three of them having a picnic lunch, a signature scene featured on the poster for the documentary (Fig. 8.2). This scene is first shot from a distance. We see a natural, quintessential Chinese-style one-child "family" having a picnic lunch under a full-blooming peach tree in an open field against a vast mountain range. This utopian, picture-perfect scene seems to remind the audience that human beings in the form of family are the center of the universe. As the camera moves closer, the conversation among the members of the "family" became audible. To the audience's surprise, the conversation is about how much time is left for each of them to live.

The most tragic and ironic thing they find is that twelve-year-old Taotao is likely to have the shortest time to live—"I could live for probably one more year, the year 2012," Taotao announced, as cool as if he were talking about someone he didn't know at all. This is a moment charged with immense tragic irony. What we saw earlier as natural turned awry: people of this "family" were not talking about the familiar family topics in this spring day, but withering of their lives and untimely death. The future is drastically foreshortened—everyone, though in the prime of life, will soon die, and the youngest one will die first. Indeed, "the future is not in the future, where it belongs, but already here and now, haunting the present with a sense of impending disaster."[33] They also talked about what they want to become in their next incarnation; they all wish there would be another chance to relive "this life" that would be soon cut off. Taotao wants to become a bird that would not be tied to the ground like human beings are, but Liu doesn't want to become anything else: "I still want to become a woman. How wonderful to be a woman…." Even living in the shadow of death, desires for life, reproduction and family are apparently dominant. Blanche DuBois is precisely right: "the opposite of death is desire."[34]

This imagined family of three largely embodies Director Zhao's utopian ideas about helping the general public to have a more sympathetic understanding of AIDS patients. The temporary proximity and unity of this pseudo-family dissolves toward the end of the documentary when Xia has to go back to the hospital due to fast deterioration from the illness. He bids farewell to the crew and staff, thanks them for treating him as a one of a big family without imposing prejudices against him, and then walks to the train station accompanied by the other two members of his "family." Though many biological families of PWAs turned their back on the infected one, Zhao nonetheless hopes to create via his documentary social "families," exemplified by the "family" of Xia, Liu and Taotao, or family-like communities, like the crew and staff of *Love for Life*.

Yet, this utopianism for "family" and "togetherness" is but wishful and imaginary, and it makes the ending of Zhao's project open to more questions about the grim reality rather than bringing closure to the problems. *Together*

33 Chambers, "Untimely Interventions," 334.

34 DuBois' epigraph is cited in Clum, "And Once I Had It All," in Murphy and Poirier, *Writing AIDS*, 209.

ends by recording encounters between various people on the street with Liu Jiulong 刘九龙, a PWA street artist. The artist labels himself as an *aizi bingren* 爱滋病人 (an AIDS patient) and upholds a banner with a challenging request: "Please give me a hug!" People pass him from all directions on the busy street, but few pay any attention to his existence. He stops a girl, asking her whether she has heard of PWA. The girl quickly throws him a contemptuous reply without even stopping: "They are those who indulge themselves in deviant sex…." The artist, apparently looking rather awkward, shrugs his shoulders and murmurs: "Do you really think so?" Later on, as a young couple is passing by, the artist stops them: "Have you heard about AIDS?" The couple look rather embarrassed simply by being asked this question, and the girl throws some money on the ground and tries to walk away. The artist picks up the money and returns it to the girl, stating: "This is not what I want—I want…understanding!" Eventually, an older lady is passing by and the artist asks her: "Can you give me a hug?" The woman pauses for a moment, obviously notices the existence of the camera, and then gives a full hug to the artist. This ending seems to force us, in essence, to repeat the experience of the film in miniature.

Conclusion

Zhao Liang's intent in making this documentary is neither conservative, caving to State pressure, nor liberal, striving to legitimize gay rights. It is primarily pragmatic. The core effort of *Together* lies in "demystifying" the popular imagination of AIDS by bringing out a full range of coming-out stories. It demonstrates that the epidemic is not only associated with the gay lifestyle and illicit acts, such as prostitution and drug abuse, but also intermingles with "normal" people's everyday lives. Among the many dangerous attributes of AIDS, the biggest is its latency—the fact that, in many cases, the patient can "pass it to others even before knowing one has it…." Thus, the biggest threat the AIDS epidemic has imposed on society is public denial and a secretive silence. Yet, the silence cannot be broken and the denial cannot be rectified without detaching the socially invented meanings surrounding the epidemic. The hope seems to lie in the detachment of the illness from its meanings, as Teacher Liu repeatedly tells us: "An AIDS patient should be treated simply as a patient (*bingren*), not a criminal (*zuiren* 罪人)—no matter what caused one's infection." "But the metaphors cannot be distanced just by abstaining from them. They have to be exposed, criticized, belabored, used up,"[35] and *Together* is a renewed effort in all these directions.

---

35 Sontag, *Illness as Metaphor and AIDS and Its Metaphors*, 182.

References

Berry, Chris. *Chinese Films in Focus II*. New York: Palgrave Macmillan, 2008.

Brophy, Sarah. *Witnessing AIDS: Writing, Testimony, and the Work of Morning*. Toronto: University of Toronto Press, 2004.

Chambers, Ross. *Untimely Interventions: AIDS Writing, Testimonial, & the Rhetoric of Hunting*. Ann Arbor: University of Michigan Press, 2004.

Davison, Nicola. "Zhao Liang on Gu Changwei's *Til Death Do Us Part*." *Satellite Voices*, May 3, 2011. http://www.dazeddigital.com/satellitevoices/shanghai/film/493/zhao-liang-on-gu-changweis-til-death-do-us-part (accessed Aug. 1, 2012).

Edwards, Dan. "Fear, Loathing and HIV: Zhao Liang's *Together*." *Screening China*. Jan. 19, 2010. http://screeningchina.blogspot.com/2011/01/fear-loathing-and-hiv-zhao-liangs.html (accessed Aug. 1, 2012).

———. "Zhao Liang on His New Documentary *Together*." *Screening China*, Dec. 11, 2010. http://screeningchina.blogspot.com/2010/12/zhao-liang-on-his-new-documentary.html (accessed Aug. 1, 2012).

Elwood, William N., ed. *Power in the Blood: A Handbook on AIDS, Politics, and Communication*. Mahwah, N.J.: Lawrence Erlbaum Associates, 1999.

Erwin, Kathleen. "The Circulatory System: Blood Procurement, AIDS, and the Social Body in China." *Medical Anthropology Quarterly* 20. 2 (2006): 139–59.

Fei Xiaotong. *The Soil: The Foundations of Chinese Society*. Trans. Gay Hamilton and Wang Zheng. Berkeley: University of California Press, 1992.

Gao Yaojie 高耀洁. *Zhongguo aizibing diaocha* 中国爱滋病调查 [The Investigation of the AIDS Epidemic in China]. Guilin: Guangxi shifan daxue chubanshe, 2005.

Humes, Bruce. "The Transparent Translator: Cindy Carter on 'Dream of Ding Village'." *Ethnic ChinaLit*. http://www.bruce-humes.com/?=6871 (accessed Aug. 23, 2012).

Lee, Kevin B. "The New Yorker's Richard Brody on Zhao Liang, Jia Zhangke, Ai Weiwei." *dGenerate Films*, Aug. 23, 2011. *dgeneratefilms*.com./page/24 (accessed Aug. 1, 2012).

Murphy, Timothy, and Susanne Poirier, eds. *Writing AIDS: Gay Literature, Language, and Analysis*. New York: Columbia University Press, 1993.

Pickowicz, Paul G., and Yingjin Zhang, eds. *From Underground to Independent: Alternative Film Culture in Contemporary China*. Lanham: Rowan & Littlefield, 2006.

Rosenthal, Elisabeth. "AIDS Visits Rural China, While Many Look the Other Way." *The New York Times*, Oct. 28, 2000.

———. "Silent Plague: Deadly Shadow Darkens Remote Chinese Village." *The New York Times*, May 28, 2001.

Sontag, Susan. *Illness as Metaphor and AIDS and Its Metaphors*. New York: Anchor Books, 1990.

Spielberg, Steven. *Time* 172.26 (2008): 96.

Tatlow, Didi Kirsten. "Anderson Cooper's Coming Out Rattles China's Closet." *The New York Times*, July 5, 2012. http://rendezvous.blogs.nytimes.com/2012/07/05/anderson-coopers-coming-out (accessed Sept. 13, 2012).

Treichler, Paula A. *How to Have Theory in an Epidemic: Cultural Chronicles of AIDS*. Durham: Duke University Press, 1999.

Tsai, Chien-hsin. "In Sickness or in Health: Yan Lianke and the Writing of Autoimmunity." *Modern Chinese Literature and Culture* 23.1 (Spring 2011): 77–104.

Wong, Edward. "Chinese Director's Path from Rebel to Insider." *The New York Times*, Aug. 14, 2011.

Yan Lianke. *Dream of Ding Village*. Trans. Cindy Carter. New York: Grove Press, 2009.

Yu Hua. *Chronicle of a Blood Merchant*. Trans. Andrew Jones. New York: Pantheon, 2003.

CHAPTER 9

The Unknown Virus: The Social Logic of Bio-conspiracy Theories in Contemporary China*

Kevin Carrico

Following a long night of drinking with colleagues in early 2010, Chen made what he claims was his first and only visit to a sex worker, at a sauna in Guangzhou.[1] After a semi-sobering shower, he proceeded to a back room. A young woman with a Northeastern accent soon entered, and after a bit of suggestive massaging, the true intention of his visit began. Aware of the potential risks involved, Chen wore a condom; however, he was unable to perform and left in embarrassment after some awkward embraces and even more awkward dialogue. On his walk home, where his wife and daughter were already fast asleep, Chen began to feel itchy, and claimed that he could feel his organs swelling inside of him. When he awoke the next morning, he had a throbbing headache and diarrhea, and vomited a number of times. Overlooking the possibility of an intense hangover after a long night of drinking, Chen's mind immediately raced to his liaison, or rather his attempted liaison, the night before, and then raced onward to AIDS, where everything suddenly made quite anxiety-inducing sense: he had contracted AIDS during his sauna visit. When his first HIV test came back negative just a few days later, he did not feel relief: instead, he was certain that it was wrong.[2] In the weeks and months that followed, Chen experienced chills, sweating, diarrhea, uncontrollable muscular spasms, depression, weight loss, and impotence; furthermore, he underwent one HIV test after another, completing a total of fourteen at various medical institutions around

* I would like to thank the Comparative Literature Section at Sun Yat-sen University, particularly Ai Xiaoming 艾晓明 and Ke Qianting 柯倩婷, for providing me with such an intellectually exciting home during my fieldwork. I would also like to thank Magnus Fiskesjö, TJ Hinrichs, Gail Hershatter, Ronald Knapp, and Tiantian Zheng for their thoughtful comments on earlier drafts and presentations of this project.

1 Pseudonyms are used throughout this chapter to protect the anonymity of interviewees.

2 Numerous aspects of "unknown virus" narratives, from the nearly immediate onset of "AIDS" to its easy passage through condoms to the assumed accuracy of HIV tests taken within days of presumed exposure, stand in stark contrast to the biological realities of the actual HIV virus. While recognizing and indeed analyzing these incongruent moments, this chapter nevertheless aims to present this illness as experienced by patients, despite apparent biological inaccuracies and logical shortcomings.

 | DOI 10.1163/9789004319219_011

the city in the year that followed, all with the same "wrong" result: negative. While attempting to hide his secret anguish from everyone around him, he gradually became convinced that he had unintentionally infected his family and coworkers, tying their occasional complaints of headaches, chills, and other forms of discomfort to that fateful night at the sauna. When I got to know Chen, he had largely withdrawn from society.

Yang, a twenty-four-year-old real-estate agent and longstanding virgin, spent most of his waking hours on the popular chatting portal QQ. But in late 2010, his life took an unexpected turn when he began chatting with a quite open-minded female acquaintance known as Lonely Soul (Jimo de Linghun 寂寞的灵魂). Their chats became quite intimate and eventually led to an agreement to meet in person; Yang soon found himself in a seedy hourly motel room enjoying his first sexual experience. Yet he was shocked to find, he tells me, that his companion acted "like a damn animal," panting and screaming throughout their encounter, scratching his back, kissing him aggressively, and even biting his lip so hard that she left teeth marks. Returning to his parents' apartment after this overwhelming evening, Yang first lay in bed and ran his fingers over the interior of his mouth, the object of Lonely Soul's untamed aggression and the subsequent object of Yang's fascination over the months to come. Convinced that the once-smooth interior of his mouth had suddenly grown rough and bumpy, he spent endless hours that night anxiously staring into a mirror, inspecting his tongue, gums, and the inner surface of his cheeks, all of the while growing increasingly anxious about Lonely Soul's sexual aggression, presumed promiscuity, and the risks that such behavior brings. Reading the bumps in his mouth like a fortune of impending doom, the physiological changes that he perceived presented an unambiguous and painful truth to Yang: he had been infected with AIDS during his one-night stand. Yang took one HIV-test after another in the months that followed, refusing, like Chen, to accept his repeated negative results. As he perceived his condition worsening, Yang quit his job and gathered the courage to admit his illness to his parents: his mother broke down in tears and cursed him repeatedly, he tells me, while his father sat in silence, staring blankly ahead. Since then, Yang has spent much of his time in bed in his parents' apartment, increasingly distant even from those physically closest to him.

Despite their self-isolation, Chen and Yang are not alone. A few months into each of their infections, they both discovered an online community of thousands of people in cities across China, particularly in the Pearl River (Guangzhou, Zhuhai, Dongguan, and Shenzhen) and Yangtze River (Shanghai, Suzhou, Nanjing) delta regions, who, over the past five years, have similarly become convinced that they are infected with a terrifying AIDS-like disease, which has an almost immediate onset of symptoms after sex, proceeds to destroy one's immune system and bodily organs, but which continually produces negative results in HIV testing. Dozens of online groups and forums have emerged in which those who have been infected share their symptoms, experiences, anxieties, and hope for a cure, gathering around the contradictory name "HIV-negative AIDS" (*yinxing aizibing* 阴性艾滋病 or simply *yinzibing* 阴滋病) or the ominously elusive term "the unknown virus" (*weizhi bingdu* 未知病毒).[3] Bringing their cases to a number of media outlets in recent years, particularly Guangzhou's *Southern Metropolis Daily* (*Nanfang dushi bao* 南方都市报), patients have not only succeeded in generating public discussion and growing concern about this new illness but have also seen a rapid expansion in their ranks from 2009 through 2010.[4] Drawing the attention of the authorities, the Ministry of Public Health responded in the beginning of 2011 by conducting a characteristically non-transparent study of sixty patients in six provinces and municipalities.[5] Announcing its findings in early April 2011, to the surprise

---

3 Information related to this illness began spreading over such popular forums as dzh.mop.com 猫扑大杂烩, Baidu 百度 info pages, and QQ chat in 2008. This eventually led to the formation of a number of QQ groups dedicated to the discussion of HIV-negative AIDS, many of which have been erased by censors since the official state response of April 2011. However, since mid-2010, these multiple sources have been consolidated into one main website, www.life-voice.org, which serves as a very lively central forum for discussion of all aspects of this illness (along with the recent emergence, following life-voice.org's block by the Great Firewall of China in late June, of an unblocked mirror site www.life-voice.info), and one QQ mega-group which has been able to survive state crackdowns by registering under a relatively innocuous name. In the ever-tightening Internet environment of 2013, these sites and groups have been shut down for an extended period.

4 The *Southern Metropolis Daily* is known for its relatively open approach to reporting, compared to most Chinese media. One of the paper's more influential early reports on this illness is Bao Xiaodong's 鲍小东 "Huo zai 'weizhi bingdu' yinying xia 活在'未知病毒'阴影下 [Life in the Shadows of the 'Unknown Virus']," Nanduwang 南都网 (nddaily), Oct. 14, 2009, http://gcontent.oeeee.com/d/fb/dfb84a11f431c624/Blog/d2e/3889b7.html (accessed Nov. 4, 2013).

5 At other times, the government has also claimed that ninety-nine patients were involved according to a CCTV report viewed in Zhengzhou, April 8, 2011. In a thought-provoking attempt to allay doubts and prove the thoroughly scientific nature of this investigation, the PRC Ministry of Public Health claims that patients' samples were also sent to a laboratory in the United States for final analysis. See "Zhongguo bao shu qian ren ran 'yinzibing' 中国爆数千人染'阴滋病' [Thousands in China Infected with HIV-Negative AIDS]," *Taiwan Pingguo ribao* 台湾苹果日报 (Taiwan Apple Daily), April 6, 2011, http://www.appledaily.com.tw/appledaily/article/international/20110406/33298142/(accessed Nov. 4, 2013). However, no evidence has been presented to support this claim, and the speed with which results were concluded and released has led to widespread skepticism amongst patients.

of self-proclaimed carriers, the Ministry asserted that there was in fact no such thing as HIV-negative AIDS, no new virus that had infected this group, and that their primary problem was psychological, namely AIDS-phobia.[6] One researcher from the Ministry of Public Health even went so far as to joke that the only means of transmitting this virus was the popular chatting portal QQ, which has hosted numerous HIV-negative AIDS discussion groups.[7] Dismissing patients' concerns, they were advised to steer clear of pernicious rumors and pursue a more "sunny" life.

Considering the idiosyncrasies and fundamental biological inconsistencies of patients' illness narratives, the Ministry of Public Health's assertion that HIV-negative AIDS is primarily phobic or imaginary seems eminently reasonable. Yet this does not mean, as the ministry and other government departments assume, that this illness can be casually dismissed and forgotten. The fact that HIV-negative AIDS is psychological, or an imaginary illness, does not make it any less significant, particularly considering that this "virus" continues to spread and to greatly affect the lives and wellbeing of so many young people across China. Recognizing the importance of making sense of this illness, this paper asks: what is HIV-negative AIDS? How does this illness develop, and how is it experienced? Why has it become so "infectious"? And what are its

---

6 Li Xiuting 李秀婷, "Weishengbu tongbao 'yinzibing' diaocha jieguo, meiyou zhengju zhichi ran aizibing 卫生部通报"阴滋病"调查结果 没有证据支持染艾滋病 [Ministry of Public Health Reports Results of 'HIV-Negative AIDS' Investigation, No Evidence to Support AIDS Claims]," *Nanfang ribao* 南方日报 [Southern Daily], April 7, 2011, http://www.southcn.com/nfdaily/china/content/2011-04/07/content_22396517.htm (accessed Nov. 4, 2013); Bai Jianfeng 白剑峰, Wang Junping 王君平, and Jia Linping 贺林平, "Yinxing aizibing' shi shenme bing '阴性艾滋病'是什么病? [What is 'HIV-Negative AIDS'?]" *Renmin ribao* 人民日报 [People's Daily], April 7, 2011, http://paper.people.com.cn/rmrb/html/2011-04/07/nw.D110000renmrb_20110407_7-04.htm?div=-1 (accessed Nov. 4, 2013); Bi Lei 毕磊, "Weishengbu: 'yinzibing' bingdu bu cunzai 卫生部:'阴滋病'病毒不存在 Ministry of Public Health: The 'HIV-Negative AIDS' Virus Does Not Exist," Renminwang 人民网 (people), April 12, 2011, http://scitech.people.com.cn/GB/14363375.html (accessed November 10, 2013); and a month later, Zeng Liming 曾利明, "Weishengbu: Jianyi meiti buyao zai yong 'yinzibing' yi ci 卫生部:建议媒体不要再用'阴滋病'一词 [Ministry of Public Health Recommends that Media Should Not Use the Term 'HIV-Negative AIDS'']," Renminwang 人民网 (people), May 10, 2011, http://health.people.com.cn/GB/14598459.html (accessed Nov. 4, 2013).

7 Wang Weiwei 王维维, "Zhuanjia cheng 'yinxing aizibing' shi kongaizheng, duo you yiyeqing jingli" 专家称'阴性艾滋病'是恐艾症 多有一夜情经历 "[Experts Assert that 'HIV-Negative AIDS' is AIDS-Phobia, the Majority of Patients Had One-Night Stands]," interview with Ministry of Public Health researcher Zeng Guang 曾光, Xinhuawang 新华网 [New China Net], April 7, 2011, http://news.xinhuanet.com/health/2011-04/07/c_121275425.htm (accessed Nov. 4, 2013).

implications for sufferers, and by extension for contemporary Chinese society? In pursuit of these questions, I followed relevant media reports, online forums, and discussion groups, and conducted unstructured, open-ended interviews with twenty-three "patients" between late 2010 and late 2011. Listening in an open, unrestricted environment to the illness narratives of sufferers like Chen and Yang, so as to better grasp their experiences, symptoms, and concerns, I have attempted to enter their world to find the social and personal truths behind this imaginary virus.[8]

Knowing the Unknown Virus

In light of the almost instinctive dismissal of imaginary illness, the question of how to go about taking such illness seriously remains for serious consideration. Toward this goal, I propose a new analytical rubric that traces the unknown virus's articulation at the intersection of symbolic expression, social change, and individual experience and anxiety. Beyond illness as a purely biological phenomenon, Susan Sontag's work has importantly brought attention to the associative thinking encompassing illness, which she calls "illness as metaphor." Drawing upon her personal experience as a cancer patient, Sontag critiques the erroneous notions of culpability and even guilt surrounding the biological phenomenon of cancer.[9] Yet, inverting Sontag's analysis of the metaphorical imaginaries tied to biological illness, might it be possible to analyze imaginary illnesses as expressions of internal conflicts through biological metaphor: rather than illness as metaphor, perhaps metaphorical illness? In this direction, Paula Treichler's discussion of the AIDS crisis reveals, along with Sontag's later analysis of AIDS, the uniquely rich symbolic elements surrounding this virus, which constitute AIDS as not only a very real "epidemic of a transmissible lethal disease" but also as an "epidemic of meanings or signification."[10] Treichler's examination of the succession of irrational myths through which people have "understood" AIDS, from toxic cock syndrome to the shock of

8 Rita Charon defines narrative medicine as "medicine practiced with the narrative competence to recognize, absorb, interpret, and be moved by the stories of illness." See Rita Charon, *Narrative Medicine: Honoring the Stories of Illness* (Oxford: Oxford University Press, 2006), vii. As the unknown virus is an illness composed of narrative, I argue that it is accordingly only through patients' illness narratives that it can be fully understood.

9 Susan Sontag, *Illness as Metaphor and AIDS and Its Metaphors* (New York: Picador, 1989), 57–58.

10 Paula A. Treichler, *How to Have Theory in an Epidemic: Cultural Chronicles of AIDS* (Durham: Duke University Press, 1999), 11.

celebrity AIDS, highlights the centrality of social imaginaries and personal anxieties in our vision of this biological reality, or the double life of AIDS as both a epidemiological and cultural-linguistic phenomenon.[11] Illness can thus be metaphorical, and no illness in contemporary society is more symbolically charged than HIV/AIDS. The recent emergence of HIV-negative AIDS in China presents a new addition to this series of irrational myths and social imaginings: a new imagining in which social and personal anxieties are articulated through the idea of a simultaneously destructive and elusive illness.

Such interplay of anxiety, imagination, and illness has played an important role at other moments in modern Chinese history, producing what has been called a "dialectic between symptom and society."[12] The Republican period, wherein a metaphorical relationship between the individual and the national body brought new emphasis upon personal purity and hygiene,[13] saw the proliferation of such symptomatically vague yet symbolically rich illnesses as spermatorrhea (*yijinglao* 遗精痨), which combined this period's political instability, socioeconomic pressures, and sexual anxiety into the telling symptom of the involuntary loss of semen.[14] Later, in the post-Mao era, "neurasthenia" (*shenjing shuairuo* 神经衰弱) became a common diagnosis in mental institutions in the 1980s, labeling depressive disorders as products of the "degeneration of the nervous system." Yet Arthur Kleinman has instead found the roots of many such biologized depressive cases in the extreme social and political suffering of the Maoist years.[15] Much like spermatorrhea, neurasthenia was, despite its biochemical facade, a somatic expression of the social tensions and anguish that people faced, emerging as the mental illness of its era.

Similarly, according to my analyses of patients' illness narratives, HIV-negative AIDS is the illness of the present era in China, in that it is a highly contagious metaphorical articulation of personal conflicts in contemporary society through the vocabulary of biological illness.[16] The very real sources of this imaginary illness, as will be demonstrated below, are the contradictory

---

11 Treichler, *How to Have Theory in an Epidemic*, 13, 15, 19.

12 Arthur Kleinman, *Social Origins of Disease and Distress: Depression, Neurasthenia, and Pain in Modern China* (New Haven: Yale University Press, 1986), 2.

13 Frank Dikötter, *Sex, Culture, and Modernity in China* (Honolulu: University of Hawai'i Press, 1995).

14 Hugh Shapiro, "The Puzzle of Spermatorrhea in Republican China," *positions* 6.3 (Winter 1998): 565–71.

15 Kleinman, *Social Origins of Disease and Distress*, 14–15, 123–42.

16 For studies of illness narrative, see Arthur Kleinman, *The Illness Narratives: Suffering, Healing, and the Human Condition* (New York: Perseus Books, 1989); and Charon, *Narrative Medicine*.

duality of self, sex, society, and government, located at a tenuous point between purity and pollution, articulated through the symptoms and indeed the very idea of the "unknown virus." Expanding upon this volume's theme of discourses of disease, HIV-negative AIDS is a disease woven of discourse, generating a self-reproducing and highly infectious symptomatic-symbolic chain giving voice to the pressures and uncertainties of the present.

A *Epidemiology*

Who, then, is contracting HIV-negative AIDS? My research has provided me with the opportunity to speak with a total of twenty-three patients, consisting of twenty-one men and two women. This seemingly skewed sample in fact reflects the population of sufferers quite accurately: amongst all of the forums and groups visited throughout the course of my research, easily ninety-five percent of patients are self-described heterosexual males.[17] The means of transmission are similarly homogeneous across cases: twenty patients, the overwhelming majority, report having been infected via contact with female sex workers. The other three, including the two female interviewees and one male interviewee (Yang, featured above), were infected during one-night stands with acquaintances met online.

Transmission data thus immediately highlights the intertwinement of this personal illness with society, and particularly the sociosexual change that has been called "China's sexual revolution."[18] Despite such revolutionary rhetoric, sexual license and pleasure have an immensely uncertain place in Chinese society today, an uncertainty manifested in unknown virus experiences and narratives. On the one hand, sex for money and anonymous one-night stands, the two main sources of HIV-negative AIDS transmission, are increasingly ubiquitous. Despite an ostensible crackdown on the sex trade (*saohuang* 扫黄) in infamously "open" Guangzhou for the 2010 Asian Games,[19] on my downtown

---

17 This notable trend in sexual preferences has led to occasional questioning and puzzlement at the apparent lack of homosexuals patients, widely presumed in China to be "HIV carriers." See, for example, "Tongxinglian huanzhe you meiyou 同性恋患者有没有? [Do We Have Any Homosexual Sufferers?]" Life-Voice HIV-Negative AIDS Forum, May 15, 2011, http://www.life-voice.info/redirect.php?tid=1935&goto= lastpost&styleid=4 (last accessed Jan. 2012, no longer available).

18 Everett Yuehong Zhang, "China's Sexual Revolution," in Arthur Kleinman et al., *Deep China: The Moral Life of the Person, What Anthropology and Psychiatry Tell Us about China Today* (Berkeley: University of California Press, 2011).

19 "Ying Yayun quanguo 'saohuang dafei', Guangdong wei xingdong zhongdian diqu 迎亚运全国'扫黄打非'广东为行动重点地区 [Nationwide Crackdown on Prostitution and Other Illegal Activities for the Asian Games: Guangdong Is the Campaign's

apartment block less than two kilometers from the site of the Games' opening ceremonies, at least four establishments which were not at all subtle about their provision of sexual services remained open; elsewhere, the few samples of nightlife that I experienced during my year of research were surprisingly bawdy, particularly in comparison to the far more familiar China nightlife scene of the late 1990s and early 2000s, usually characterized by dice games and Richard Marx covers. On the other hand, alongside the rapid proliferation of sex—both commoditized and spontaneous—throughout society and the accompanying diversification of sexual lives, a quite extreme degree of unrelenting sexual repression remains present: sex work remains illegal; a cult of female virginity continues unabated; one-night stands and other forms of unsanctioned sexual activity are still widely frowned upon, at least in public; and sexually transmitted diseases are perceived as a mark of guilt.[20] I have chosen the term sociosexual duality to describe this contradictory situation: although sex is literally everywhere, it is not something that one talks about; and although boundaries are repeatedly transgressed on a daily, or rather perhaps nightly, basis, they remain largely intact on the social surface. This contradictory duality of sex in society, a simultaneous ubiquity and inexpressibility, produces at the personal level a similarly conflicted combination of desire, easy access, and shame. The symbolic symptomatology of the "unknown virus," to which we now turn, reveals the personal experiences of these social contradictions, triggered by highly ambivalent sexual situations.

B *Transmission and Symptomatology*

How does HIV-negative AIDS emerge and develop in a patient? Almost all interviewees reported an onset of symptoms immediately or very soon after the completion of the sexual act; unlike HIV/AIDS as a biological phenomenon, there is no seroconversion lag or latency period for this strain of imaginary AIDS. Initial symptoms include shortness of breath, itchiness, sweating, chills and shivers, diarrhea, weak legs, fever, and lightheadedness. Similar symptoms

Focal Point]," *Xin kuaibao* 新快报 [New Express Daily], Sept. 29, 2010, http://2010.163.com/10/0929/08/6HO1Q9HE00863AUC.html (accessed Nov. 4, 2013).

20 There is an ironically resilient virginity complex amongst my male interviewees, likely contributing to their paranoid concerns about pollution and infection following contact with non-virginal sex workers. On the complex and indeed contradictory place of virginity in contemporary Chinese society and interpersonal relations, see James Farrer, "Virginity: Purity of Purpose," in his *Opening Up: Youth Sex Culture and Market Reform in Shanghai* (Chicago: University of Chicago Press, 2002), 223–57.

continue to develop in the months that follow, expanding to include thrush,[21] swollen glands, sore throat, fatigue, declining eyesight, weight loss, hair loss, loss of appetite, subcutaneous bleeding, bloodshot eyes, insomnia, abundant dreams, a growling or noisy stomach, perpetually weak legs, erectile dysfunction, foul-smelling fecal matter, stuffy nose, uncontrollable muscle spasms or contractions, stiff and painful joints, persistently bad body odor, and darkening of the skin on the hands and surrounding the genitalia.

Although this might at first appear to be an illogical medley of vague and at times mutually contradictory symptoms,[22] a certain logic can be read from this list to explain symptoms' persistence and indeed "contagion." Yet to begin such an interpretation, it is imperative that we return to their point of origin in the immediate aftermath of the sexual act. All but two interviewees assert that they were infected during their first visit to a sex-worker or first one-night stand, and every interviewee claims to have used a condom in his or her sexual act: patients are thus clearly new to the worlds of sex-for-money or anonymous sex, yet are also informed enough about the potential risks of unsafe sexual behavior to use protection.[23] This awareness of potential risks, however, combines with misinformation to produce fundamental misunderstandings and exaggeration of risk. For example, patients unanimously characterize safe sex with a condom as "high-risk sexual behavior" (*gaowei xing xingwei* 高危性行为), a key term in "unknown virus" discourse.[24] Such labeling suggests a simultaneous awareness of the risks of sexually transmitted infections alongside a glaring and anxiety-inducing lack of knowledge about the ways in which these infections are transmitted or prevented, insofar as sex with a condom is the definition of "safe sex." Mirroring the contradictory duality of sex in society described above, we thus find a similarly ambivalent duality in

21 Thrush is a white buildup on the tongue resulting from an oral yeast infection, which is a common condition in AIDS patients. Much smaller degrees of white substance on the tongue are a fairly widespread human trait, explaining the frequent misrecognition of common buildup as "thrush" in HIV-negative AIDS patients.

22 For example, weak legs following sexual intercourse are not an uncommon experience and would not be viewed as a symptom of an underlying illness by most people. Later symptoms such as a stuffy nose, growling stomach, and foul-smelling fecal matter attest to the commonality of purported "symptoms of HIV-negative AIDS," a commonality which clearly works to this imaginary illness's advantage as a logically unfounded yet experientially convincing affirmation of the presence of "symptoms."

23 "DT" in unknown virus parlance, which stands for *dai tao* 戴套, meaning "to wear a condom."

24 This is such a common term in unknown virus discourse that it is frequently abbreviated for "insiders" as simply "high-risk" (*gaowei*).

patients' sexual experiences: on the one hand, patients were trying new and presumably enjoyable activities; but on the other hand, they were aware, and even perhaps too aware, of the potential risks associated with such activities.[25]

This original duality of the sexual experience is further compounded by the duality of the pre-coital and post-coital self. Within such an ambivalent sexual situation, the pre-coital lure of enjoyment is often able to override one's concerns; a certain buildup of energy creates what Wilhelm Reich memorably calls the "genital magnet effect," leading one to overlook any potential risks for the moment.[26] However, within a mixed situation of pleasure and perceived risk, enjoyment quickly fades upon the conclusion of the sexual act, and all that one has left is concern; the post-coital self, burdened with worry, can look back in puzzlement upon the alien self prior to and during the act, bursting with sexual tension and energy, transgressing social boundaries and indeed the boundaries of self and other. This moment of post-coital split experience and uncertain selfhood is in fact precisely when symptoms tend to emerge in patients. On one level, standing outside of this experience, initial symptoms such as shortness of breath, diarrhea, or nausea clearly appear to be nervous reactions or "hysterical materializations" of post-coital anxiety.[27] However, they are not interpreted as such by patients; instead, internal to this experience, they are invested by the anxiety that they represent with imaginary biological meaning as "AIDS symptoms," turning an initially irrational and anxiety-producing

25 It is likely not just a coincidence that the first reports of HIV-negative AIDS in China appeared around the time of the first nationwide television campaign promoting condom use to prevent the spread of HIV in 2007. As anyone who was a teenager in the post-Magic era can attest, the incorporation of AIDS education into sex education can be just as terrifying as informative, reinforcing sexual guilt through the stigma of a gradually fatal disease that would reveal one as a sexual transgressor, even equating sex and death. Cf. Sontag, *Illness as Metaphor and AIDS and Its Metaphors*, 112. For more information on this Chinese ad campaign and to view a television clip, see Scott Hensley, "Jackie Chan to Fight AIDS in Chinese Condom Ad," *The Wall Street Journal*, Nov. 14, 2007, http://blogs.wsj.com/health/2007/11/14/jackie-chan-to-fight-aids-in-chinese-condom-ad/(accessed Nov. 5, 2013).

26 Wilhelm Reich, *The Bioelectrical Investigation of Sexuality and Anxiety* (New York: Farrar, Strauss, and Giroux, 1982), 13–14. Similar pre-coital sentiments have been recorded in João Biehl et al., "Technology and Affect: HIV/AIDS Testing in Brazil," *Culture, Medicine and Psychiatry* 25.1 (Mar. 2001): 87–129, an ethnography of a HIV/AIDS Testing and Counseling Center in Brazil, where one client noted, for example: "when one likes the other person one thinks that he does not have any disease."

27 Sándor Ferenczi, "The Phenomenon of Hysterical Materialization," in his *Further Contributions to the Theory and Technique of Psychoanalysis* (New York: Brunner/Mazel Publishers, 1926).

concern about contamination into a self-reproducing feedback cycle of initial AIDS-panic and the experience of panic-induced imaginary "AIDS symptoms" seemingly confirming this panic, in turn further aggravating symptoms.[28] This "semi-erudite" cyclical experience of anxiety and meaning,[29] appearing to provide a complete explanation of patients' imagined infections, is then validated through the "truth-seeking" group psychology of online forums and reproduced experientially on a daily basis, continually reaffirming patients' anxiety and resulting diagnosis.

At another level, however, symptoms of the "unknown virus" can also be read as symbolic expressions of the alienated nature of one's body and oneself in this initial moment of split experience. The HIV virus, in which "the body's own cells become the invader"[30] and distressingly participate in the breakdown of one's own immune system,[31] metaphorically captures the post-coital sense of having lost control over oneself and having transgressed boundaries that should not have been broken down, making it an ideal medium for the internalization of sexual guilt through imaginary punishment.[32] Yet such

---

28 In my interviews, I inquired about individual interviewees' means of transmission, as well as other known means of transmission. Seemingly "impure" and thus anxiety inducing sexual practices were almost unanimously recognized as the primary source of infection. The only exception that I have heard secondhand was one interviewee's online acquaintance, who had been infected via needles. According to the narrative as reported to me, this female patient's live-in boyfriend was an intravenous drug user; once, while going through a closet in their apartment, she encountered a container of used needles and felt a prick. She then had an immediate onset of symptoms including fever, vomiting, chills, and sweat while vigorously scrubbing her pricked finger with soap in the bathroom: she supposedly ended up scrubbing until her skin was raw. This outlying example, while distinct from other cases of infection via sexual activity, nevertheless affirms the role of self-reproducing anxiety in the emergence and cyclical escalation of this illness.

29 According to Adorno, "the semi-erudite vaguely wants to understand and is also driven by the narcissistic wish to prove superior to the plain people but he is not in a position to carry through complicated and detached intellectual operations. To him, astrology, just as other irrational creeds like racism, provides a short-cut by bringing the complex to a handy formula and offering at the same time the pleasant gratification that he who feels to be excluded from educational privileges nevertheless belongs to the minority of those who are 'in the know'." See Theodor Adorno, *The Stars Down to Earth: And Other Essays on the Irrational in Culture* (New York: Routledge, 1994), 61.

30 Sontag, *Illness as Metaphor and AIDS and Its Metaphors*, 106.

31 Peter Sloterdijk, *Sphéres* [Spheres], vol. 3, *Écumes*: *Sphérologie plurielle* [Foam: Plural Spherology], trans. Olivier Mannoni (Paris: Hachette Litteratures, 2005).

32 AIDS is often portrayed in the popular imagination as a "death sentence" for sexual transgression. The guilty symbolic weight accompanying the AIDS virus is so plentiful that

viral symbolism has been given a unique and highly contagious twist in the case of HIV-negative AIDS. From the start, the first symptoms, including shortness of breath, diarrhea, nausea, and shivering, signal a loss of control over one's most basic bodily functions: breathing, the abilities to stand still and to exercise control over one's stomach and bowels. Later symptom clusters continue this symbolism through the decline of otherwise automatic organ functions, such as appetite, sight, and the use of one's legs; swelling and growths on the body, such as thrush (self-incriminating white buildup on the tongue revealing itself and thus marking carriers in all subsequent acts of social communication) and swollen glands or organs, which signal the fundamental uncontrollability and foreignness of the body; and finally an increasingly all-encompassing dissolution of one's body and one's sovereignty over it, in the form of uncontrollable muscle contractions, potent rotting odors, and the darkening of one's skin.

The final two symptoms of decay and darkening are tellingly reminiscent of the most anxiety-inducing and uncontrollable of processes, the decomposition of the body in death; yet this darkening of the skin around the genitalia and hands is a particularly evocative symbol on another level. Within Chinese society, dark skin is a longstanding symbol of inferiority and even pollution.[33] Tellingly, numerous interviewees remembered that their sexual partners' "cunts" were "very dark" (*ta de B hao hei* 她的B好黑), not only signaling their perceived lower and polluted social and sexual status but also enacting an anatomical "geography of blame."[34] In hindsight, they claim, such darkness should have been a warning sign, but they failed to turn away from these simultaneously despised and desired sources of pollution.[35] Intimate contact then leads

---

early in the course of the epidemic, psychiatrist Casper G. Schmidt analyzed this then little understood illness as a group fantasy of scapegoating enacted by the "Moral Majority" against disenfranchised groups, which (according to his theory) produced depression amongst targeted groups that in turn led to autoimmune disorders. Cf. Casper G. Schmidt, "The Group-Fantasy Origins of AIDS," *The Journal of Psychohistory* 12.1 (Summer 1984): 37–78. Although Schmidt's analysis of the cultural symbolism surrounding AIDS and its social context is telling, his denial of AIDS as a biological phenomenon presents a dangerous line of analysis—Schmidt, in fact, died of complications from AIDS in 1994.

33 Frank Dikötter, *The Discourse of Race in Modern China* (Stanford: Stanford University Press, 1992), 38–39.

34 Paul Farmer, *AIDS and Accusation: Haiti and the Geography of Blame* (Berkeley: University of California Press, 1992).

35 The abbreviated name for HIV-negative AIDS, namely, *yinzibing* 阴滋病, could alternatively be read as "genital moisture illness" or even "feminine moisture illness," perhaps subconsciously reminding sufferers of the perceived origins of their illness.

one to be marked by the darkening of one's own genitalia, a largely unseen (i.e., "private parts") yet inescapable mark of guilt, followed by the inevitable spread of such pollution to the physically remotest yet also nearest extremities of one's hands, a highly visible form of self-stigmatization.[36] The virulence of this pollution, spreading from one set of genitalia to another, and eventually onward across the body, is further attested to by its eventual spread to one's family members and colleagues: interviewees were either convinced that they had passed this illness to their closest friends and family members, or were immensely concerned about the potential for such transmission. Such inescapable concerns invert the naming of the witch interpreted by James Siegel as a means of formulating and understanding the causes of such unknowable and uncontrollable aspects of life as misfortune and death, in that the attribution to the self of witch-like polluting powers that are nevertheless fundamentally "unknown" and clearly uncontrollable leads to an absolute uncertainty and anxiety about what one may do next, without even knowing.[37]

In this regard, the notion of "black hands" (*hei shou* 黑手) has other far more illuminating symbolic connotations. Unharmonious events in contemporary China are conspiratorially attributed by officialdom to intricate planning and orchestration by so-called "black hands"; the term is shorthand for a person guilty of manipulating and disturbing an otherwise harmonious society. The imagined transfer of darkness to one's hands and beyond then expresses guilt, revealing oneself caught in the act between the moralistic ideals of society and the harsh realities of interpersonal relations in actual society. The onset and development of a seemingly confusing array of symptoms in unknown virus patients is then in fact a symbolically logical expression of the duality of self, derived from the contradictory duality of sex in society, and eventually leading to many sufferers' guilty withdrawal from society altogether.

The duality reflected in symptomatology is further apparent in descriptions of the virus itself. On the one hand, interviewees characterize the HIV-negative AIDS virus as infinitely small, allowing it to penetrate through condoms; in a colorful sports simile, one interviewee described the virus passing through condoms like a ping-pong ball sliding through the netting of a basketball net. But on the other hand, despite its tiny size, this virus is also infinitely powerful: if other "known" viruses are like lions or tigers, one interviewee told me, this virus is like a tick, a parasite capable of living on top of other viruses. One can kill a lion or a tiger with the right weapon, but the tick living on its body

36 Erving Goffman, *Stigma: Notes on the Management of Spoiled Identity* (Edgewood Cliffs: Prentice Hall, 1963).

37 James Siegel, *Naming the Witch* (Stanford: Stanford University Press, 2006).

will still be able to survive; it lives on by simply moving on to another body. This tick metaphor also tellingly and troublingly relates to imaginings of the perceived sources of "infection." Normally, the sex workers believed to have infected patients would naturally be presumed to also be ill. However, patients who visit their infectors (including six of my interviewees) are surprised to see absolutely no signs of illness. One interviewee from Wuhan told me that he had spoken to his presumed infector in early February of 2011, and was surprised to find that she was still wearing her usual "work uniform," a very short skirt and a tight shirt. Although she had to be ill according to his interpretation of his illness, he also concluded that in order to dress like she did in the cold of winter, her immune system had to be much stronger than his: her resilience, he told me, shocked him. This image of the undying and even unaffected super-infector, able to live on and move like a tick from one body to another, embodies the impure yet infinite power capable of drawing in the self to do things which one cannot comprehend, projecting self-duality outward onto a despised yet desired scapegoat.[38]

Viral Politics: The Sick Man of East Asia, Redux

> *The People's Daily* is screwing the people, and the nation's cadres are fucking the nation (Renmin ribao *ri renmin, guojia ganbu gan guojia* 《人民日报》日人民,国家干部干国家).
>
> HIV-negative AIDS sufferer, male, age 25

A similarly simultaneous object of desire and disgust in unknown virus discourse is the government, imagined as at once a potential savior as well as the ultimate culprit behind the "cover-up" and continued spread of this illness. On the one hand, resembling the passionate energy in the run-up to the sexual encounter, there have been a number of instances in which ambiguous official announcements, such as the initial state-sponsored clinical project of early 2011 or the subsequent intervention by Guangzhou-based "model" medical researcher Zhong Nanshan 钟南山 in May of the same year,

38 This is a common feature of sexually transmitted disease discourse in that sex workers are perceived not as victims of illness, but rather as guilty agents of infection. For further discussion of this phenomenon, see Treichler, *How to Have Theory in an Epidemic*. See also Tiantian Zheng's thought-provoking discussion of sex work, gender relations, nationalist disease imaginaries, and safe (or unsafe) sex in *Ethnographies of Prostitution in China: Gender Relations, HIV/AIDS, and Nationalism* (New York: Palgrave MacMillan, 2009).

have created an optimistic hope that the illness from which patients believe they suffer will finally be revealed and resolved.[39] On the other hand, however, resembling the onset of post-coital anxiety, there is perpetual disappointment of these hopes, and discontent at each of the government's attempts to re-territorialize the unknown-ness of the unknown virus, whether as AIDS-phobia or once, extremely anti-climactically, as reactive arthritis. As much as patients determinedly believe that they are infected with a virus, they seem equally determined to keep its unknown-ness for themselves, maintaining a self-reproducing and collectively infectious symbolic chain of anxiety that intertwines symptoms and selfhood.[40] And much as paranoid concern takes over in the aftermath of sexual excitement, paranoid anger takes over from disappointed hope,[41] eventually leading patients to the appropriately

39 After the Ministry of Public Health's announcement that HIV-negative AIDS does not exist failed to silence patients, Guangzhou-based model medical researcher and hero in the "people's war against SARS" Zhong Nanshan 钟南山 was brought out to reassure sufferers that their concerns were being taken seriously. Articles from the period prior to the release of Zhong's findings demonstrate the vague yet high hopes created for patients: Guo Xiaoyan 郭晓燕, "Yangguang xia de 'guai bing' zhuizong: Zhong Nanshan jiang gongbu diaocha jieguo 阳光下的'怪病'追踪:钟南山将公布调查结果 [Tracking a 'Strange Virus' in the Open: Zhong Nanshan to Release Results of Investigation Soon]," *Yangcheng wanbao* 羊城晚报 [Guangzhou Evening News], May 4, 2011, http://news.ycwb.com/2011-05/04/content_3424448.htm (accessed Nov. 7, 2013); and Li Heng 黎蘅 and Liu Dan 刘丹, "Zhong Nanshan jiang gongbu shu shi zishu yinxing aizibingzhe jiance jieguo 钟南山将公布数十自述阴性艾滋病者检测结果 [Zhong Nanshan Will Soon Release the Test Results of Dozens of Self-described HIV-Negative AIDS Sufferers]," *Guangzhou ribao* 广州日报 [Guangzhou Daily], May 5, 2011, http://gd.news.sina.com.cn/news/2011/05/05/1133854.html (accessed Nov. 7, 2013). However, Zhong's attempt to attribute patients' illness to a combination of the EB virus, best known for its association with mononucleosis, and reactive arthritis was destined to disappoint. His results, vehemently rejected amongst unknown virus sufferers, can be read at: Wu Peng 吴鹏, "Zhong Nanshan cheng 'yinxing aizibing' duoshu you yizhi bingdu yinqi 钟南山称'阴性艾滋病'多数由已知病毒引起 [Zhong Nanshan Asserts that 'HIV-Negative AIDS' Is Primarily the Product of a Number of Already Known Viruses]," *Xin Jingbao* 新京报 [Beijing News], May 7, 2011, http://health.sina.com.cn/news/2011-05-07/011922419917.shtml (accessed Nov. 7, 2013).

40 Sigmund Freud, *Inhibitions, Symptoms, and Anxiety* (New York: W. W. Norton, 1959), 21.

41 Particular vitriol is reserved for Ministry of Public Health researcher Zeng Guang, who made the aforementioned joke about HIV-negative AIDS being spread via QQ: he is frequently discussed by patients in a language of violent denunciation reminiscent of the Cultural Revolution (e.g., "the #1 Chinese traitor of the 21st century") and his—or perhaps some other very unlucky person's—office and cell phone numbers are repeatedly leaked in forums and QQ groups, so that patients can "educate" him about their illness.

contradictory belief that only this destructive virus from which they suffer can provide the final cure.

In the course of their illness narratives, interviewees repeatedly reference such political slogans as "serving the people" (*wei renmin fuwu* 为人民服务) as a simultaneous source of hope and grounds for accusing the government of failing to live up to its ideals. One interviewee commented: "For all these years, all that they have ever talked about is 'serving the people'. But when have they actually served the people?" Another focused on the blatantly contradictory use of "the people" in modern China, telling me: "They say that it is *The People's Daily*, but in fact it is *The Party's Daily*. All that they do on their *The People's Daily* website is block us, the people, from spreading information about our illness. Clearly, the Party would rather sacrifice all of their beloved people than sacrifice any of its power." Here, recognition of the real and reliably disappointing products of affective investments in state power mirror the downward spiral of post-coital anxiety, producing provocative and at times revealing associations, despite their passing through imaginary viral rhetoric.

Most patients with whom I have spoken believe that the government refuses to acknowledge widespread infections by HIV-negative AIDS simply because they have yet to find a cure that would allow the state to cast itself as the hero in this saga of sickness. Despite the omnipresent and unchanging motto of "serving the people," they tell me, officials' sole concern is promotion and self-interest: without a cure, and without having anyone close to them who is infected, officials have no interest (or, rather, self-interest) in "serving the people" and facing this problem. The government's repeatedly proven tendency to cover up anything and everything that does not conform to official narratives, whether they be critical writings, pollution, protests, or most ominously for patients, large-scale epidemics like SARS, undoubtedly further compounds such concerns.[42] Some interviewees even believe that their lives are being sacrificed simply to protect the local dining and sauna industries and associated GDP, the ultimate arbiter of political correctness in China today, which would supposedly suffer severe economic losses if the full extent of the "unknown virus" was revealed: this common suspicion, while appearing irrational at first glance,

42 This pattern of denial also likely plays an essential role in one of the central moments of this illness: disbelief at the negative results of one's HIV test. João Biehls' ethnography of HIV testing in Brazil in his "Technology and Affect" identifies the test as an attempt to find jouissance in the bio-technical production of truth in blood. Yet within the context of contemporary Chinese politics and the current state of the medical profession, the fundamental inability to achieve such "psychological prophylaxis" or even to find certain truth anywhere is central to patients' experience and illness.

is in fact a revealing metaphorical expression of the all-too-real experience of being held hostage to the whims of self-serving "servants of the people."[43]

Just as sexually transmitted infections are imagined as judgments upon or punishment for one's purportedly deviant behavior, so plagues have frequently been interpreted as judgments upon sickly societies[44]: patients accordingly see HIV-negative AIDS as a judgment upon contemporary China's paradoxical sociopolitical situation. One interviewee told me, "everyone knows what the root of China's real problems is, from SARS to corruption to inflation to pollution to HIV-negative AIDS. You just can't say it so directly." This assertion that "you just can't say it so directly" indirectly acknowledges the immunitary structures through which the government protects itself against popular criticism and rebellion, from the extensive state-controlled media and rapidly expanding online censorship apparatuses, to the People's Liberation Army and the People's Armed Police, to such ideologies as "stability" (*wending* 稳定), "harmony" (*hexie* 和谐), and "tradition" (*chuantong* 传统). Breaking through such ideological immune structures in the aftermath of the state's dismissive accusations of AIDS-phobia just like the unknown virus breaks down individual immune structures, patients tellingly stopped referring to the Ministry of Public Health according to its proper Chinese name *weishengbu* 卫生部, calling it instead *weishengjin* 卫生巾, the term for maxi pads, conjuring images of an impure entity drenched in the people's blood: again, not unlike a tick. Further playing upon Deng Xiaoping's 邓小平 once path-breaking and now canonical motto that "development is the iron rule" (*fazhan caishi ying daoli* 发展才是硬道理), unknown virus sufferers have begun promoting an alternative apocalyptic motto for a new era: "infection is the iron rule" (*chuanran caishi ying daoli*

43 It is precisely such politicized conspiracy theories that led to the sudden block of the Life Voice forum, the main site for unknown virus discussions, in late June of 2011, as the celebration of the 90th anniversary of the Chinese Communist Party approached on July 1, 2011. Although censorship is never a sensible approach to problems, the failings of such heavy-handed censorship were particularly glaring in this case. First, the site's block only further added to the paranoia of patients. Second, it drove another constituency in contemporary Chinese society to learn how to scale the Great Firewall (roughly half of interviewees had not attempted this feat prior to the block). The third and most concerning aspect of this approach is that it has only resulted in the radicalization of unknown virus patients' rhetoric about the government, a quite unfortunate development which is nevertheless understandable within the context of virus narratives: patients believe that the virus destroying their lives and those of their families is being covered up and suppressed by powerful political interest groups, resulting in growing calls for violent action.

44 Sontag, *Illness as Metaphor and AIDS and Its Metaphors*, 132–34, 148–49.

传染才是硬道理). Enacting a new vision of "the people" as the heroic enactors of history in a mixture of altruism, consumption, and "relationships" (*guanxi* 关系), patients have proposed donating blood, visiting sex workers en masse, and drawing upon their *guanxi* to find chances to wine and dine cadres, in hopes of further spreading this illness to important officials or other high-profile individuals, so that the diligently reinforced immunitary structures protecting and sustaining the prevailing unhealthy sociopolitical situation might also be broken down by this illness, and the state might finally be forced to "serve the people."[45] Beginning from the private transgression of sex and opening onto the ultimate transgression of politics, the spread of this unknown pollution is then apocalyptically envisioned as an opportunity to wipe the slate clean of the omnipresent sociopolitical duality that generates and feeds this virus, and to seek a fresh start in the ashes of today's society.

Hence, our analysis has come full circle, from society producing imaginary illness to illness imaginarily curing society. The duality of increasingly amorphous sexual lives and an unabated culture of conservative sexual guilt have fueled the emergence of this unknown virus, which symbolically expresses tensions of enjoyment and control, and purity and pollution, within oneself and one's body. Yet the continued spread of this illness is ironically envisioned by sufferers as providing a final cure for society, forcing officials to live up to their stated ideals through infection. Rather than seeing illness as a "call to arms" and seeking out diligent treatments to "save China," as has been fashionable since Lu Xun 鲁迅 viewed the famous lantern slide in his bacteriology course, unknown virus sufferers propose a completely unexpected approach, expressing the paradoxes of social experience, wherein illness provides an answer. Abandoning the search for yet another false panacea with the inevitable side effects that overpower its benefits, they instead embrace this virus and all that it represents, taking this disease to its logical conclusion of complete destruction towards a "new life" (*xin shenghuo* 新生活). Coming full circle through a string of contradictory doublings of self, society, sex, and government, then, infection by the unknown virus, ironically, becomes the certain cure.

---

45 During the course of my research, high-profile figures who have been hopefully suspected of infection include Hong Kong actress Cecilia Pak-Chi Cheung 张柏芝, who is widely regarded as an unnaturally sex-charged figure following her implication in the Edison Koon-hei Chan 陈冠希 photo scandal of 2008, and who was reportedly "not feeling well" on the set of her most recent film; and, in the aftermath of her victory in the 2011 Australian Open, tennis star Li Na 李娜, for no apparent reason other than the fact that the attention focused upon her at the time might be redirected towards the virus.

References

Adorno, Theodor. *The Stars Down to Earth: And Other Essays on the Irrational in Culture*. London: Routledge, 1994.

Anonymous. "Ying Yayun quanguo 'saohuang dafei', Guangdong wei xingdong zhongdian diqu 迎亚运全国 '扫黄打非' 广东为行动重点地区 [Nationwide Crackdown on Prostitution and Other Illegal Activities for the Asian Games: Guangdong Is the Campaign's Focal Point]." *Xin kuaibao* 新快报 [New Express Daily], Sept. 29, 2010. http://2010.163.com/10/0929/08/6HO1Q9HE00863AUC.html (accessed Nov. 4, 2013).

———. "Zhongguo bao shu qian ren ran 'yinzibing' 中国爆数千人染 '阴滋病' [Thousands in China Infected with HIV-Negative AIDS]." *Taiwan Pingguo ribao* 台湾苹果日报 (Taiwan Apple Daily), April 6, 2011. http://www.appledaily.com.tw/appledaily/article/international/20110406/33298142/(accessed Nov. 4, 2013).

———. "Tongxinglian huanzhe you meiyou 同性恋患者有没有? [Do We Have Any Homosexual Sufferers?]" Life-Voice HIV-Negative AIDS Forum, May 15, 2011. http://www.life-voice.info/redirect.php?tid=1935&goto=lastpost&styleid=4 (last accessed Jan. 2012, no longer available).

Bai Jianfeng 白剑峰, Wang Junping 王君平, and Jia Linping 贺林平. "'Yinxing aizibing' shi shenme bing '阴性艾滋病' 是什么病? [What is 'HIV-Negative AIDS'?]" *Renmin ribao* 人民日报 [People's Daily], April 7, 2011. http://paper.people.com.cn/rmrb/html/2011-04/07/nw.D110000renmrb_20110407_7-04.htm?div=-1 (accessed Nov. 4, 2013).

Bao Xiaodong 鲍小东. "Huo zai 'weizhi bingdu' yinying xia 活在 '未知病毒' 阴影下 [Life in the Shadows of the 'Unknown Virus']." Nanduwang 南都网 (nddaily), Oct. 14, 2009. http://gcontent.oeeee.com/d/fb/dfb84a11f431c624/Blog/d2e/3889b7.html (accessed Nov. 4, 2013).

Bi Lei 毕磊. "Weishengbu: 'yinzibing' bingdu bu cunzai 卫生部: '阴滋病' 病毒不存在 Ministry of Public Health: The 'HIV-Negative AIDS' Virus Does Not Exist." Renminwang 人民网 (people), April 12, 2011. http://scitech.people.com.cn/GB/14363375.html (accessed Nov. 10, 2013).

Biehl, João, with Denise Coutinho and Ana Luzia Outerio. "Technology and Affect: HIV/AIDS Testing in Brazil." *Culture, Medicine and Psychiatry* 25.1 (Mar. 2001): 87–129.

Charon, Rita. *Narrative Medicine: Honoring the Stories of Illness*. Oxford: Oxford University Press, 2006.

Dikötter, Frank. *The Discourse of Race in Modern China*. Stanford: Stanford University Press, 1992.

———. *Sex, Culture, and Modernity in China*. Honolulu: University of Hawai'i Press, 1995.

Farmer, Paul. *AIDS and Accusation: Haiti and the Geography of Blame*. Berkeley: University of California Press, 1992.

Farrer, James. *Opening Up: Youth Sex Culture and Market Reform in Shanghai*. Chicago: University of Chicago Press, 2002.

Ferenczi, Sándor. "The Phenomenon of Hysterical Materialization." In Ferenczi, *Further Contributions to the Theory and Technique of Psychoanalysis*. New York: Brunner/Mazel Publishers, 1926.

Freud, Sigmund. *Inhibitions, Symptoms, and Anxiety*. New York: W. W. Norton, 1959.

Goffman, Erving. *Stigma: Notes on the Management of Spoiled Identity*. Edgewood Cliffs: Prentice Hall, 1963.

Guo Xiaoyan 郭晓燕. "Yangguang xia de 'guai bing' zhuizong: Zhong Nanshan jiang gongbu diaocha jieguo 阳光下的 '怪病' 追踪:钟南山将公布调查结果 [Tracking a 'Strange Virus' in the Open: Zhong Nanshan to Release Results of Investigation Soon]." *Yangcheng wanbao* 羊城晚报 [Guangzhou Evening News], May 4, 2011. http://news.ycwb.com/2011-05/04/content_3424448.htm (accessed Nov. 7, 2013).

Hensley, Scott. "Jackie Chan to Fight AIDS in Chinese Condom Ad." *The Wall Street Journal Blog*, Nov. 14, 2007. http://blogs.wsj.com/health/2007/11/14/jackie-chan-to-fight-aids-in-chinese-condom-ad/(accessed Nov. 5, 2013).

Kleinman, Arthur. *Social Origins of Disease and Distress: Depression, Neurasthenia, and Pain in Modern China*. New Haven: Yale University Press, 1986.

———. *The Illness Narratives: Suffering, Healing, and the Human Condition*. New York: Perseus Books, 1989.

Li Heng 黎蘅 and Liu Dan 刘丹. "Zhong Nanshan jiang gongbu shu shi zishu yinxing aizibingzhe jiance jieguo 钟南山将公布数十自述阴性艾滋病者检测结果 [Zhong Nanshan Will Soon Release the Test Results of Dozens of Self-described HIV-Negative AIDS Sufferers]." *Guangzhou ribao* 广州日报 [Guangzhou Daily], May 5, 2011. http://gd.news.sina.com.cn/news/2011/05/05/1133854.html (accessed Nov. 7, 2013).

Li Xiuting 李秀婷. "Weishengbu tongbao 'yinzibing' diaocha jieguo, meiyou zhengju zhichi ran aizibing 卫生部通报 '阴滋病' 调查结果 没有证据支持染艾滋病 [Ministry of Public Health Reports Results of 'HIV-Negative AIDS' Investigation, No Evidence to Support AIDS Infection Claims]." *Nanfang ribao*南方日报 [Southern Daily], April 7, 2011. http://www.southcn.com/nfdaily/china/content/2011–04/07/content_22396517.htm (accessed Nov. 4, 2013).

Reich, Wilhelm. *The Bioelectrical Investigation of Sexuality and Anxiety*. New York: Farrar, Strauss, and Giroux, 1982.

Schmidt, Casper. "The Group-Fantasy Origins of AIDS." *The Journal of Psychohistory* 12.1 (Summer 1984): 37–78.

Shapiro, Hugh. "The Puzzle of Spermatorrhea in Republican China." *positions* 6.3 (Winter 1998): 565–71.

Siegel, James. *Naming the Witch*. Stanford: Stanford University Press, 2006.

Sloterdijk, Peter. *Sphéres* [Spheres]. 3 vols. Vol. 3, *Écumes: Sphérologie plurielle* [Foam: Plural Spherology]. Trans. from German to French by Olivier Mannoni. Paris: Hachette Litteratures, 2005.

Sontag, Susan. *Illness as Metaphor and AIDS and Its Metaphors*. New York: Picador, 1989.

Treichler, Paula A. *How to Have Theory in an Epidemic: Cultural Chronicles of AIDS*. Durham: Duke University Press, 1999.

Wang Weiwei 王维维. "Zhuanjia cheng 'yinxing aizibing' shi kongaizheng, duo you yiyeqing jingli 专家称 '阴性艾滋病' 是恐艾症 多有一夜情经历 [Experts Assert that 'HIV-Negative AIDS' is AIDS-Phobia, the Majority of Patients Had One-Night Stands]." Xinhuawang 新华网 [New China Net], April 7, 2011. http://news.xinhuanet.com/health/2011-04/07/c_121275425.htm (accessed Nov. 4, 2013).

Wu Peng 吴鹏. "Zhong Nanshan cheng 'yinxing aizibing' duoshu you yizhi bingdu yinqi 钟南山称 '阴性艾滋病' 多数由已知病毒引起 [Zhong Nanshan Asserts that 'HIV-Negative AIDS' Is Primarily the Product of a Number of Already Known Viruses]." *Xin Jingbao* 新京报 [Beijing News], May 7, 2011. http://health.sina.com.cn/news/2011-05-07/011922419917.shtml (accessed Nov. 7, 2013).

Zeng Liming 曾利明. "Weishengbu: Jianyi meiti buyao zai yong 'yinzibing' yi ci 卫生部:建议媒体不要再用 '阴滋病' 一词 [Ministry of Public Health Recommends that the Media Should Not Use the Term 'HIV-Negative AIDS']." Renminwang 人民网 (people), May 10, 2011. http://health.people.com.cn/GB/14598459.html (accessed Nov. 4, 2013).

Zhang, Everett Yuehong. "China's Sexual Revolution." In Arthur Kleinman et al, *Deep China: The Moral Life of the Person, What Anthropology and Psychiatry Tell Us about China Today*. Berkeley: University of California Press, 2011.

Zheng Tiantian. *Ethnographies of Prostitution in Contemporary China: Gender Relations, HIV/AIDS, and Nationalism*. New York: Palgrave McMillan, 2009.

Index